The Role of Nutrition in Maintaining Health in the Nation's Elderly

Evaluating Coverage of Nutrition Services for the Medicare Population

Committee on Nutrition Services for Medicare Beneficiaries

Food and Nutrition Board

INSTITUTE OF MEDICINE

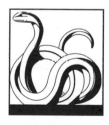

NATIONAL ACADEMY PRESS
Washington, DC

NATIONAL ACADEMY PRESS • 2101 Constitution Avenue, N.W. • Washington, DC 20418

NOTICE: The project that is the subject of this report was approved by the Governing Board of the National Research Council, whose members are drawn from the councils of the National Academy of Sciences, the National Academy of Engineering, and the Institute of Medicine. The members of the committee responsible for the report were chosen for their special competences and with regard for appropriate balance.

This project was funded by the U.S. Department of Health and Human Services, Health Care Financing Administration Contract No. 500-98-0275. Any opinion, findings, conclusions, or recommendations expressed in this publication are those of the Institute of Medicine committee and do not necessarily reflect the view of the funding organization.

International Standard Book Number 0-309-06846-0
Library of Congress Card Number 00-103252

This report is available for sale from the National Academy Press, 2101 Constitution Avenue, N.W., Box 285, Washington, DC 20055; call (800) 624-6242 or (202) 334-3313 (in the Washington metropolitan area), or visit the NAP's on-line bookstore at **www.nap.edu**.

For more information about the Institute of Medicine or the Food and Nutrition Board, visit the IOM home page at **www.iom.edu**

The serpent has been a symbol of long life, healing, and knowledge among almost all cultures and religions since the beginning of recorded history. The image adopted as a logotype by the Institute of Medicine is based on a relief carving from ancient Greece, now held by the Staatliche Museen in Berlin.

THE NATIONAL ACADEMIES

National Academy of Sciences
National Academy of Engineering
Institute of Medicine
National Research Council

The **National Academy of Sciences** is a private, nonprofit, self-perpetuating society of distinguished scholars engaged in scientific and engineering research, dedicated to the furtherance of science and technology and to their use for the general welfare. Upon the authority of the charter granted to it by the Congress in 1863, the Academy has a mandate that requires it to advise the federal government on scientific and technical matters. Dr. Bruce M. Alberts is president of the National Academy of Sciences.

The **National Academy of Engineering** was established in 1964, under the charter of the National Academy of Sciences, as a parallel organization of outstanding engineers. It is autonomous in its administration and in the selection of its members, sharing with the National Academy of Sciences the responsibility for advising the federal government. The National Academy of Engineering also sponsors engineering programs aimed at meeting national needs, encourages education and research, and recognizes the superior achievements of engineers. Dr. William A. Wulf is president of the National Academy of Engineering.

The **Institute of Medicine** was established in 1970 by the National Academy of Sciences to secure the services of eminent members of appropriate professions in the examination of policy matters pertaining to the health of the public. The Institute acts under the responsibility given to the National Academy of Sciences by its congressional charter to be an adviser to the federal government and, upon its own initiative, to identify issues of medical care, research, and education. Dr. Kenneth I. Shine is president of the Institute of Medicine.

The **National Research Council** was organized by the National Academy of Sciences in 1916 to associate the broad community of science and technology with the Academy's purposes of furthering knowledge and advising the federal government. Functioning in accordance with general policies determined by the Academy, the Council has become the principal operating agency of both the National Academy of Sciences and the National Academy of Engineering in providing services to the government, the public, and the scientific and engineering communities. The Council is administered jointly by both Academies and the Institute of Medicine. Dr. Bruce M. Alberts and Dr. William A. Wulf are chairman and vice chairman, respectively, of the National Research Council.

COMMITTEE ON NUTRITION SERVICES FOR MEDICARE BENEFICIARIES

VIRGINIA A. STALLINGS *(Chair)*, Division of Gastroenterology and Nutrition, The Children's Hospital of Philadelphia, Pennsylvania

LAWRENCE J. APPEL, Welch Center for Prevention, Epidemiology and Clinical Research, John Hopkins School of Hygiene and Public Health, Baltimore, Maryland

JULIA A. JAMES, Principal, Health Policy Alternatives, Washington, D.C.

GORDEN L. JENSEN, Division of Gastroenterology and Nutrition, Vanderbilt University Medical Center, Nashville, Tennessee

ELVIRA Q. JOHNSON, Clinical Nutrition Services, Cambridge Health Alliance, Massachusetts

JOYCE K. KEITHLEY, Rush University College of Nursing, Rush-Presbyterian-St. Luke's Medical Center, Chicago, Illinois

ESTHER F. MYERS, 60th Diagnostics and Therapeutics Squadron/ SGOD, United States Air Force, Travis Air Force Base, California

F. XAVIER PI-SUNYER, Division of Endocrinology, Diabetes, and Nutrition, St. Luke's/Roosevelt Hospital Center, Columbia University College of Physicians and Surgeons, New York

HAROLD POLLACK, Health Management and Policy, University of Michigan, Ann Arbor

CAROL PORTER, Nutrition Services and Dietetic Internship, University of California at San Francisco

DAVID B. REUBEN, Division of Geriatrics, University of California, Los Angeles

ROBERT S. SCHWARZ, Division of Geriatrics Medicine, University of Colorado, Denver

ANNALYNN SKIPPER, Nutrition Consultation Service, Rush-Presbyterian-St. Luke's Medical Center, Chicago, Illinois

LINDA G. SNETSELAAR, Department of Preventive Medicine and Environmental Health, University of Iowa, Iowa City

Staff

ROMY GUNTER-NATHAN, Study Director
GERALDINE KENNEDO, Project Assistant
CARMIE CHAN, Project Assistant
EDEN RAUCH, Intern (June to August 1999)

v

Acknowledgments

Appreciation is due to the many individuals and groups who were instrumental in the development of this report. First and foremost, many thanks are extended to the committee who volunteered countless hours to the research, deliberations, and preparation of the report. Their dedication to this project and to a very stringent time line was commendable, and the basis of our success.

Many consultants also provided assistance and reviewed drafts of specific chapters. In particular, appreciation and thanks are extended to Rowan Chlebowski, MD, Division of Medical Oncology and Hematology, Harbor UCLA Medical Center, Torrance, CA; Bess Dawson-Hughes, MD, Calcium and Bone Metabolism Laboratory, Tufts University, Boston; Rosanna Gibbons, MS, RD, Consultant Dietitian in Home Care, Baltimore, Maryland; Talat Alp Ikizler, MD, Division of Nephrology, Vanderbilt University Medical Center, Nashville; John Kostis, MD, University of Medicine and Dentistry of New Jersey; and Andrew S. Levey, MD, Division of Nephrology, New England Medical Center, Boston.

The report was also independently reviewed in its entirety by many individuals who were chosen for their diverse perspectives and technical expertise to assure that the report meets institutional standards for objectivity, evidence, and responsiveness to the study charge. These individuals included Bruce R. Bistrian, MD, PhD, Division of Clinical Nutrition, Beth Israel Deaconess Medical Center, Boston; Ronni Chernoff, PhD, RD, FADA, Geriatric Research Education and Clinical Center, John L. McClellan Memorial Veterans Hospital, Little Rock; Cutberto Garza, MD,

PhD, Vice-Provost, Cornell University; Stanley Gershoff, PhD, Professor of Nutrition, Emeritus, Tufts University, Boston; Margaret M. Heitkemper, PhD, RN, FAAN, Department of Biobehavioral Nursing and Health Systems, University of Washington School of Nursing, Seattle; Jerome P. Kassirer, MD, Editor in Chief Emeritus, *New England Journal of Medicine*, Boston; Penny Kris-Etherton, PhD, RD, Department of Nutrition, Pennsylvania State University, University Park; Lauren LeRoy, PhD, Grantmakers in Health, Washington, DC; John E. Morley, MD, Division of Geriatric Medicine, St. Louis Veterans Affair Medical Center; Henry Riecken, PhD, Professor of Behavioral Sciences, Emeritus, University of Pennsylvania, Philadelphia; Louise B. Russell, PhD, Institute for Health, Health Care Policy, and Aging Research, Rutgers University, New Jersey; and Philip J. Schneider, RPh, MS, College of Pharmacy, The Ohio State University, Columbus.

Many individuals also volunteered significant time and effort to address and to educate the committee at its workshop and public meeting. Workshop speakers included Bess Dawson-Hughes, MD and Ernest Schaefer, MD of Tufts University, Boston; Linda Delahanty, MS, RD of the Massachussets General Hospital, Boston; V. Annette Dickinson, PhD of the Council for Responsible Nutrition, Washington DC; Marion Franz, MS, RD of the International Diabetes Center, Minneapolis; Samual Klein, MD of Washington University, School of Medicine, St. Louis; William Mitch, MD of Emory University, Atlanta; Tom Prohaska, PhD of the University of Chicago; Dennis Sullivan, MD of the University of Arkansas, Little Rock; and Mackenzie Walser, MD of Johns Hopkins University, Baltimore.

In addition, organizations that provided either oral or written testimony to the committee included the American College of Health Care Administrators; the American College of Nutrition; the American Dietetic Association; the American Society for Clinical Nutrition; the American Society for Enteral and Parenteral Nutrition; Fresnisus Medical Care, North America; and the National Kidney Foundation.

Other individuals who deserve special thanks are Tate Erlinger, PhD of Johns Hopkins University for his special assistance with the NHANES III database, Lisa Prosser, MS of Harvard University for sharing her prepublication data on cost analysis of dietary interventions, Marilyn Field, PhD of the Health Care Services Division, Institute of Medicine for her guidance throughout the report process, and Joan DaVanzo, PhD, Allen Dobson, PhD, and Namrata Sen, MHA of The Lewin Group for their patience and number-crunching abilities.

So, it is apparent that many individuals from a variety of clinical and scientific backgrounds provided timely and essential support for this project. Yet, we would have never succeeded without the efforts, skills, and grace that was provided in large measure by Romy Gunter-Nathan, MPH, RD, our study director for this project, from Geraldine Kennedo, Project Assistant, and from Allison Yates, PhD, RD, Director, Food and Nutrition Board, Institute of Medicine.

Lastly, as the chair, may I express my sincere appreciation to each member of this committee for your extraordinary commitment to the project and for the wonderful opportunity to work with you on this important task for the medical and nutrition community and for the Medicare beneficiaries whose care we were asked to consider.

Virginia A. Stallings, MD
Chair
Committee on Nutrition Services
for Medicare Beneficiaries

Contents

xi

SECTION II
THE ROLE OF NUTRITION IN THE
MANAGEMENT OF DISEASE

SECTION III
NUTRITION SERVICES ALONG THE CONTINUUM OF CARE

SECTION IV
PROVIDERS AND COSTS OF NUTRITION SERVICES

The Role of Nutrition in Maintaining Health in the Nation's Elderly

Executive Summary

Poor nutrition is a major problem in older Americans. Inadequate intake affects approximately 37 to 40 percent of community-dwelling individuals over 65 years of age (Ryan et al., 1992). In addition, the vast majority of older Americans have chronic conditions in which nutrition interventions have been demonstrated to be effective in improving health and quality-of-life outcomes. Eighty-seven percent of older Americans have either diabetes, hypertension, dyslipidemia, or a combination of these chronic diseases (NCIIS, 1997). These conditions all have adverse outcomes that can be ameliorated or reduced with appropriate nutrition intervention. Yet for the vast majority of Medicare beneficiaries, nutrition therapy by a nutrition professional is not a covered benefit. Although varying amounts of basic nutrition services are included in reimbursement payments in hospital, home health, and post-acute care settings, services have been largely inconsistent or inadequate to meet the needs of the growing elderly population.

The Medicare program has traditionally not covered preventive services. Nutrition therapy in the ambulatory or outpatient setting has been considered a preventive service and, therefore, given its original intent to provide only reasonable and necessary services for the diagnosis and treatment of disease, Medicare has explicitly not covered nutrition therapy, or any other type of health education or counseling. In 1980 Congress approved its first exception to the exclusion of preventive services by approving coverage for the pneumococcal pneumonia vaccine. In 1997, recognizing the need for education and counseling in the management of diabetes, Congress approved Medicare coverage for diabetes self-management training as part of the Balanced Budget Act.

In addition to the recent coverage for diabetes education, the Balanced Budget Act of 1997 also required that the Department of Health and Human Services contract with the National Academy of Sciences, Institute of Medicine to examine the benefits and costs associated with extending Medicare coverage for certain preventive and other services. The services specifically targeted for examination included screening for skin cancer; medically necessary dental services; elimination of time restrictions on coverage for immunosuppressive drugs after transplants; routine patient care for beneficiaries enrolled in approved clinical trials; and nutrition therapy, including the services of a registered dietitian. This report addresses the benefits and costs associated with extending Medicare coverage specifically for nutrition therapy.

THE COMMITTEE AND ITS CHARGE

In early 1999, the Institute of Medicine appointed an expert committee charged with the task of analyzing available information, hearing from other experts, and developing recommendations regarding technical and policy aspects of the provision of comprehensive nutrition services, delineated as follows:

- coverage of nutrition services provided by registered dietitians and other health care practitioners for inpatient medically necessary parenteral and enteral nutrition therapy;
- coverage of nutrition services provided by registered dietitians and other health care practitioners for patients in home health and skilled nursing facility settings; and
- coverage of nutrition services provided by registered dietitians and other trained health care practitioners in individual counseling and group settings, including both primary and secondary preventive services.

In addition, the committee was charged with evaluating, to the extent data were available, the cost and benefit of such services to Medicare beneficiaries as well as the research issues needed to provide additional understanding of the relationship between provision of quality nutrition services and quality-of-life outcomes.

The expert committee was composed of 14 individuals and represented the areas of geriatric medicine, clinical nutrition and metabolism, epidemiology, clinical dietetics, nursing, evidence-based medicine, outpatient counseling, nutrition services management, nutrition support, health economics, and health policy. Committee members held a variety of science and professional degrees and were representative of a geographical cross section of the nation.

Although the majority of committee members were medical or nutrition professionals, in order to avoid a potential conflict of interest, committee members were limited to those who were employed in areas that would not be directly affected by any changes in legislation with regard to nutrition services (i.e., management, research, education). One member of the committee had experience in, but was not primarily responsible for, the evaluation of reimbursement for nutrition services within the professional association, the American Dietetic Association. On the other end of the spectrum, another member had no medical or nutrition background but rather had experience in legislation associated with Medicare policy and its statutory limitations.

For the purposes of this report, the committee considered the term "nutrition services" to consist of two tiers. The first tier of services is *basic nutrition education or advice*, which is generally brief, informal, and typically not the focal reason for the health care encounter. More often than not, its aim is to promote general health and/or the primary prevention of chronic diseases or conditions. The second tier of nutrition services is the provision of *nutrition therapy*, which includes individualized assessment of nutritional status; evaluation of nutritional needs; intervention, which ranges from counseling on diet prescriptions to the provision of enteral (tube feeding) and parenteral (intravenous feeding) nutrition; and follow-up care as appropriate. Nutrition therapy generally addresses nutrition interventions specific to the management or treatment of certain existing conditions and is usually individualized to meet the food habits of the patient.

Although the population of Medicare beneficiaries includes individuals younger than 65 years of age through its coverage of the disabled and those with end-stage renal disease, the focus of this report is the examination of medical evidence for people age 65 and older. However, because clinical studies focusing solely on individuals older than 65 are limited, most of the evidence examined to evaluate the extent to which nutrition therapy affects outcome included studies conducted with subjects or patients of younger ages. Renal disease has been included in this review, but with a primary focus on pre-end-stage disease. This focus was taken given the available data, which suggested that nutrition therapy could slow the progression of pre-end-stage disease and that Medicare coverage for those with renal disease now begins only when an individual is classified as having "end-stage disease."

The Committee's Approach

In approaching the charge to the committee, three distinct questions needed to be systematically addressed. The first question was—Is there evidence that the provision of nutrition services is of benefit to individuals in terms of morbidity, mortality, or quality of life? Approximately two-thirds of the committee's effort was spent in this initial phase. In gathering available evidence, systematic searches of online databases were conducted and the committee reviewed relevant medical literature with a focus on original research and systematic reviews. This literature was evaluated and categorized in terms of types of studies and preponderance of the evidence that indicated specific effects of nutrition therapy for each condition evaluated.

The committee also sought out opinions from experts in various fields. A workshop was held at which invited professionals were asked to present on requested topics and engage in discussion with the committee regarding various aspects of this report. Organizations were also contacted and invited to give both oral and written testimony. In addition, consultants were used for several fields in order to augment the committee's expertise in the areas of cancer, osteoporosis, renal disease, and heart failure. The names of all workshop speakers, organizations contacted, and consultants to the committee can be found in Appendix C.

For conditions where documentation was found to support nutrition intervention, a second question asked—Specifically, to what extent are registered dietitians, as well as other health care professionals, qualified by training and credentials to provide such services? Credentialing agencies for various health professionals involved in nutrition care were contacted for professional education and training qualifications. Evidence for nutrition interventions resulting in positive outcomes was evaluated with regard to type of health provider administering the nutrition intervention. For most conditions, the types of individuals conducting study interventions were not uniform. In the studies reviewed, although registered dietitians most often provided the nutrition-based therapy, in some studies other personnel administered the intervention evaluated, and many studies did not describe who specifically provided the intervention.

The final question to be answered was—What are the costs and possible offsets for the provision of such services? The Lewin Group, a quantitative analysis consulting firm in the Washington, D.C. area, assisted in the analysis of estimated overall costs to the Medicare program after being given the committee's recommendations on which conditions should be covered and what assumptions the analyses should be based upon. The findings of the committee with regard to the three questions follow.

NUTRITION SERVICES AND TRENDS THAT INFLUENCE THE DELIVERY OF SERVICES

Health care trends have had a significant impact on the delivery of nutrition services to Medicare beneficiaries. Nutrition professionals historically have been available primarily to the inpatient hospital population, where length of stay allowed some degree of provision of nutrition therapy. In these traditional settings, outpatient clinics were maintained as a service to the hospital community and staffed by inpatient departments. The shift from traditionally delivered inpatient care to ambulatory care has reduced the number of hospital beds and increased the acuity level of patients hospitalized. Shorter stays have reduced or eliminated the ability to provide in-depth nutrition counseling during hospitalization. Cost centers without revenue streams, such as routine nutrition counseling, within the hospital have been eliminated. This has resulted in decreased availability of continued nutrition therapy and monitoring as an ambulatory service of the hospital. Although the trends in health care have led to these changes in the availability of services, the change in practice setting is not necessarily a problem given that nutrition counseling, for many reasons, is likely to be more effective in the ambulatory or home health setting than in the complex environment of today's hospitals. The changes in where the service of nutrition therapy is provided and how it is financed however, have led to significant barriers to access for many Medicare beneficiaries.

NUTRITIONAL HEALTH IN THE OLDER PERSON

In reviewing the importance of nutrition to the health of older Americans, both malnutrition and the role of nutrition in the management of health conditions must be considered. As a population, older adults are more likely than younger ones to have a variety of chronic conditions and functional impairments that may interfere with the maintenance of good nutritional status. In turn, lack of attention to dietary intake and poor nutritional status can impact the progression of many chronic diseases and contribute to declining health.

Malnutrition as a term is defined more specifically by nutrition professionals as *poor nutrition*; thus, it encompasses not only inadequate intake (e.g., lack of adequate calories, protein, and vitamins), but also excess intake of nutrients (e.g., obesity or conditions caused by taking too much of a nutrient, such as hypercholesterolemia or hypervitaminosis).

Obesity, a condition of overnutrition, is the most common nutritional disorder in the U.S. population and in the elderly. In the older population, obesity often occurs linked with other clinical conditions such as hypertension, diabetes, and dyslipidemia. In all of these conditions, the treatment of obesity in itself can produce improvements in diagnosis-specific outcomes. However, in older persons, it has been demonstrated that obesity or excess body fat alone does not necessarily predict mortality and, indeed, may even be protective against early death. For these reasons, the committee felt that generalizations regarding weight reduction in the older population should be individualized and would best be addressed only as it pertained to other specific conditions examined in this report.

Undernutrition, although much less common than obesity, can be of significant prognostic importance among older adults. Among hospitalized and nursing home patients, undernutrition is especially prevalent. Many older adults are admitted to hospitals already undernourished; others become undernourished during hospitalization as a result of poor nutritional intake and higher-than-normal energy requirements. The committee found supporting, but limited, data showing that outcomes were improved by nutrition therapy in the acute care setting. The absence of data likely reflects the short lengths of hospital stays, which preclude appropriate efforts to intervene. Nonetheless, the assessment of dietary intake and the implementation of interventions in such settings are encouraged, when possible, if only to prevent further deterioration in the patient's nutritional status and to serve as a baseline for interventions to be initiated in other settings.

In the nursing home setting, undernutrition has received widespread attention and is particularly complicated. When problems such as chronic disease, multiple medications, depression, functional limitations, limited cognitive ability, and self-feeding deficits are superimposed on dependence on institutionalized food service and staffing issues, overt undernutrition is likely to occur.

In considering the provision of nutrition therapy across the continuum of care, the committee examined evidence for specific diseases and conditions that frequently impact Medicare beneficiaries and produce significant morbidity and mortality, and for which nutrition interventions have generally been recommended. In addition, nutrition services in each of the following distinct patient care settings were evaluated: acute care, short-stay facilities (hospitals); ambulatory services (outpatient); home care; and skilled nursing and long-term care facilities.

FINDINGS AND RECOMMENDATIONS FOR MEDICARE COVERAGE OF NUTRITION THERAPY

Recommendation 1. Based on the high prevalence of individuals with conditions for which nutrition therapy was found to be

of benefit, nutrition therapy, upon referral by a physician, should be a reimbursable benefit for Medicare beneficiaries.

Although few randomized clinical trials have directly examined the impact of nutrition therapy, there is consistent evidence from limited data to indicate that nutrition therapy is effective as part of a comprehensive approach to the management and treatment of the following conditions: dyslipidemia, hypertension, heart failure, diabetes, and kidney failure. Conditions evaluated for which data at this time are lacking or insufficient to support a recommendation for nutrition therapy included cancer and osteoporosis. In the case of osteoporosis, although nutrition intervention through calcium and vitamin D supplementation has clearly been found to improve health outcomes, there is a lack of available evidence to suggest that nutrition therapy, as opposed to basic nutrition education from various health care professionals, would be more effective. For cancer treatment, however, with the exception of the role of enteral and parenteral nutrition therapy, a preliminary review of the literature revealed insufficient data at this time regarding the role of nutrition therapy, specifically nutrition counseling, in the treatment of cancer and the management of its symptoms. For this reason, only evidence pertaining to enteral and parenteral nutrition therapy in the management and treatment of cancer was extensively reviewed.

Summaries of the evidence for conditions which were extensively reviewed can be found in Box ES.1. In addition, a summary of the types of evidence available for these conditions can be found in Table ES.1. It was beyond the scope of this report to examine all possible medical conditions for which nutrition therapy may be indicated. There are likely other conditions that were not specifically reviewed but may warrant coverage. Likewise, medical conditions which individually might not warrant nutrition therapy may well require intervention from a trained nutrition professional when these conditions occur in combination.

An underlying factor for the recommendation that coverage be included for nutrition therapy upon physician referral for any condition, including those not reviewed in this report, is that 87 percent of Medicare beneficiaries over 65 years of age have diabetes, hypertension, and/or dyslipidemia alone. This estimate does not include those individuals with heart failure, chronic renal insufficiency, or undernutrition. Thus, it may be administratively more efficient for the Health Care Financing Administration (HCFA) (the unit of the Department of Health and Human Services responsible for administering the Medicare program) to base coverage on physician referral rather than on specific diagnoses. In addition, while physicians may not necessarily be trained in nutrition therapy, they are trained to gauge which conditions warrant referral to a nutrition pro-

---

BOX ES.1 Summary of Evidence Supporting the Use of Nutrition Therapy in Selected Prevalent Diagnoses

Dyslipidemia Substantial evidence from observational studies and from randomized trials supports the use of nutrition therapy as a means to improve lipid profiles and thereby prevent cardiovascular disease in the elderly. Furthermore, numerous professional organizations including the American Heart Association, the National Cholesterol Education Program of the National Heart, Lung, and Blood Institute, and the Second Joint Task Force of European and Other Societies on Coronary Prevention advocate nutrition therapy as an integral part of medical therapy for persons with dyslipidemia. Recommendations for nutrition therapy extend to those individuals not on cholesterol-lowering therapy as well as persons on medications such as statins.

Hypertension Available evidence from several trials conducted in the elderly and from numerous studies conducted in other populations strongly supports nutrition-based therapy as an effective means to reduce blood pressure in older-aged persons with hypertension. At a minimum, such therapy can be an adjuvant to medication. In selected individuals, medication stepdown and potentially medication withdrawal are feasible. Nutrition therapy is recommended as part of the standard of care by the Joint National Committee on Prevention, Detection, Evaluation, and Treatment of High Blood Pressure and the National Heart, Lung, and Blood Institute Working Group report on Hypertension in the Elderly.

Heart Failure Available evidence from several small clinical trials and a few observational studies supports the use of nutrition therapy in the context of multidisciplinary programs. Such programs can prevent readmissions for heart failure, re-

---

fessional, just as they are trained to recognize any other conditions which require referral for sub-specialty care. Additionally, by basing nutrition therapy on referral from a physician, it will prevent self-referral for conditions for which evidence of efficacy is not available. For these reasons it is recommended to Congress that reimbursement for nutrition therapy be based on physician referral rather than on a specific medical condition.

Recommendations regarding the number of nutrition therapy visits for various conditions, other than for the necessary purpose of producing cost estimates, were not made because it is within the appropriate role of HCFA to establish reasonable limits in accordance with accepted practice.

> **Recommendation 2. With regard to the selection of health care professionals to provide nutrition therapy, the registered dietitian is currently the single identifiable group with standardized education, clinical training, continuing education, and national credentialing requirements necessary to be directly reimbursed as a provider of nutrition therapy. However, it is rec-**

duce subsequent length of stay, and improve functional status and quality of life. Nutrition therapy is recommended as part of the standard of care in guidelines prepared by the American College of Cardiology-American Heart Association and by the Agency for Healthcare Research and Quality.

Diabetes Available evidence from randomized clinical trials, including data in substantial numbers of individuals over the age of 65, supports the use of nutrition therapy as part of the overall multidisciplinary approach to the management of diabetes, which also includes exercise, medications, and blood glucose monitoring. Nutrition therapy is also recommended as part of the standard of care by the American Diabetes Association and the World Health Organization.

Pre-Dialysis Kidney Failure Research findings from a randomized clinical trial and two meta-analyses suggest that nutrition therapy may have a beneficial effect, over the long term, in delaying the progression of kidney disease. A National Institutes of Health consensus conference has recommended nutrition therapy as part of the management for chronic renal insufficiency.

Osteoporosis Enhanced intake of calcium and vitamin D for both the prevention and treatment of osteoporosis in the at-risk elderly population is strongly supported by a considerable body of evidence including multiple randomized controlled trials. Increased calcium and vitamin D intake is recommended as part of the standard of care by the National Osteoporosis Foundation as well as the World Health Organization. Whether or not nutrition therapy by a trained nutritional professional is needed depends on the individual's desired mode of calcium and vitamin D intake, specifically supplements versus foods, as well as other potential nutrient restrictions or unique meal planning circumstances.

ognized that other health care professionals could in the future submit evidence to be evaluated by HCFA for consideration as reimbursable providers.

The congressional language which initiated this study requested not only an analysis of the extent to which nutrition services might be of benefit to Medicare beneficiaries but also "an examination of nutritional services provided by registered dietitians...". Available evidence regarding the education and training of registered dietitians as well as other health professionals needed to adequately provide nutrition services was systematically reviewed (see chapter 13). A summary of this information can be found in Table 13.1. The committee however, found a paucity of literature that compared the roles of specific providers of nutrition services to patient outcome or efficacy of treatment.

The committee determined that in the spectrum of health care settings and patient conditions, two tiers of nutrition services exist. The first tier is basic nutrition education and advice, which is generally provided

TABLE ES.1 Summary of Evidence Supporting the Use of Nutrition Therapy for Medicare Beneficiaries in Specific Conditions or Diseases

Conditions[a]	Types of Evidence					Overall Strength of Evidence Supporting Nutrition Therapy
	Observational Studies[b]	Consensus Document	Systematic Review	Some Clinical Trial Evidence	Extensive Clinical Trial Evidence	
Dyslipidemia	✓	✓	✓		✓	Strongly supportive[c]
Hypertension	✓	✓	✓		✓	Strongly supportive[c]
Heart failure	✓	✓	✓	✓		Supportive[c]
Diabetes	✓	✓	✓		✓	Strongly supportive[c]
Pre-dialysis kidney failure	✓		✓	✓		Supportive[d]
Osteoporosis[e]	✓	✓	✓		✓	Strongly supportive[c]
Undernutrition	✓			✓		Supportive[d]

[a] Conditions listed are those for which evidence supports the use of nutrition therapy. Obesity was evaluated in the context of conditions related to it (dyslipidemia, hypertension and diabetes) rather than as a separate condition.

[b] This category includes case series, case-control studies, cohort studies and nonrandomized trials of nutrition-based therapies including nonhuman studies.

[c] From studies of the elderly as well as studies conducted in broader population age groups.

[d] Predominantly from studies in broad population age groups rather than from studies in elderly.

[e] Evidence for the intake of calcium and vitamin D in the prevention and treatment of osteoporosis is strongly supportive. However, at this time it is unclear whether an equivalent and consistent intake of calcium and vitamin D can be achieved through foods as has been demonstrated in trials in which supplements were given.

incidental to other health services. This type of nutrition service, "nutrition education," can generally be provided by most health care professionals who have had basic academic training in food, nutrition, and human physiology (e.g., physicians, nurses, pharmacists). The second tier of nutrition services is nutrition therapy, which involves the secondary and tertiary prevention and treatment of specific diseases or conditions.

The provision of nutrition therapy was found to require significantly more training in food and nutrition science than is commonly provided in typical medical, nursing, pharmacy, or chiropractic education curricula. Nutrition science requires components of biochemistry, biology, medicine, behavioral health, human physiology, genetics, anatomy, psychology, sociology, economics, and anthropology. Food science requires knowledge of food chemistry, food selection, food preparation, food processing, and food economics (see chapter 13). In summary, nutrition therapy involves a comprehensive working knowledge of food composition, food preparation, and nutrition and health sciences, in addition to components of behavior change. This broad knowledge base is necessary to translate complex diet prescriptions into meaningful *individualized* dietary modifications for the layperson.

The committee therefore finds that, with regard to the selection of health care professionals, the registered dietitian is currently the single identifiable group of health care professionals with standardized education, clinical training, continuing education, and national credentialing requirements necessary to be a directly reimbursable provider of nutrition therapy. This recommendation is in line with the U.S. Preventive Services Task Force (1995) rating of professionals to deliver dietary counseling which indicated that, based on available evidence, counseling performed by a trained educator such as a dietitian is more effective than by a primary care clinician.

It is recommended, however, that other health care professionals within certain subspecialty areas of practice may be knowledgeable in particular areas of nutrition intervention through individual training and experience and should be considered for reimbursement on a case-by-case basis. Some health professionals may be knowledgeable with regard to nutrition intervention for specific categories of patients (e.g., certified diabetes educators). These health professionals serve as excellent reinforcers of nutrition interventions and behavior modification following individualized nutrition therapy by a dietitian. While their involvement contributes to the nutritional management of diabetes, it is considered basic nutrition education and should continue to be viewed as incidental to routine medical care and not specifically reimbursable as nutrition therapy.

In addition to providing reimbursable nutrition therapy directly to clients and patients, a registered dietitian should be involved in educating other members of the health care team regarding nutrition interventions and practical aspects of nutrition care. This is of particular importance in the areas of home care, ambulatory (outpatient) care, and care given in skilled nursing and long-term care facilities, where basic nutrition advice or reinforcement of nutrition plans will likely be provided by other health care professionals.

In the congressional conference report that described the areas to be reviewed by the requested study, the effectiveness of group versus individual counseling was also identified. A lack of scientific data comparing the effectiveness of individual versus group nutrition counseling sessions was apparent. While group education can provide elderly individuals with opportunities for discussion and support, it may be a suboptimal environment for many elderly individuals with learning barriers such as vision or hearing loss. Individualized counseling can better take into account the multiple diagnoses frequently encountered in older individuals when relating dietary interventions, food preferences, life-style, and cultural factors—all of which are important factors in achieving and sustaining dietary changes. For these reasons, it was concluded that at least one session of *individualized* nutrition therapy is necessary and should be included for optimal effectiveness. However, given that learning styles vary among individuals, it may not be possible to generalize as to whether group or individual counseling is more effective in specific disease states for the remainder of the educational process.

> **Recommendation 3. Reimbursement for enteral and parenteral nutrition-related services in the acute care setting should be continued at the present level. A multidisciplinary approach to the provision of this care is recommended.**

The provision of enteral and parenteral nutrition in the acute care setting is currently covered for Medicare beneficiaries as part of the prospective payment system. Medical conditions for which enteral and parenteral nutrition regimes may be warranted were reviewed and it was concluded that their use in preventing complications and overt malnutrition has been shown to be effective for many conditions. A summary of supporting evidence for various conditions can be reviewed in Table ES.2.

The delivery and oversight of enteral and parenteral nutrition therapy is best carried out by a multidisciplinary team including a physician, pharmacist, nurse, and dietitian. Although a multidisciplinary team is optimal, a variety of formal and informal multidisciplinary models have utility, and ultimately the composition and administration should depend on the institutional setting and available resources. However, the critical involvement of an individual trained in the progression of patients from enteral nutrition to solid food needs to be ensured.

ADMINISTRATIVE RECOMMENDATIONS REGARDING THE PROVISION OF NUTRITION SERVICES

Recommendation 4. HCFA as well as accreditation and licensing groups should reevaluate existing reimbursement systems and regulations for nutrition services along the continuum of care (acute care, ambulatory care, home care, skilled nursing and long-term care settings) to determine the adequacy of care delineated by such standards.

The committee found numerous inconsistencies with regard to regulations and reimbursement systems related to the provision of nutrition services across the continuum of care. The most pronounced inconsistency is the variation in coverage of nutrition services between the acute care inpatient setting and the ambulatory care (outpatient) setting. Patients are often discharged from a short-stay, acute care setting in need of nutrition therapy. However, although nutrition services are part of the bundled payment system in the acute care setting, coverage is no longer available upon discharge to the ambulatory setting. Ironically, it is the ambulatory (outpatient) setting in which patients may benefit most from nutrition counseling. In the home care setting, weak regulations with regard to nutrition therapy result in inadequate services being provided.

HCFA relies on accrediting agencies to enforce standards of nutrition care. Although the Joint Commission on Accreditation of Healthcare Organizations (JCAHO) designates the geriatric population as a high-risk group and has emphasized nutrition in its on-site inspections during the past few years, increased attention still has to be drawn to developing and implementing standards related to the process of assessing the nutritional and functional status of elders as well as identifying and correcting inadequacies of care.

Nutrition services for Medicare beneficiaries in acute care, home care, and long-term care settings are covered largely through bundled payment systems. Reimbursement systems must be strengthened to ensure provision of adequate nutrition care in acute care, home care, dialysis centers, and skilled nursing and long-term care facilities. It is recommended that HCFA as well as accreditation and licensing groups reevaluate all existing reimbursement systems and regulations for nutrition care in acute care, ambulatory care, home care, and long-term care settings. Several areas have been identified that should specifically be addressed and are included in the following recommendations.

TABLE ES.2 Hospital Settings: Evaluation of Nutrition Support Interventions

Intervention	Observational Studies[a]		Consensus Document		Systematic Review	
	GP[b]	Elderly	GP	Elderly	GP	Elderly
Gastrointestinal						
Short bowel						
Enteral	✓	–	✓	–	✓	–
Parenteral	✓	–	✓	–	✓	–
Fistulas						
Enteral	✓	–	✓	–	✓	–
Parenteral	✓	–	✓	–	✓	–
Inflammatory bowel disease						
Enteral	✓	–	✓	–	✓	–
Parenteral	✓	–	✓	–	✓	–
Pancreatitis						
Enteral	✓	–	✓	–	✓	–
Parenteral	✓	–	✓	–	✓	–
Liver disease						
Enteral	✓	–	✓	–	✓	–
Parenteral	✓	–	✓	–	✓	–
HIV/AIDS						
Enteral	✓	–	–	–	–	–
Parenteral	✓	–	–	–	–	–
Cancer Therapy						
Chemotherapy						
Enteral	✓	–	✓	–	✓	–
Parenteral	✓	–	✓	–	✓	–
Radiation Therapy						
Enteral	✓	–	✓	–	✓	–
Parenteral	✓	–	✓	–	✓	–
Renal Failure						
Acute						
Enteral	–	–	–	–	–	–
Parenteral	✓	–	–	–	–	–
Chronic						
Enteral	✓	–	–	–	–	–
Parenteral	✓	–	–	–	–	–
Critical Illness						
Enteral	✓	–	✓	–	–	–
Parenteral	✓	–	✓	–	✓	–
Perioperative						
Abdominal						
Enteral	–	✓	–	–	✓	–
Parenteral	✓	✓	–	–	✓	–
Hip fracture						
Enteral	–	✓	–	–	–	–
Parenteral	–	–	–	–	–	–

[a] This category includes case series, case-control studies, cohort studies and nonrandomized trials of nutrition-based therapies including nonhuman studies.

[b] GP = general population.

Some Clinical Trial Evidence		Extensive Clinical Trial Evidence		Overall Strength of Evidence Supporting Nutrition Therapy for Elderly Persons
GP	Elderly	GP	Elderly	
–	–	–	–	Efficacious
–	–	–	–	Efficacious
–	–	–	–	Insufficient data
–	–	–	–	Efficacious
✓	–	–	–	Insufficient data
✓	–	–	–	Not primary therapy
✓	–	–	–	Insufficient data
✓	–	–	–	Insufficient data
✓	–	–	–	Insufficient data
✓	–	–	–	Insufficient data
✓	–	–	–	Insufficient data
✓	–	–	–	Insufficient data
✓	–	–	–	Not supported
✓	–	–	–	Not supported
✓	–	–	–	Not supported
✓	–	–	–	Not supported
–	–	–	–	Insufficient data
✓	–	–	–	Insufficient data
–	–	–	–	Insufficient data
–	–	–	–	Not supported
✓	–	–	–	Insufficient data
✓	–	–	–	Insufficient data
✓	–	–	–	Selected efficacy
✓	–	–	–	Selected efficacy
–	✓	–	–	Efficacious
–	–	–	–	Insufficient data

Screening for Malnutrition in Acute Care Settings

Recommendation 4.1. While screening for nutrition risk in the acute care setting is crucial, the JCAHO requirement that nutrition screening be completed within 24 hours of admission is not evidence-based and may produce inaccurate and misleading results. It is recommended that validation of nutrition screening methodologies as well as the optimal timing of nutrition screening be reviewed.

Although the committee recognizes that the optimal method of identification of undernutrition in the hospitalized older patient has not been determined, the current JCAHO requirement of nutrition screening within 24 hours of admission to a hospital lacks sensitivity and specificity. Though screening within the first 24 hours of admission may help identify older persons with undernutrition prior to hospitalization, the medical instability of these patients precludes an accurate assessment of how well they will be able to meet their nutritional needs in the hospital. Undernutrition indicators, when available in this time frame, may be altered by acute illness and hence may be inaccurate. Moreover, the acute illness or procedure precipitating hospitalization may result in a transient inability to eat.

Screening within 24 hours of hospital admission, when accomplished, uses resources which may be better utilized helping elderly patients select food they can eat, helping them to eat, and monitoring food intake. In addition, with decreased lengths of stay in acute care settings, patients found to be at risk for malnutrition are often discharged before interventions to improve nutritional status can take place. The most appropriate and clinically useful method of nutritional screening of hospitalized older persons remains an unanswered question and should be a high priority for further research.

Provision of Nutrition Services in the Home Care Setting

Recommendation 4.2. The availability of nutrition services should be improved in the home health care setting. Both types of nutrition services are needed in this setting: nutrition education and nutrition therapy. A registered dietitian should be available to serve as a consultant to health professionals providing basic nutrition education and follow-up, as well as to provide nutrition therapy, when indicated, directly to Medicare beneficiaries being cared for in a home setting.

Medicare beneficiaries are often discharged from hospitals to home care settings with, or at high risk for, overt malnutrition. Yet there is currently no HCFA regulation that requires a nutrition professional to participate in the nutritional management of homebound patients. The adequate provision of services and the staffing of appropriately credentialed nutrition professionals in home care are essential for the training and education of home health nurses and nurses aides so that they may adequately provide appropriate basic nutrition screening and other services. In addition, nutrition professionals should provide nutrition therapy directly to homebound patients when indicated.

Enteral and Parenteral Nutrition in the Ambulatory Care and Home Health Care Settings

Recommendation 4.3. In ambulatory and home care settings, the regulation that excludes coverage for enteral and parenteral nutrition if the gut functions within the next 90 days needs to be reevaluated.

The committee identified a major gap in the coverage of enteral and parenteral nutrition for undernourished ambulatory and home care patients. The current regulation, which excludes coverage for enteral and parenteral nutrition unless the gut is expected to be dysfunctional for at least 90 days, needs to be reevaluated. To avoid the complications of extended semistarvation and possible rehospitalization, reimbursement for enteral or parenteral nutrition in selected Medicare beneficiaries who would otherwise be unable to eat or to assimilate adequate nutrition due to gastrointestinal dysfunction or neurological impairment for longer than 7 days, must be evaluated as a prudent, potentially cost-saving, alternative. Patients who are already malnourished or highly stressed due to infection or response to trauma may not even tolerate this duration of starvation or semistarvation.

In addition, monitoring of patients while on enteral and parenteral nutrition regimes is crucial to avoid both the under- and the overuse of this type of expensive therapy. The registered dietitian is an integral member of the multidisciplinary team and should be involved in the transition of feeding from enteral and parenteral therapies to oral or other modalities, when appropriate or indicated by the referring physician.

Nutrition Services in Skilled Nursing and
Long-Term Care Facilities

Recommendation 4.4. HCFA, as well as accrediting and licensing agencies, should improve requirements and standards for food and nutrition services in skilled nursing and long-term care facilities.

As Medicare shifts to a prospective payment system for skilled nursing and long-term care facilities, the nutrition services provided must not be compromised, but should be improved beyond the current pattern of practice. Some states require that long-term care facilities employ dietitians for so little time (8 hours per month) that little can be accomplished when nutrition problems are identified. Staffing must be adequate, and staff members should be well trained and professionally supervised by nutrition professionals so that patients are fed sensitively and appropriately. Efforts to improve quality of care should be aimed at improving staffing patterns, the quality of food services, the incorporation of appropriate feeding techniques into patient services, and the education and training of staff on feeding techniques for patients with functional limitations. Nutrition professionals should be available to educate and train nursing staff and aides on the prevention, detection, and treatment of malnutrition in elderly patients. In addition, registered dietitians, along with other members of the multidisciplinary team, should also be available for the provision and monitoring of enteral and parenteral nutrition regimes.

Research Agenda

Recommendation 4.5. Federal agencies such as the National Institute on Aging, the Agency for Healthcare Research and Quality, and HCFA should pursue a research agenda in the area of nutrition in the older person.

Throughout this study, the committee found a paucity of usable data with regard to nutritional status of the older person, particularly in the area of evaluating the success of interventions with regard to treatment of nutritionally related multiple diseases and conditions. In some instances, issues had not been studied, and in others, previously conducted research did not provide definitive answers. The committee identified numerous areas for research, which can be found at the end of relevant chapters of this report.

ECONOMIC POLICY ANALYSIS

Cost to the Medicare program of expanded coverage for nutrition therapy will be directly determined by the specific design of the reimbursement benefit, patient demand, and other factors. Forecasts of these costs are thus imprecise given currently available data. However, because of the comparatively low treatment costs and ancillary benefits associated with nutrition therapy, expanded coverage will improve the quality of care and is likely to be a valuable and efficient use of Medicare resources.

The committee's approach to cost estimation used generic practices consistent with the Congressional Budget Office process (e.g., not discounting estimates to present value). A more detailed description of the cost estimate process is provided in chapter 14. Data from other cost studies, current accepted practice guidelines, clinical studies, and Medicare cost data were used in the cost estimates. Previous studies show that from 5 to 20 percent of beneficiaries would likely use a nutrition therapy service if it were a covered benefit. The Medicare portion of estimated charges for coverage of nutrition therapy during the 5-year period, 2000 to 2004, is $1.43 billion. However, due to uncertainty about the actual utilization of a nutrition therapy benefit, two additional scenarios were calculated to reflect a low utilization estimate and a high utilization estimate. The range is from $873 million (low utilization scenario) to $2.63 billion (high utilization scenario) with diagnosis-specific utilization rates ranging from 5 to 30 percent. Some of these costs will be passed on to Medicare beneficiaries through associated premium increases.

Expanded coverage for nutrition therapy is likely to generate economically significant benefits to beneficiaries, and in the short term to the Medicare program itself, through reduced healthcare expenditures. Nutrition therapy, in the context of multidisciplinary care, has a potential short-term cost savings for specific populations such as those with hypertension, dyslipidemia, and diabetes. While these effects have been expressed in economic terms, detailed budget forecasts of these effects require a more extensive actuarial analysis that is beyond the scope of this study. Initial estimates for potential cost avoidance for individuals with hypertension, elevated lipids, and diabetes have been included. The estimates were provided in ranges corresponding to the utilization scenarios and are $52 million to $167 million for hypertension, $54 million to $164 million for those with elevated lipids, and $132 million to $330 million for those with diabetes. It is not appropriate to add these estimates together since beneficiaries have overlapping diagnosis. Estimates were not made for the 5.62 million beneficiaries likely to receive nutrition therapy for other diagnoses such as chronic renal insufficiency and heart failure. Expanded coverage may be cost saving in these broader patient groups, although data are inadequate to reliably establish these patterns.

Whether or not expanded coverage reduces overall Medicare expenditures, it is recommended that these services be reimbursed given the reasonable evidence of improved patient outcomes associated with such care.

In addition to decreased mortality and morbidity, nutrition therapy can have an impact on quality of life in less tangible ways that cannot be measured quantitatively. Meals provide the social context for important religious and family experiences across the life course. Because food is central to an individual's social attachment and role, dietary problems that require significant behavior change or interfere with long-established social relationships can have a significant impact on patient well-being independent of their impact on mortality or morbidity. Nutrition therapy translates the desired treatment goals into daily life skills such as grocery shopping, food preparation, and selecting from restaurant menus. Nutrition therapy that assists homebound patients to participate in family meals may have a greater impact on subjective well-being than many other interventions that have equal impact on physical health.

CONCLUDING REMARKS

In summary, evidence exists to conclude that nutrition therapy can improve health outcomes for several conditions that are highly prevalent among Medicare beneficiaries while possibly decreasing costs to Medicare. Basic nutrition advice for healthy living and the primary prevention of disease can often be provided by a multitude of health care professionals who have had less extensive academic preparation in nutrition science and/or clinical training than a registered dietitian. This is not considered a service that should be a separately covered benefit to Medicare beneficiaries. However, the provision of nutrition therapy requires in-depth knowledge of food and nutrition science. Registered dietitians are currently the primary group of health care professionals with the necessary type of education and training to provide this level of nutrition service. It is recognized that there may be others within medical subspecialties who may have particularly strong levels of expertise and could in the future be evaluated by HCFA as a certified provider. The committee found numerous inconsistencies in current health care regulations and standards. Agencies responsible for oversight need to reevaluate regulations associated with the provision of quality nutrition care to ensure that policies and standards are based on evidence and represent the best use of resources. In addition, reimbursement policies must be reevaluated to ensure that the nutritional needs of Medicare beneficiaries are met consistently across the continuum of care.

REFERENCES

NCHS (National Center for Health Statistics). 1997. *Third National Health and Nutrition Examination Survey* (Series 11, No. 1, SETS version 1.22a). [CD-ROM]. Washington, D.C.: U.S. Government Printing Office.

Ryan AS, Craig LD, Finn SC. 1992. Nutrient intakes and dietary patterns of older Americans: A national study. *J Gerontol* 47:M145–M150.

U.S. Preventive Services Task Force. 1995. *Guide to Clinical Preventive Services, 2nd Ed. Report of the U.S. Preventive Services Task Force.* Washington, D.C.: U.S. Department of Health and Human Services, Office of Public Health, Office of Health Promotion and Disease Prevention.

Section I

Introduction and Overview

1

Introduction

Provision of adequate food, which in turn supplies the needed nutrients and energy, is essential to the health and well-being of all people. In healthy, independently living adults, this process is based on food availability, food intake, and life-style choices, and generally results in an acceptable range of health and nutritional status. The relationship of food, nutrition, and health often changes with aging; with age-related alterations in nutrient requirements; with the acquisition of acute and chronic illnesses; and, in many elderly, with the loss of personal and financial independence.

These age-related changes are in part the basis of the significant nutritional risks associated with the older population of Medicare beneficiaries. In the current U.S. health care environment, these personal changes in age, health, and living status are highly influenced by the availability of quality health care and health care funding policy. The number of Medicare beneficiaries is increasing and the cost of medical care is rising. Yet there is a recognition that the currently available Medicare coverage may need to be expanded to include new services previously not covered, including nutrition services.

Changes in health care since the inception of Medicare in 1965 have had a significant impact on the delivery of nutrition services to Medicare beneficiaries. The shift from traditionally delivered inpatient care to ambulatory care has reduced the number of hospital beds and increased the severity of illness in the remaining hospitalized patients. Shorter lengths of hospital stays have reduced or eliminated the ability to provide in-depth nutrition counseling, including life-style change counseling, necessary to prevent or treat chronic diseases during the hospital admission.

Rapid discharge from the acute care hospital setting has created new dimensions in the continuum of care—transitional or subacute care, home health, and hospice care. In these settings, the provision of nutritional services is not required and monitored with the same rigor as in the acute care setting. The resulting services provided to Medicare beneficiaries often do not adequately address nutrition and lifestyle issues (Posner and Krachenfels, 1987). Yet, with careful planning, these non-acute care settings may be better suited, along with the traditional outpatient office setting, to deliver the nutrition services needed by Medicare beneficiaries.

Scientific advances in medical care have increased the need for a multidisciplinary team approach to patient care and a shift from the individual provider model. The need for medical cost containment has led to various approaches to managing care, as well as an increased focus on health promotion, disease prevention, and patient self-management skills for some conditions. The self-management effort has moved to center stage with the development of formal self-management programs in several settings, particularly for diabetes.

With increasing emphasis on disease prevention, there has been a proliferation of nutrition-related disease prevention and screening programs targeted at increasing dietary intake of fiber, fruits, and vegetables; reducing the fat content of foods; and increasing specific nutrients such as folate or calcium. In addition, among the fastest-growing areas of the food, pharmaceutical, and related industries are nutrition supplements and herbal products. Older consumers are often among the primary target groups for these companies and are often poorly informed as to the risks, benefits, and costs of including such products in their health care plans.

THE COMMITTEE AND ITS CHARGE

In accordance with the Institute of Medicine committee process, an expert committee was appointed to undertake the congressionally mandated study looking at nutrition services for Medicare beneficiaries. Financial support for the committee was provided through a contract between the Institute of Medicine (IOM), National Academy of Sciences (NAS) and the Health Care Financing Administration (HCFA), as mandated in the Balanced Budget Act of 1997.

The committee was charged with the task of analyzing available information, holding a workshop, and making recommendations regarding technical and policy aspects of the provision of comprehensive nutrition services, including the following:

• coverage of nutrition services provided by registered dietitians and other health care practitioners for inpatient care of medically necessary parenteral[1] and enteral[2] nutrition therapy;

• coverage of nutrition services provided by registered dietitians and other health care practitioners, including registered dietitians, for patients in home health and skilled nursing facility settings; and

• coverage of nutrition services provided by registered dietitians and other trained health care practitioners in individual counseling and group settings, including both primary and secondary preventive services.

In addition, the committee was charged with evaluating, to the extent data were available, the cost and benefit of such services to Medicare beneficiaries and to identify the research issues needed to provide a better understanding of the relationship between the provision of quality nutrition services and quality-of-life outcomes. The Lewin Group, a quantitative analysis consulting firm in the Washington, D.C. area, provided an analysis of the financial impact on the Medicare program given the committee's recommendations on coverage for nutrition services under contract with the NAS.

The committee was composed of 14 individuals with expertise in the areas of geriatric medicine, clinical nutrition and metabolism, epidemiology, clinical dietetics, evidence-based medicine, outpatient counseling, nutrition services management, nutrition support, nursing, health economics, and health policy. Committee members held a variety of professional degrees and represented a geographical cross section of the nation. A complete roster of committee members, including a description of their background and expertise, is included in Appendix I.

The committee met over a 5-month period to consider its scope of work; review the relevant scientific evidence; and develop its findings, conclusions, and recommendations. In all, four meetings were held. One meeting included a workshop open to the public. Experts in areas selected by the committee were invited to make presentations and discuss evidence related to particular elements of nutrition services as well as behavioral considerations in the elderly population. During the workshop, a public comment period was held, and interested individuals and organizations were invited to present both oral and written testimony to the committee. Several consultants to the committee participated either through presentations and/or critical review of report sections. The names

---

[1]Delivery of nutrients intravenously rather than through the gastrointestinal tract.
[2]Delivery of nutrients through a feeding tube into the gastrointestinal tract.

of workshop speakers, organizations contacted, and consultants to the committee can be found in Appendix C.

Once the committee had completed its initial draft report, a set of reviewers familiar with the issues under discussion and approved by the National Research Council's Report Review committee individually reviewed and commented on the draft report. These reviewers remained anonymous until the report was finalized. The review process is intended to ensure that the report addresses the committee's charge, that the conclusions and recommendations are based on scientific evidence, and that the report is presented in an effective and impartial manner.

OVERVIEW OF THE REPORT

In evaluating nutrition services for the elderly, the committee adopted definitions for common terms which are often referred to in the report. Nutrition services is a broad term which encompasses varied approaches to improving the nutritional health of the elderly from informal nutrition advice and community programs to intensive nutrition counseling and the provision of intravenous feedings. Nutrition services can be divided into two levels. The first tier is *basic nutrition services*, which includes informal nutrition advice and education. The second tier is more complex and is referred to as *nutrition therapy*.

For the purposes of this report, the term nutrition therapy is defined as the treatment of a disease or condition through the modification of nutrient or whole-food intake. Nutrition therapy encompasses the assessment of an individual's nutritional status, the evaluation of nutritional needs, interventions or counseling to achieve optimal clinical outcomes, and follow-up care as appropriate. The assessment of nutritional needs takes into consideration the individual's medical and dietary histories, as well as physical, anthropometric, and laboratory data. Nutrition therapy includes oral, enteral, and parenteral nutrition interventions and takes into consideration the cultural, socioeconomic, and food preferences of the individual.

Even though the population of Medicare beneficiaries includes a significant number of individuals younger than 65 years of age with disabilities (about 13 percent) and with end-stage renal disease (about 0.8 percent), this report was designed to focus on the examination of evidence and the role of nutrition services for those age 65 and older. Renal disease was reviewed, but with a more in-depth focus on pre-end-stage disease. Since there were often limited clinical studies on individuals older than 65 years, most of the evidence examined includes study subjects of younger ages.

The report reviews evidence related to the role of nutrition in several chronic conditions which significantly impact on the morbidity, mortality, and quality of life of the nation's elderly. While there are likely other conditions for which evidence regarding the role of nutrition exists, it was beyond the scope of this report to review evidence related to all medical conditions. The conditions which the committee chose to review in depth—dyslipidemia, heart failure, hypertension, diabetes mellitus, renal failure, and osteoporosis—do not imply that other conditions were of less importance. The conditions chosen were those that the committee felt had not only a significant impact on morbidity and mortality in this population, but also had sufficient data available to evaluate.

In the elderly, obesity is common and most often occurs with other important clinical conditions for which there is significant scientific literature, such as hypertension, heart failure, diabetes, and hyperlipidemia. For reasons discussed in chapter 2, the committee chose to include and review scientific evidence of nutrition services for obesity only within each of the associated clinical conditions and chapters where applicable.

This report is organized into four sections:

- Section I (chapters 1–3) sets the stage for the report—giving an overview of the Medicare program, nutritional concerns in older persons, as well as the methods committee members used to guide them through their deliberations.
- Section II (chapters 4–8) addresses the conditions reviewed in this report which can affect elderly individuals in health care settings across the continuum of care: ambulatory (outpatient care), acute care hospitals (inpatient care), sub-acute and long-term care facilities, and home care. For this reason, the efficacy of the role of nutrition in diseases or conditions is independent of particular settings of care. Each of the condition-specific chapters addresses the strength of the evidence for the efficacy of the role of nutrition, makes recommendations regarding the provision of services to Medicare beneficiaries, and addresses research gaps in areas where evidence is needed.
- Section III (chapters 9–12) addresses the continuum of care: short-stay acute care facilities (hospitals), ambulatory care (outpatient services), home care, and skilled nursing and long-term care facilities. It also addresses the delivery of nutrition support (enteral and parenteral feedings) which may be needed and provided in any of the above settings.
- Section IV (chapters 13–15) presents the committee's findings regarding providers of nutrition services, cost estimates of providing services found to be efficacious to Medicare beneficiaries, and a summary of the committee's conclusions and recommendations.

OVERVIEW OF THE MEDICARE PROGRAM[3]

Congress created the Medicare program in 1965 to provide health insurance for Americans age 65 or over. It later extended coverage to some individuals with disabilities or permanent kidney failure. From the outset, the program has focused on hospital, physician, and certain other services that are "reasonable and necessary for the diagnosis or treatment of illness or injury or to improve the functioning of a malformed body member" (section 1862 of the Social Security Act). With certain exceptions, Congress explicitly excluded coverage for preventive services, outpatient prescription drugs, dental care, and long-term nursing home care and other supportive services for people with chronic disabling conditions.

Most sessions of Congress see proposals to expand Medicare coverage for one or more of the services that are currently excluded. For example, while this report was being drafted, Congress was debating the addition of outpatient drug benefits, which even under the most limited proposals would add substantially to the program's costs. With growth in Medicare spending and health care costs having far exceeded 1960s' estimates, the increased cost of additional services has generally discouraged coverage expansions. Moreover, Congress has set budget rules for itself requiring that decisions to increase most types of federal spending must be accompanied by explicit decisions to reduce spending elsewhere or to raise taxes. These rules underscore the reality that expanding Medicare coverage involves making trade-offs to face the resource constraints.

In the Balanced Budget Act of 1997 (Public Law 105-33), Congress called for the Department of Health and Human Services to arrange for the NAS to analyze "the short- and long-term benefits, and costs to Medicare" of extending coverage for certain preventive and other services. These services were screening for skin cancer; medically necessary dental services; elimination of time restrictions on coverage for immunosuppressive drugs after transplants; nutrition therapy; and routine patient care for beneficiaries enrolled in approved clinical trials.

This request from Congress reflects two significant developments since Medicare's beginnings: an accelerating pace of technological innovation and—partly as a consequence—a greater than anticipated escalation of program expenditures and overall health care costs. Scientific and technological advances have clearly led to a multitude of new medical procedures, drugs, devices, and other services that prolong life, protect physical and mental functioning, prevent disease, and otherwise improve

---

[3]Excerpted and adapted from the companion report *Extending Medicare Coverage for Preventive and Other Services* (IOM, 2000).

people's health and well-being. Of course, not all innovations perform as promised. Moreover, most new—and established—technologies have risks that must be weighed against expected benefits. Cost constraints also require that trade-offs be made.

Historical Background

When Congress—following years of debate—created Medicare as Title XVIII of the Social Security Act (SSA), it was responding to the growing availability of effective medical services and the difficulty faced by older people in either paying for these services directly or obtaining private health insurance.[4] At the same time, Congress also created the federal–state Medicaid program (Title XIX of the SSA), which provided health insurance for certain categories of low-income individuals (especially low-income mothers and children and low-income aged, blind, or disabled people). Reflecting the needs of these lower-income beneficiaries, Medicaid covers a generally broader array of services (e.g., well-baby visits, extended nursing home care). It also provides states some flexibility in deciding what to cover (e.g., certain dental services, outpatient prescription drugs). Certain low-income people, called "dual eligibles," qualify for full or partial Medicaid benefits as well as regular Medicare coverage. Their Medicaid benefits cover many of the Medicare program's cost-sharing requirements and "fill-in" some of the gaps in Medicare benefits. In 1972, Congress expanded Medicare to cover certain disabled persons and created a unique entitlement to coverage for people who suffer from end-stage renal disease (ESRD).

Continuing a division that had emerged earlier in private health insurance, the Medicare program as initially created had two parts: hospitalization insurance, also known as HI or Part A, and supplementary medical insurance for physician and certain other services, also known as SMI or Part B.[5] Part A, which is financed by payroll taxes (1.45 percent paid by employers and employees), covers inpatient hospital care subject to an annual deductible set at $768 in 1999 and a per-day copayment after 60 days. It also covers (subject to various time limitations, cost-sharing

---

[4]This discussion draws on Ball, 1995; Feingold, 1966; Harris, 1969; Marmor, 1973; Somers and Somers, 1961, 1967, 1977a, b; Starr, 1982; Stevens, 1989.

[5]In 1997, as part of the Balanced Budget Act, Congress created Part C (also known as Medicare+Choice), which restructured and expanded options for Medicare beneficiaries to enroll in approved health maintenance organizations and other private health insurance plans. These plans, which are paid a fixed monthly amount per enrolled beneficiary, must provide Medicare-covered services but may also offer additional benefits.

requirements, and other restrictions) services provided by other institutional providers including skilled nursing facilities and hospices. One rationale for covering these kinds of services has been that such coverage may encourage the use of alternatives to more expensive hospital care. Part B covers physician and certain other professional services provided in the hospital, office, and selected other settings. It also covers a number of additional services such as outpatient hospital care, outpatient dialysis services, clinical laboratory tests, durable medical equipment, ambulance services and, since 1997, most home health care services. For part B coverage, beneficiaries pay a monthly premium (set to cover 25 percent of Part B expenditures or $45.50 per beneficiary in 1999) and coinsurance of 20 percent for most services. Part A coverage is virtually automatic for those eligible, but enrollment in Part B is voluntary, although nearly all of those eligible do enroll.

As noted above, the legislation creating Medicare excluded coverage for services not deemed "reasonable and necessary" for the diagnosis or treatment of an illness or injury or to improve the functioning of a malformed body member. Preventive services, dental care (except in very limited situations related to serious medical problems), and outpatient prescription drugs were among the services categorically excluded in 1965.

One rationale for excluding preventive services from Medicare was that they did not fit the traditional insurance model of providing coverage for expenses that are unpredictable (and thus cannot be budgeted) and substantial (and thus are a serious financial burden for individuals and families). When Medicare was created, hospitalization and other major expenses related to care for acute illnesses fit the model; expenses for most preventive services then available, outpatient prescription drugs, and dental care did not. In addition, insurance principles also discouraged coverage for "broad and ill-defined" services such as routine physicals and health education or counseling (Breslow and Somers, 1977; OTA, 1990).

Since 1965, Congress has authorized a few exceptions to the coverage exclusions just described. After rejecting 350 bills to make one or more exceptions to Medicare's exclusion of preventive services, Congress approved its first exception—for pneumococcal pneumonia vaccine—in 1980 (Schauffler, 1993), and more exceptions have followed. Congress has waived the application of the Part B deductible and coinsurance provisions for some covered preventive services.

Because of gaps in Medicare coverage, about 80 percent of beneficiaries purchase or otherwise obtain some form of supplemental coverage to help pay for certain excluded services, deductibles, and copayments or coinsurance (HCFA, 1998a). This coverage may be provided through an employer-sponsored program, an individually purchased "Medigap" policy, or a state Medicaid program. Medicare beneficiaries covered by health maintenance organizations (HMO) may be eligible for additional preventive and other services, sometimes by paying an additional premium, but HMOs vary greatly in the extent to which they offer benefits not required by Medicare (Kaiser Family Foundation, 1998).

Enrollment and Expenditure Trends

Since the program was implemented, the number of Medicare beneficiaries has roughly doubled, from 19.1 million when the program began in 1966 to approximately 38.4 million for 1997 (about 4.8 million of whom qualify for Medicare due to disability and about 0.3 million due to ESRD) (HCFA, 1999a). The growth in Medicare enrollment will accelerate as the baby boom generation begins to reach age 65 (and becomes eligible for coverage) in 2011. By 2015, the population age 65 years and over is projected to reach 56.3 million. Unless age or other eligibility requirements change, virtually all will be covered by Medicare. Those qualifying because of disability or ESRD are expected to constitute a somewhat larger fraction of the total beneficiary population by 2015 (about 16 percent compared to 13 percent in 1997).

Initial forecasts of program spending proved to be gross underestimates of actual spending. While the number of beneficiaries was doubling, Medicare net outlays grew from $2.7 billion in 1967 (the program's first full year) to $174.2 billion in 1996 (U.S. House of Representatives, 1997, 1998). (In constant 1995 dollars, 1967 expenditures would amount to about $10 billion.)

Current debates about Medicare's future revolve primarily around predictions that Part A of the program will become insolvent (spending will exceed revenues) early in the twenty-first century. Projections of long-term Medicare program costs—and health care costs more generally— have many uncertainties (White, 1999), but the predictions of future funding shortfalls are being taken seriously. Nonetheless, concerns about federal spending and program solvency have prompted discussions of major and controversial changes such as raising the age of eligibility, instituting some kind of means testing, directing more beneficiaries into capitated managed care plans, and establishing a formula for the government's contribution to program costs that would shift more of the risk for continued health care cost escalation to beneficiaries. A major component of the Balanced Budget Act of 1997 was a set of measures to slow the growth in program spending and at least delay the date at which Medicare spending is projected to exceed revenues (Kahn and Kuttner, 1999).

Solvency concerns are also shaping reactions to less comprehensive changes of the kind considered in this report.

As mentioned earlier, congressional budget rules also require that certain decisions to increase federal government spending in one area be offset with actions to reduce spending in other areas or to increase taxes or other revenues. For example, higher net spending for new nutrition services benefits would have to be matched by increasing taxes or by spending reductions either elsewhere in the Medicare program (e.g., through lower payment rates for health care providers) or in other areas (e.g., Medicaid).

MEDICARE COVERAGE DECISIONS[6]

Medicare coverage decisions range from very broad-based decisions about whole categories of services to very narrow decisions about whether a specific service will be covered for a specific individual. In between are decisions about the general circumstances under which a specific service will be covered (e.g., that bone marrow transplant will be covered for certain cancers and not others). In general, these kinds of decisions are made at three different levels with

• Congress making broad decisions about categories of coverage and coverage exceptions,
• HCFA focusing on the circumstances under which a new or established service will be covered, and
• private contractors that administer Medicare claims for the government deciding whether specific services billed for a specific beneficiary are covered and also establishing more general policies for services and circumstances for which HCFA has no policy.

Congress

Congress establishes the broad categories of covered and excluded services. It may also make coverage exceptions for individual services in otherwise excluded categories. In considering legislative proposals to extend coverage, Congress may hold hearings to solicit expert advice (including assessments of scientific evidence) and the views of patients, families, clinicians, health industry manufacturers, administrators, and other interested groups. Until it was terminated in 1995, the congressional Office of Technology Assessment (OTA) responded to congressional re-

---

[6]Excerpted and adapted from the companion report *Extending Medicare Coverage for Preventive and Other Services* (IOM, 2000).

quests for assessments of clinical preventive measures, immunosuppressive drugs, and other services. The OTA analyses considered scientific and clinical issues but were also explicitly intended to provide guidance to policymakers by examining the cost-effectiveness of clinical interventions, possible costs to Medicare of extending coverage, and other policy issues.

For categories of covered services, Congress has authorized the HCFA to establish procedures for making more specific coverage decisions about individual services within the broad categories established legislatively. It could also authorize HCFA (which is part of the Department of Health and Human Services) or a quasi-public body either to make coverage exceptions for services that now fall in the categories of generally excluded services. For example, the early 1990s discussion of health care reform saw various proposals for delegating decisions about preventive services (OTA, 1993).

Health Care Financing Administration

Within the broad coverage categories established by Congress, more specific determinations about what services are or are not covered are the responsibility of the Health Care Financing Administration (Bagley and McVearry, 1998). HCFA also provides detailed guidance to Medicare contractors regarding the application of its coverage rules and the development of local contractor medical policies for situations not dealt with by such rules.

Altogether, HCFA has issued about 700 national coverage policy decisions (John Whyte, Health Care Financing Administration, Baltimore, Maryland, personal communication, July 1999). These decisions typically involve either new services and technologies or new indications (clinical circumstances) for the use of technologies that had previously been covered for a limited set of indications. Some determinations restrict coverage of an already covered service—usually because new evidence suggests the service is unsafe or ineffective.

The coverage determination process may involve reviews of the scientific evidence, consultations with clinical experts, and comparisons with similar technologies. Some technology assessments are conducted by HCFA staff, whereas others are referred to different governmental or private organizations including the federal Agency for Healthcare Research and Quality (AHRQ) and its Evidence-Based Practice Centers (EPCs). Created by Congress in 1989, AHRQ supports an array of activities intended to increase and evaluate the evidence base for health care services. The EPCs—many of which are consortia or partnerships of universities and other institutions—produce evidence reports and technology assessments on topics as requested. If nongovernmental parties request a coverage determination from HCFA, they are expected to provide supporting documentation including reviews and analyses of the scientific evidence, unless they lack the resources to do so.

In making coverage determinations, HCFA must follow federal rulemaking procedures and requirements. After criticism that agency procedures violated federal open government rules, HCFA created a new Medicare Coverage Advisory Committee, for which administrative procedures are being developed and reviewed.[7] A typical candidate for the committee review would be a new technology or new use of an established technology relevant to an existing coverage category. Various gene therapies are examples of the former and innovative uses of lasers are examples of the latter.

HCFA has interpreted the congressional requirement that services be covered only if "reasonable and necessary" for the diagnosis or treatment of an illness or injury to mean that they must be (1) safe and effective, (2) provided in an appropriate setting, and (3) not experimental or investigational (HCFA, 1989). The criteria and processes for determining what services are medically necessary have been the subject of much debate and dissatisfaction (e.g., see Anderson et al., 1998; Bergthold, 1995; Cunningham, 1999; IOM, 1992; NHPF, 1998, 1999).

In January 1989 and as recently as 1996, HCFA proposed to consider the cost-effectiveness of technologies as part of the coverage review process (*Health Systems Review*, 1997). The proposal provoked considerable controversy and was never adopted. HCFA should shortly be issuing a new *Federal Register* notice proposing national coverage criteria.

Because individual coverage determinations by HCFA are not directly governed by the "budget neutrality" rules of Congress, new services that fit within established coverage categories face different hurdles to coverage approval than do services that require congressional action.

Administrative Contractors

In practice, many coverage determinations, perhaps 90 percent (HIMA, 1999), are made not by HCFA but by the 60-plus private contractors that the agency uses to administer payment of Medicare claims on a state, substate, or multistate basis. On the Part A side, these organizations

---

[7]This committee will operate under the Federal Advisory Committee Act (HCFA, 1998b). HCFA has also published a notice explaining the new process of making national coverage decisions (HCFA, 1999c). A notice on proposed coverage criteria is expected by the end of 1999.

are called "intermediaries." For Part B, which generates nearly all of these coverage questions, they are known as "carriers." HMOs and other private health plans approved by Medicare to serve beneficiaries must follow intermediary and carrier policies, but they also must make their own coverage determinations in the absence of such policies.

Frequently, it is these private carriers that first encounter questions about new medical services or services for which coverage is sought beyond the uses originally recognized. Their determinations are codified in the form of local medical review policies. Local medical policies may also specify more precisely the appropriate indications for established technologies for which excessive use is suspected. This is consistent with HCFA's description of medical review policy as a "program integrity" tool intended to protect the program from fraud and abuse (HCFA, 1999b).

Carriers make decisions about payment after services have been provided. HCFA uses another group of contractors, Peer Review Organizations (PROs) to conduct prior reviews of certain surgical procedures and engage in other activities intended to improve the quality of care provided to Medicare beneficiaries. Contractors administering provider claims for payment must coordinate with the appropriate PROs to assure that payments are made consistent with the PROs' decisions (HCFA, 1999b).

HCFA's new procedures for national coverage decision making make clear that local medical policy decisions cannot conflict with a national decision by HCFA. Other HCFA policies direct carriers to base policies on the best evidence available, cite the basis and references for local medical policies, submit the policies to their Carrier Advisory Committees, publish them in their provider bulletins, and consider comments submitted in response (HCFA, 1999b). Carriers may conduct their own assessments of new or established services and technologies, or they may rely on others, for example, ECRI (originally the Emergency Care Research Institute) or the Technical Evaluation Center of the Blue Cross and Blue Shield Association (both of which are designated EPCs).

Carrier coverage policies are generally prompted by the need to make determinations about coverage of a service provided to a specific individual rather than by, for example, a request for a policy or by the anticipation of claims related to an emerging technology. When the judgments are negative, such case-by-case negative decisions may readily evoke images of big, impersonal bureaucracies refusing to pay for innovative treatments that provide the last hope for desperately ill individuals. Controversies about such negative coverage decisions—and conflicting decisions from different carriers—may then prompt HCFA on its initiative or at the request of others to develop a uniform national policy. In addition to revising procedures for national coverage decision making and clarifying the role of local organizations in the coverage process, HCFA has a contractor examining variation in local medical policies.

MEDICARE COVERAGE OF NUTRITION SERVICES

A summary of current Medicare coverage of nutrition services along the continuum of care is presented in Table 1.1. The information is somewhat simplified and does not reflect all possible instances but serves as the general assumptions of current coverage by the committee.

TABLE 1.1 Medicare Coverage of Nutrition Services

Service	General Coverage	Nutrition Services Coverage
MEDICARE PART A		
Hospital inpatient care	Medicare reimburses hospitals a bundled payment, based on diagnosis, for all services provided by the facility, including bed and board, nursing and related services, diagnostic and therapeutic services, drugs, and supplies.	The hospital conditions of participation require a hospital to have a full-time employee who serves as director of the food and dietary service; is responsible for the daily management of the dietary services; and is qualified by experience and training. There must be a qualified dietitian, full-time, part-time, or on a consultant basis. There must be administrative and technical personnel competent in their respective duties. Menus must meet the needs of the patients. Therapeutic diets must be prescribed by the practitioner responsible for the care of patients. Nutritional needs must be met in accordance with orders of the practitioner responsible for the care of patients. The facility must ensure that residents receive proper treatment and care for, among other special

TABLE 1.1 Continued

Service	General Coverage	Nutrition Services Coverage
Hospital inpatient care *(continued)*		services, parenteral and enteral fluids. Nutrition services are included as part of the hospital's bundled payment and are not reimbursed as a separate charge.
Skilled nursing facility (SNF) care	Medicare pays SNFs a per diem payment that covers bed and board, nursing and related services, therapeutic services, drugs, and supplies.	Conditions of participation include the following: "The facility must assure that a resident maintains acceptable parameters of nutritional status (unless the resident's clinical condition demonstrates that this is not possible) and receives a therapeutic diet when there is a nutritional problem." In addition, section 483.35 is as follows: "The facility must provide each resident with a nourishing, palatable, well-balanced diet that meets his or her daily nutritional and special dietary needs." The subparagraphs of this section address (a) staffing (indicates a qualified dietitian must be employed or contracted with on a consultant basis); (b) sufficient dietary staff; (c) menus and nutritional adequacy; (d) food; (e) therapeutic diets; (f) frequency of meals; (g) assistive devices; and (h) sanitary conditions. Nutrition services are included as part of the SNFs per diem payment and are not reimbursed as a separate charge.

continued on next page

TABLE 1.1 Continued

Service	General Coverage	Nutrition Services Coverage
Home health care	Medicare Part A covers up to 100 visits of home health care following a 3-day hospital stay if rendered within 14 days of discharge. Home health agencies are paid on a cost basis, up to certain limits. Beginning in 2001, home health services will be paid under a prospective payment system. While each covered home health service will be bundled into the rate, each covered service will appear in the consolidated billing provided to patients.	Although very limited, administrative costs associated with the provision of nutrition services are included in the benefit. While home health agencies are required to have specialized nutrition expertise in order to be Medicare certified, nutrition services are not reimbursed as a separate charge.
Hospice care	The Medicare hospice benefit is limited to patients with a life expectancy of 6 months or less. Hospices are paid per diem rates for provision of pain relief, symptom management, and support services.	Part of the core services that must be provided by Medicare certified hospices is dietary counseling. Rural hospices may obtain a waiver, which will allow hospices to contract out for counseling. Dietary counseling is included in the per diem rate and is not reimbursed as a separate charge.
MEDICARE PART B Health care provider visits	Medicare pays physicians and certain other health care professionals (e.g., dentists, chiropractors, optometrists, podiatrists, advanced practice nurses, physician assistants, psychologists, social workers, physical and occupational therapists) according to the Medicare fee schedule. Some nonphysician practitioners	Nutrition services provided by health professionals recognized by Medicare as "certified providers" may receive reimbursement if the service is deemed reasonable and medically necessary. For example, a physician may counsel a patient regarding a diet and bill for the time spent with the patient under an office visit

TABLE 1.1 Continued

Service	General Coverage	Nutrition Services Coverage
Health care provider visits *(continued)*	may be reimbursed only for certain procedures (e.g., chiropractors may be reimbursed by Medicare only for spinal manipulation). Some nonphysician practitioners may receive less than the full Medicare fee schedule amount (e.g., advanced practice nurses and physician assistants receive 85% of the payment that would be made to a physician for the same service).	"evaluation and management" code. Nutrition services may also be reimbursed by Medicare when nutrition services are provided "incident to" a physician's service if deemed reasonable and medically necessary. *All* requirements of "incident to" must be met. The physician must perform the initial service and subsequent services with a frequency that reflects the active participation of or management by the physician during the course of treatment. "Incident-to" services must be provided by an employee of a physician or physician group practice and must be directly supervised by the physician billing for the services. Registered dietitians in independent practice are not authorized by Medicare to receive reimbursement for providing nutrition services.
Hospital outpatient department care	Medicare has in the past reimbursed hospital outpatient departments on a cost basis. Effective in 2000, hospital outpatient departments will be paid on a prospective payment basis and receive bundled payments based on the classification of the procedure performed. The payments will cover all facility costs, diagnostic	Nutrition services provided as part of a patient educational program, such as a diabetes education or cardiac rehabilitation program may be covered if they are furnished "incident to" a physician's service and if deemed reasonable and medically necessary for the individual patient. Nutrition counseling by a

continued on next page

TABLE 1.1 Continued

Service	General Coverage	Nutrition Services Coverage
Hospital outpatient department care (continued)	tests, drugs, supplies, etc., necessary for the procedure.	qualified dietitian, which does not meet the "incident to" medically necessary requirements for the individual patient, is not covered. Payment is made to the facility for the whole program.
Diabetes self-management training	A new benefit effective in 1998. Regulations for reimbursement and qualifications of certified programs are currently under development.	The nutrition component of the benefit is reimbursed as part of the total payment. Dietitians are required to be involved with a certified program; however, they cannot sponsor a program or receive Medicare reimbursement because they are not recognized independent providers under the Medicare program.
Routine preventive services	Medicare covers only certain preventive services: flu, hepatitis B, and pneumonia vaccines; mammography; pelvic exams and Pap smears; colorectal cancer screening; bone mass measurements; and prostate screening. Payment is made for professional services or for laboratory tests according to the applicable fee schedule.	In general, nutrition services provided for primary prevention are not covered.
Home health care	Home health services reimbursed under Part B include those not related to an inpatient stay or visits in excess of 100 following an inpatient stay. Reimbursement methods are the same as for Part A (see above).	See home health services under Part A above.

TABLE 1.1 Continued

Service	General Coverage	Nutrition Services Coverage
Prosthetic device benefit	Medicare covers reasonable and necessary prosthetic devices and reimburses based on a fee schedule.	Parenteral and enteral nutrition provided on an outpatient basis is covered to a limited degree under the prosthetic device benefit.
Outpatient renal dialysis facilities	Medicare pays a composite rate for dialysis services furnished in outpatient renal dialysis facilities.	Nutritional services are included under the composite rate. Under the conditions for coverage, each facility must provide dietetic services to meet the needs of patients; employ or have a contractual relationship with a qualified dietitian who, in consultation with the attending physician, assesses the nutritional and dietetic needs of each patient, recommends therapeutic diets, counsels patients and their families on prescribed diets, monitors adherence and response to prescribed diets, and records findings in the patient's medical record. The full range of dialysis services, including personnel services for dietitians, is covered under the composite rate.

MEDICARE+CHOICE (M+C)

Private health plans	M+C plans are paid global capitated amounts by Medicare and must provide all Medicare-covered benefits to enrollees.	M+C plans make their own arrangements for payment of providers and may provide nutrition services over and above Medicare requirements as an extra benefit to enrollees.

REFERENCES

Anderson G, Hall MA, Smith TR. 1998. When courts review medical appropriations. *Med Care* 36:1295–1302.

Bagley GP, McVearry K. 1998. Medicare coverage for oncology services. *Cancer* 8210:S1991–S1994.

Ball RM. 1995. What Medicare's architects had in mind. *Health Aff* 14:62–72.

Bergthold LA. 1995. Medical necessity: Do we need it? *Health Aff* 14:180–190.

Breslow L, Somers AR. 1977. The lifetime health monitoring program: A practical approach to preventive medicine. *N Engl J Med* 296:601–608.

Cunningham R. 1999. Perspective. Policymakers grapple with foundations of process for coverage decisions, appeals. *Med Health* 53:S1–S4.

Feingold E. 1966. *Medicare: Policy and Politics.* San Francisco: Chandler Publishing Company.

Harris R. 1969. *A Sacred Trust.* Baltimore: Penguin Books.

HCFA (Health Care Financing Administration, U.S. Department of Health and Human Services). 1989. Criteria and procedures for making medical services coverage decisions that relate to health care technology. *Fed Regis* 54:4302–4318.

HCFA (Health Care Financing Administration, U.S. Department of Health and Human Services). 1998a. *A Profile of Medicare: Medicare Chartbook.* Baltimore: U.S. Department of Health and Human Services.

HCFA (Health Care Financing Administration, U.S. Department of Health and Human Services). 1998b. Medicare program; Establishment of the Medicare Coverage Advisory Committee and request for nominations for members. *Fed Regis* 63:68780.

HCFA (Health Care Financing Administration, U.S. Department of Health and Human Services). 1999a. Information clearinghouse: Medicare national enrollment trends, 1966–1998. Available at: http://www.hcfa.gov/stats/stats.htm. Accessed August 17, 1999.

HCFA (Health Care Financing Administration, U.S. Department of Health and Human Services). 1999b. Medicare and Medicaid program manuals. Available at: http://www.hcfa.gov/pubforms/htmltoc.htm. Accessed various dates from June 1, 1999 to November 1, 1999.

HCFA (Health Care Financing Administration, U.S. Department of Health and Human Services). 1999c. Medicare program; Procedures for making national coverage decisions. *Fed Regis* 64:22619–22625.

HIMA (Health Industry Manufacturers Association). 1999. *Overview of Change in the National Medicare Coverage Process.* Washington, D.C.: HIMA.

Health Systems Review. 1997. A technology anthology: Recent writings and remarks on the state of the state-of-the-art. *Health Syst Rev* 30:58–62.

IOM (Institute of Medicine). 1992. *Guidelines for Clinical Practice: From Development to Use.* Washington, D.C.: National Academy Press.

IOM (Institute of Medicine). 2000. *Extending Medicare Coverage for Preventive and Other Services.* Washington, D.C.: National Academy Press.

Kahn CN, Kuttner H. 1999. Budget bills and Medicare policy. *Health Aff* 18:37–47.

Kaiser Family Foundation. 1998. Medicare managed care. Available at: http://www.kff.org/content/archive/2052/mngcare.html. Accessed July 9, 1999.

Marmor T. 1973. *The Politics of Medicare.* Chicago: Aldine Publishing Company.

NHPF (National Health Policy Forum). 1998. *Medicare Coverage and Technology Diffusion: Past, Present and Future.* Washington, D.C.: The George Washington University.

NHPF (National Health Policy Forum). 1999. *Medical Necessity and Evolving Standards of Care.* Washington, D.C.: The George Washington University.

OTA (Office of Technology Assessment). 1990. *Preventive Health Services for Medicare Beneficiaries: Policy and Research Issues*. Washington, D.C.: U.S. Government Printing Office.

OTA (Office of Technology Assessment). 1993. *Benefit Design in Health Care Reform: Clinical Preventive Services*. Washington, D.C.: U.S. Government Printing Office.

Posner BM, Krachenfels MM. 1987. Nutrition services in the continuum of health care. *Clin Geriatr Med* 3:261–274.

Schauffler HH. 1993. Disease prevention policy under Medicare: A historical and political analysis. *Am J Med* 9:1226–1230.

Somers AR, Somers HM. 1997a. National health insurance: Criteria for an effective program and a proposal. Pp. 192–203 in *Health and Health Care: Policies in Perspective*, Somers AR, Somers HM, eds. Germantown, Md.: Aspen Systems Corporation.

Somers AR, Somers HM. 1977b. National health insurance: Story with a past, present, and future. Pp. 179–197 in *Health and Health Care: Policies in Perspective*, Somers AR, Somers HM, eds. Germantown, Md.: Aspen Systems Corporation.

Somers HM, Somers AR. 1961. *Doctors, Patients, and Health Insurance*. Washington, D.C.: The Brookings Institution.

Somers HM, Somers AR. 1967. *Medicare and the Hospitals: Issues and Prospects*. Washington, D.C.: The Brookings Institution.

Starr P. 1982. *The Social Transformation of American Medicine*. New York: Basic Books.

Stevens R. 1989. *In Sickness and in Wealth: American Hospitals in the Twentieth Century*. New York: Basic Books.

U.S. House of Representatives, Committee on Ways and Means. 1997. *1997 Medicare and Health Care Chartbook*. Washington, D.C.: U.S. Government Printing Office.

U.S. House of Representatives, Committee on Ways and Means. 1998. *1998 Green Book: Overview of Entitlement Programs*. Washington, D.C.: U.S. Government Printing Office.

White J. 1999. Uses and abuses of long-term Medicare cost estimates. *Health Aff* 18:63–79.

2

Overview:
Nutritional Health in the Older Person

As a population, older adults are more likely than younger ones to be afflicted with a variety of age-related diseases and functional impairments that may interfere with the maintenance of good nutritional status. Members of this population are also at increased risk of drug-induced nutritional deficiencies due to the number of prescription drugs they take. As a result of these potential risks of malnutrition, the Department of Health and Human Services has identified nutrition as a priority area in the health goals for the nation in *Healthy People 2010* (USDHHS, 2000). Although this overview focuses on older persons, other Medicare beneficiaries, particularly those with end-stage renal disease, also have high rates of nutritional disorders.

When considering the importance of nutrition in the health of Medicare beneficiaries, both the primary prevention of malnutrition and the role of nutrition in the management of health conditions prevalent in this population (secondary prevention) must be considered. Brief overviews of these two issues are presented here, and details are discussed in subsequent sections.

MALNUTRITION

There is no universally accepted clinical definition of malnutrition (Klein et al., 1997). In fact, the term "malnutrition" has been used to refer to a wide range of deficiencies (e.g., protein–energy, vitamins, fiber, water) and excesses (e.g., obesity, hypervitaminosis), which may or may not be clearly associated with adverse health outcomes (Reuben et al., 1995). The concept of malnutrition among older persons is more complicated because of the many settings along the continuum of care in which the elderly receive care.

- community dwelling (including those receiving home care and Programs of All Inclusive Care (PACE),
- hospitalized,
- post-acute hospitalization,
- institutionalized (nursing home) long-term care, and
- hospice.

The burden of acute and chronic disease differs across these settings, and nutritional requirements vary as a result. Moreover, an individual older person may move through many of these settings over the course of a single illness. Some measures of nutritional status vary in their degree of specificity for malnutrition across care settings. For example, changes in serum proteins among hospitalized older persons may be more reflective of inflammation and the acute-phase reaction than of malnutrition per se, whereas such changes may be more likely to indicate protein–energy undernutrition in community-dwelling persons. In addition, nursing home residents may have chronic inflammation, which complicates both the diagnosis and the management of malnutrition. Nevertheless, changes in these traditional indicators frequently have prognostic and clinical meaning and are therefore addressed in this chapter.

Obesity

The most common nutritional disorder in older persons is obesity. Obesity has been defined variably by different organizations. Based on data from the Second National Health and Nutrition Examination Survey (NHANES II) (1976–1980), the threshold for obesity was defined as having a body mass index (BMI)[1] exceeding 27.8 for men and 27.3 for women (NIH, 1985). Today, a BMI of 25 to 29.9 is considered to be overweight and a BMI of greater than or equal to 30 is considered obese (Meisler and St. Jeor, 1996; Mokdad et al., 1999; NHLBI, 1998).

The prevalence of overweight increases with age between the ages of 22 and 55 years but then stabilizes in women and declines in men (Van Itallie, 1985). The percentage of overweight and obese persons in the 65 to

---

[1]BMI is a ratio of height to weight: BMI = wt(kg)/ht(cm)^2.

74 year age range remains substantial however. Data from the Third National Health and Nutrition Examination Survey (NHANES III) (1988–1994) indicate that in the 65 to 74 year age range, approximately 34 percent of women and 44 percent of men are considered overweight (BMI 25 to 29.9) and an additional 27 percent of women and 24 percent of men are considered obese (BMI greater than or equal to 30) (NCHS, 1999). Older African-American and poor women have higher rates of obesity.

An important characteristic of adiposity accompanying aging is the distribution of fat, which is more likely to be centrally distributed in older persons. This central obesity is commonly associated with insulin resistance, hypertension, and lipid abnormalities (Schwartz, 1997).

Data on the risks associated with obesity in older persons are less consistent than for those with undernutrition. A substantial body of evidence links overweight to hypertension, dyslipidemia, heart disease, insulin resistance and diabetes, cholelithiasis, respiratory impairment, gout, and osteoarthritis (Pi-Sunyer, 1993). However, the relation between obesity and occurrence rates of specific diseases or overall mortality in persons over 65 years has received limited study. There is some evidence that the obesity-associated relative risk of disease occurrence is less in older than in younger persons. Although some data support the association of obesity and premature mortality in older persons (Calle et al., 1999), this evidence is inconsistent. Several cohort studies have demonstrated that a high BMI does not predict mortality, and, indeed, may even be protective against early death in older persons (Diehr et al., 1998; Fried et al., 1998; Stevens et al., 1998). In addition, overweight has been identified as a protective factor for hip fracture (independent of its relation to bone density) (Greenspan et al., 1994). However, other studies indicate that obesity is related to the development of functional impairment (Galanos et al., 1994; Vita et al., 1998). Thus, perhaps unique to the geriatric population, benefits versus risks of weight reduction should be analyzed on an individual basis. A recent Institute of Medicine report, *Weighing the Options: Criteria for Evaluating Weight-Management Programs*, reviewed the health benefits of weight loss in obesity (IOM, 1995). For this reason and those addressed above, obesity is not addressed separately, but only as it relates to specific conditions (e.g., hypertension, dyslipidemia, diabetes).

Undernutrition

Although energy undernutrition and protein–energy undernutrition are much less common, these disorders have major prognostic importance. Conditions of energy undernutrition include adult marasmus (energy undernutrition), in which normal serum proteins are maintained, and adult kwashiorkor (protein–energy undernutrition).

Protein–energy undernutrition (PEU) is defined as the presence of clinical (physical signs such as wasting, low BMI) *and* biochemical (albumin or other serum protein) evidence of insufficient intake. The most commonly used threshold to define PEU, albumin less than 3.5 g/dL, was derived in hospitalized patients (Bistrian et al., 1974). More recently, it has also been recognized that this threshold may be too high, even among hospitalized patients (Del Savio et al., 1996). Among outpatients, using the 3.5 g/dL threshold may miss older persons at substantial risk. For example, in the Established Populations for the Epidemiologic Studies of the Elderly (EPESE) cohort, the adjusted relative risk of mortality over 5 years for men who met the traditional criterion (<3.5 g/dL) was 1.9 and for women 3.7. However, that study also noted significantly increased relative risks (1.9 for men and 2.5 for women) among persons with more modest hypoalbuminemia (3.5–3.8 g/dL) (Corti et al., 1994). In the MacArthur Studies of Successful Aging, which enrolled older persons who had little or no functional impairment at the study's onset, those with albumin levels less than or equal to 3.8 g/dL had an adjusted relative risk of 3-year mortality of 1.8 (Reuben et al., 1999). Moreover, in the general population, few older persons (approximately 1 percent) meet the traditional criterion, whereas approximately 8 percent meet the more liberal criterion of 3.8 g/dL (Reuben et al., 1997). Thus, there is evidence that this threshold is associated with substantial risk and also is prevalent.

Weight loss has commonly been used to define undernutrition. In fact, a history of weight loss from middle to old age may be more important than actual low body weight per se. An analysis of data from the EPESE cohort noted that after exclusion of participants who lost more than 10 percent of their weight after age 50 and adjustment for health status, the higher risk of death associated with low weight was eliminated (Losonczy et al., 1995). Objectively determined weight change has prognostic significance. In one sample of elderly persons admitted to a geriatric rehabilitation unit, weight loss (derived from medical records) predicted whether complications would develop on the unit as well as 1-year mortality (Sullivan et al., 1990, 1991). A Department of Veterans Affairs (VA) study of outpatients defined 4 percent or greater weight loss over 1 year as having the best test characteristics (sensitivity and specificity) in predicting subsequent mortality during a 2-year follow-up period; 28 percent of those with involuntary weight loss died compared to 11 percent of those without weight loss (Wallace et al., 1995). In that study, the annual incidence of involuntary weight loss of 4 percent or more was 13.1 percent. Of note, those with voluntary weight loss had no better prognosis (36 percent had a 2-year mortality) than those who had involuntary weight loss.

The prevalence of undernutrition is considerably higher among hospitalized patients. A VA's case series defined malnutrition as meeting two of the following four criteria:

1. weight–height ratio <90 percent of normal,
2. mid-arm muscle circumference (MAMC) <90 percent of normal,
3. albumin <3.5 g/dL, and
4. transferrin <200 mg/dL.

Of the 59 male patients age 65 or older in the study, 61 percent met at least two of these criteria, compared to 28 percent of the 93 younger patients admitted during the same time period (Bienia et al., 1982). Of those who met the criteria for malnutrition, 64 percent experienced infections during their illness (compared to 26 percent of those who were not malnourished), and 28 percent died (compared to 4 percent of those who were not malnourished). More recently, a VA study found that 21 percent of hospitalized older persons consumed less than half of their energy requirements; these patients with poor intake had higher in-hospital and 90-day mortality rates (Sullivan et al., 1999). Numerous studies have associated low serum albumin in hospitalized older persons (measured at various times during the hospitalization) with in-hospital complications, longer hospital stays, more frequent readmissions, in-hospital mortality, and increased mortality at 90 days and at 1 year (Agarwal et al., 1988; Anderson et al., 1984; Burness et al., 1996; Cederholm et al., 1995; D'Erasmo et al., 1997; Ferguson et al., 1993; Friedmann et al., 1997; Harvey et al., 1981; Herrmann et al., 1992; Incalzi et al., 1998; Marinella and Markert, 1998; McClave et al., 1992; Patterson et al., 1992; Sullivan and Walls, 1995; Volkert et al., 1992). When considering mortality, the lower the albumin level, the higher is the risk of death. Using Subjective Global Assessment (see below) as a measure of undernutrition, 40 percent of hospitalized older persons are moderately (24 percent) or severely (16 percent) malnourished; severely malnourished patients are more likely to die within 1 year of hospital discharge (adjusted odds ratio [OR] = 2.83) and to spend time in a nursing home during the year after discharge (adjusted OR = 3.22) (Covinsky et al., 1999). However, as discussed in chapter 4, the relationship between hypoalbuminemia and adverse outcomes may not necessarily be related to nutrition.

Undernutrition in the nursing home is a particularly complex issue because of the burden of chronic disease and medications affecting nutritional status in this population and logistical difficulties in providing adequate food intake, in large part due to staffing issues (Kayser-Jones and Schell, 1997). A review of 14 surveys of nutritional status conducted among chronically institutionalized older persons concluded that only 5 to 18 percent of nursing home residents had energy intakes below their estimated requirement on the basis of body weight, but up to 30 percent ate less than 0.8 g protein/kg body weight per day; 15 to 60 percent had substandard MAMC, serum albumin, or both (Rudman and Feller, 1989). A Canadian study of one nursing home, which used a rating system that included seven anthropometric measurements, identified severe undernutrition in 18 percent of residents, moderate undernutrition in 27 percent, and mild-to-moderate overnutrition in 18 percent (Keller, 1993). Data from 26 VA nursing homes indicated that 12 percent of residents had body weights less than 80 percent of standard, and 28 percent had albumin levels less than 3.5 g/dL (Abbasi and Rudman, 1993). Several emerging concepts of nutritional disorders of older persons have been identified that fall outside the traditional classifications of malnutrition. Among these have been "failure to thrive" (which carries its own International Classification of Diseases, 9th Revision [ICD-9] code), cachexia, wasting, and sarcopenia. Attempts have been made to apply standardized nomenclature for these syndromes (Roubenoff et al., 1997; Sarkisian and Lachs, 1996), but there has been little validation research supporting these proposed definitions. Nevertheless, these syndromes incorporate constructs such as cytokine production, immune defense, and functional status. Thus, they expand the traditional concepts of nutrition to include pathophysiologic pathways and physiologic and functional outcomes. These are described in greater detail in chapter 4.

PREVALENCE OF NUTRITION RELATED CONDITIONS

Nutrition therapy may be a key element in managing many of the most common and important disorders of older persons including hypertension, congestive heart failure, diabetes, dyslipidemia, coronary artery disease, osteoporosis, malignancies, and renal failure. These diseases are particularly common in the elderly population. The estimated prevalence of certain disorders among persons 65 years of age or older who may benefit from nutrition therapy can be found in Table 2.1. Moreover, 87 percent of the population 65 years or older has at least one of these conditions (NCHS, 1997). The effectiveness of nutrition therapy for each of these disorders is described in subsequent chapters.

SCREENING FOR NUTRITION RISK

Over the past several decades, numerous attempts have been made to develop screening instruments that identify older persons who need more comprehensive nutritional assessment (Reuben et al., 1995). These can be categorized as follows:

TABLE 2.1 Estimated Prevalences of Conditions
Among U.S. Individuals Age 65 Years and Older

Medical Disorder	Prevalence (%)
Hypertension[a]	60.9
Chronic renal insufficiency[b]	0.6
Diabetes[c]	9.3
Hyperlipidemia (LDL >130 or on medication)[d]	62.1

[a] Hypertension is defined as having a systolic blood pressure ≥140 mm Hg and/or diastolic blood pressure ≥90 mm Hg or taking blood pressure medication.

[b] Chronic renal insufficiency includes a creatinine level of >2.5 in women and >3.0 in men.

[c] Elevated low-density lipoprotein (LDL) cholesterol is defined as having a serum LDL cholesterol ≥130 mg/dl and/or taking cholesterol lowering medication.

[d] The prevalence of diabetes was based on self-report.
SOURCE: NCHS (1997).

- brief self-reported screening instruments (e.g., the Nutrition Screening Initiative's DETERMINE Checklist, the Mini-Nutritional Assessment);
- clinician-determined brief screening instruments (e.g., Subjective Global Assessment); and
- multimethod techniques (e.g., Prognostic Nutritional Index, Hospital Prognostic Index).

Because few of these are in common usage, the topic is not reviewed in depth. However, the Nutrition Screening Initiative's Determine Your Nutritional Health Checklist has received wide attention and has been incorporated into screening instruments in many health care settings. The Mini-Nutritional Assessment and Subjective Global Assessment have also received increased attention. Accordingly, brief descriptions and discussions of the properties of these instruments are provided.

Nutrition Screening Initiative

The Nutrition Screening Initiative (NSI), a partnership of the American Academy of Family Physicians, the American Dietetic Association, and the National Council on Aging, Inc., has developed a tiered approach to nutrition screening. The first tier consists of the Determine Your Nutritional Health Checklist. The Determine Checklist was originally developed as a tool to increase consumer's nutrition awareness. It is a brief 10-item questionnaire that can be administered and scored by older Americans and/or their caregivers. The Determine Checklist scores range from 0 (lowest risk) to 21 (highest risk). Those found to be at risk of poor nutritional status based on the checklist are thought to need further screening.

The second tier consists of the Level I and Level II screening tools. The Level I screening tool is designed for use in any setting in which older Americans come into contact with professionals in the health care and social service system. It includes height and weight measurement (and calculated BMI), as well as questions about 10-pound weight gain or loss within the prior 6 months, eating habits, living environment, and functional status. The Level II screening tool is designed to obtain more diagnostic information in clinical settings. It includes anthropometric measurements (BMI, midarm circumference, MAMC, triceps skinfold), laboratory data (serum albumin and cholesterol), information on therapeutic drug use, and information on clinical problems that might affect eating, eating habits, living environment, functional status, and cognitive and affective status (Lipschitz et al., 1992).

A study using a stratified random sample of Medicare beneficiaries age 70 and older living in six New England states was conducted to calibrate the Determine Checklist. After reviewing the data from the study, NSI's technical review committee selected a score of 6 as the threshold for identifying older persons at high nutritional risk. The study estimated that 24 percent of all Medicare beneficiaries would fall into this high-risk group, and it found that those at high risk were more likely to have been hospitalized overnight during the prior year (Posner et al., 1993).

Using a score of 6 as a cut point to predict inadequate nutrition, the study found that the sensitivity, specificity, and positive predictive value of the Determine Checklist were 36, 85, and 38 percent, respectively. Using the same cut point, the sensitivity, specificity, and positive predictive value for identifying perceived fair or poor health status were 46, 85, and 56 percent, respectively. When examining individual items, the strongest predictors of inadequate nutrition were "not enough money," "eating fewer than two meals per day," and "eating few fruits and vegetables." The only items significantly associated with fair or poor perceived health were "taking three or more drugs per day" and "having changed one's diet because of illness."

A longitudinal study found that several individual items of the Determine Checklist predicted 8- to 12-year mortality, but the summary score for the entire instrument had a considerably lower predictive value than the individual items (Sahyoun et al., 1997).

The Determine Checklist has been criticized for having poor test characteristics, retaining items that are not significantly associated with outcomes of interest, and using outcomes that are not well-defined pathologic states and do not have proven treatments (Rush, 1993). In addition, the methodology of the validation study by Posner et al. (1993) is questioned for relying on a single 24-hour recall as the criterion of validity (Rush, 1993), which assumes that stability in dietary intake is greater than is likely (Thompson and Byers, 1994).

Mini-Nutritional Assessment

The Mini-Nutritional Assessment (MNA) is an 18-item instrument, requiring 20 minutes to complete, which incorporates several anthropometric measures, dietary intake questions, and health and functional status questions (Vellas et al., 1999). The developers used discriminant analysis techniques applied to several cross-sectional samples to establish cut points for being "at risk" of malnutrition and being undernourished. The instrument has been validated against clinical judgment of nutritional status, dietary intake, and biochemical measures (Guigoz et al., 1994). Predictive validity for weight loss, the occurrence of acute disease, and the need for assistance have been demonstrated in a Danish study (Beck and Ovesen, 1997). The most recent validation study conducted by Azad et al. (1999) however, indicated poor sensitivity and specificity compared to a nutritionist's assessment. These studies indicate that the MNA has potential, but more extensive validation is needed before this instrument can be recommended for widespread use.

Subjective Global Assessment

The Subjective Global Assessment (SGA) combines weight change, dietary intake, gastrointestinal symptoms, functional capacity, and physical examination findings to classify individuals as well nourished, moderately malnourished or severely malnourished (Detsky et al., 1987b, 1994). The SGA has demonstrated predictive validity in the identification of patients at risk for postoperative complications (Detsky et al., 1987a; VA TPN Cooperative Study Group, 1991). Personnel who administer the SGA must be trained to achieve acceptable interobserver reliability. A recent study of 369 patients who were at least 70 years of age and admitted to a general medical service in a tertiary care hospital found that those patients classified as severely malnourished by SGA were more likely than well-nourished patients to die within 12 months of discharge (OR = 2.83, 95 percent confidence interval [CI] = 1.47–5.45), to be dependent in activities of daily living 3 months after discharge (OR = 2.81, CI = 1.06–7.46), and to spend time in a nursing home during the 12 months after discharge (OR = 3.22, CI = 1.05–9.87) (Convinsky et al., 1999).

REFERENCES

Abbasi AA, Rudman D. 1993. Observations on the prevalence of protein–calorie undernutrition in VA nursing homes. *J Am Geriatr Soc* 41:117–121.

Agarwal N, Acevedo F, Leighton LS, Cayten CG, Pitchumoni CS. 1988. Predictive ability of various nutritional variables for mortality in elderly people. *Am J Clin Nutr* 48:1173–118.

Anderson CF, Moxness K, Meister J, Burritt MF. 1984. The sensitivity and specificity of nutrition-related variables in relationship to the duration of hospital stay and the rate of complications. *Mayo Clin Proc* 59:477–483.

Azad N, Murphy J, Amos SS, Toppan J. 1999. Nutrition survey in an elderly population following admission to a tertiary care hospital. *Can Med Assoc J* 161:511–515.

Beck AM, Ovesen LF. 1997. Predictive value of the screening instrument "mini-assessment of nutritional status." *Ugeskr Laeger* 159:6377–6781.

Bienia R, Ratcliff S, Barbour GL, Kummer M. 1982. Malnutrition in the hospitalized geriatric patient. *J Am Geriatr Soc* 30:433–436.

Bistrian BR, Blackburn GL, Hallowell E, Heddle R. 1974. Protein status of general surgical patients. *J Am Med Assoc* 230:858–860.

Burness R, Horne G, Purdie G. 1996. Albumin levels and mortality in patients with hip fractures. *N Z Med J* 109:56–57.

Calle EE, Thun MJ, Petrelli JM, Rodriguez C, Heath CW Jr. 1999. Body-mass index and mortality in a prospective cohort of U.S. adults. *N Engl J Med* 341:1097–1105.

Cederholm T, Jägrén C, Hellström K. 1995. Outcome of protein–energy malnutrition in elderly medical patients. *Am J Med* 98:67–74.

Corti M-C, Guralnik JM, Salive ME, Sorkin JD. 1994. Serum albumin level and physical disability as predictors of mortality in older persons. *J Am Med Assoc* 272:1036–1042.

Covinsky KE, Martin GE, Beyth RJ, Justice AC, Sehgal AR, Landefeld CS. 1999. The relationship between clinical assessments of nutritional status and adverse outcomes in older hospitalized medical patients. *J Am Geriatr Soc* 47:532–538.

Del Savio GC, Zelicof SB, Wexler LM, Byrne DW, Reddy PD, Fish D, Ende KA. 1996. Preoperative nutritional status and outcome of elective total hip replacement. *Clin Orthop* 326:153–161.

D'Erasmo E, Pisani D, Ragno A, Romagnoli S, Spagna G, Acca M. 1997. Serum albumin level at admission: Mortality and clinical outcome in geriatric patients. *Am J Med Sci* 314:17–20.

Detsky AS, Baker JP, O'Rourke K, Johnston N, Whitwell J, Mendelson RA, Jeejeebhoy KN. 1987a. Predicting nutrition-associated complications for patients undergoing gastrointestinal surgery. *J Parenter Enteral Nutr* 11:440–446.

Detsky AS, McLaughlin JR, Baker JP, Johnston N, Whittaker S, Mendelson RA, Jeejeebhoy KN. 1987b. What is subjective global assessment of nutritional status? *J Parenter Enteral Nutr* 11:8–13.

Detsky AS, Smalley PS, Chang J. 1994. Is this patient malnourished? *J Am Med Assoc* 271:54–58.

Diehr P, Bild DE, Harris TB, Duxbury A, Siscovick D, Rossi M. 1998. Body mass index and mortality in nonsmoking older adults: The cardiovascular health study. *Am J Public Health* 88:623–629.

Ferguson RP, O'Connor P, Crabtree B, Batchelor A, Mitchell J, Coppola D. 1993. Serum albumin and prealbumin as predictors of clinical outcomes of hospitalized elderly nursing home residents. *J Am Geriatr Soc* 41:545–549.

Fried LP, Kronmal RA, Newman AB, Bild DE, Mittelmark MB, Polak JF, Robbins JA, Gardin JM. 1998. Risk factors for 5-year mortality in older adults: The cardiovascular health study. *J Am Med Assoc* 279:585–592.

Friedmann JM, Jensen GL, Smiciklas-Wright H, McCamish MA. 1997. Predicting early non-elective hospital readmission in nutritionally compromised older adults. *Am J Clin Nutr* 65:1714–1720.

Galanos AN, Pieper CF, Cornoni-Huntley JC, Bales CW, Fillenbaum GG. 1994. Nutrition and function: Is there a relationship between body mass index and the functional capabilities of community-dwelling elderly? *J Am Geriatr Soc* 42:368–373.

Greenspan SL, Myers ER, Maitland LA, Resnick NM, Hayes WC. 1994. Fall severity and bone mineral density as risk factors for hip fracture in ambulatory elderly. *J Am Med Assoc* 271:128–133.

Guigoz Y, Velas B, Garry PJ. 1994. Mini nutritional assessment: A practical assessment tool for grading the nutritional state of elderly patients. Pp. 15–59 in: Velas B, ed. *Facts and Research in Gerontology 1994 (Supplement: Nutrition)*. New York: Springer.

Harvey KB, Moldawer LL, Bistrian BR, Blackburn GL. 1981. Biological measures for the formulation of a hospital prognostic index. *Am J Clin Nutr* 34:2013–2022.

Herrmann FR, Safran C, Levkoff SE, Minaker KL. 1992. Serum albumin level on admission as a predictor of death, length of stay, and readmission. *Arch Intern Med* 152:125–130.

Incalzi RA, Capparella O, Gemma A, Landi F, Pagano F, Cipriani L, Carbonin P. 1998. Inadequate caloric intake: A risk factor for mortality of geriatric patients in the acute-care hospital. *Age Ageing* 27:303–310.

IOM (Institute of Medicine). 1995. *Weighing the Options: Criteria for Evaluating Weight-Management Programs*. Washington, D.C.: National Academy Press.

Kayser-Jones J, Schell E. 1997. The effect of staffing on the quality of care at mealtime. *Nurs Outlook* 45:64–72.

Keller HH. 1993. Malnutrition in institutionalized elderly: How and why? *J Am Geriatr Soc* 41:1212–1218.

Klein S, Kinney J, Jeejeebhoy K, Alpers D, Hellerstein M, Murray M, Twomey P. 1997. Nutrition support in clinical practice: Review of published data and recommendations for future research directions. *Am J Clin Nutr* 66:683–706.

Lipschitz DA, Ham RJ, White JV. 1992. An approach to nutrition screening for older Americans. *Am Fam Physician* 45:601–608.

Losonczy KG, Harris TB, Cornoni-Huntley J, Simonsick EM, Wallace RB, Cook NR, Ostfeld AM, Blazer DG. 1995. Does weight loss from middle age to old age explain the inverse weight mortality relation in old age? *Am J Epidemiol* 141:312–321.

Marinella MA, Markert RJ. 1998. Admission serum albumin level and length of hospitalization in elderly patients. *South Med J* 91:851–854.

McClave SA, Mitoraj TE, Thielmeier KA, Greenburg RA. 1992. Differentiating subtypes (hypoalbuminemic vs. marasmic) of protein–calorie malnutrition: Incidence and clinical significance in a university hospital setting. *J Parenter Enteral Nutr* 16:337–342.

Meisler JG, St. Jeor S. 1996. Summary and recommendations from the American Health Foundation's Expert Panel on Healthy Weight. *Am J Clin Nutr* 63:474S–477S.

Mokdad AH, Serdula MD, Dietz WH, Bowman BA, Marks JS, Kaplan JP. 1999. The spread of the obesity epidemic in the United States, 1991–1998. *J Am Med Assoc* 282:1519–1522.

NCHS (National Center for Health Statistics). 1997. *Third National Health and Nutrition Examination Survey* (Series 11, No. 1, SETS version 1.22a). [CD-ROM]. Washington, D.C.: U.S. Government Printing Office.

NCHS (National Center for Health Statistics). 1999. *Health, United States, 1999 With Health and Aging Chartbook*. Hyattsville, Md.: NCHS.

NHLBI (National Heart, Lung, and Blood Institute). 1998. *Clinical Guidelines on the Identification, Evaluation, and Treatment of Overweight and Obesity in Adults. The Evidence Report*. Bethesda, Md.: NHLBI.

NIH (National Institutes of Health). 1985. Health implications of obesity. National Institutes of Health Consensus Development Conference Statement. *Ann Intern Med* 103:147–151.

Patterson BM, Cornell CN, Carbone B, Levine B, Chapman D. 1992. Protein depletion and metabolic stress in elderly patients who have a fracture of the hip. *J Bone Joint Surg* 74:251–260.

Pi-Sunyer FX. 1993. Medical hazards of obesity. *Ann Intern Med* 119:655–660.

Posner BM, Jette AM, Smith KW, Miller DR. 1993. Nutrition and health risks in the elderly: The nutrition screening initiative. *Am J Public Health* 83:972–978.

Reuben DB, Greendale GA, Harrison GG. 1995. Nutrition screening in older persons. *J Am Geriatr Soc* 43:415–425.

Reuben DB, Moore AA, Damesyn M, Keeler E, Harrison GG, Greendale GA. 1997. Correlates of hypoalbuminemia in community-dwelling older persons. *Am J Clin Nutr* 66:38–45.

Reuben DB, Ix JH, Greendale GA, Seeman TE. 1999. The predictive value of combined hypoalbuminemia and hypocholesterolemia in high functioning community-dwelling older persons: MacArthur studies of successful aging. *J Am Geriatr Soc* 47:402–406.

Roubenoff R, Heymsfield SB, Kehayias JJ, Cannon JG, Rosenberg IH. 1997. Standardization of nomenclature of body composition in weight loss. *Am J Clin Nutr* 66:192–196.

Rudman D, Feller AG. 1989. Protein–calorie undernutrition in the nursing home. *J Am Geriatr Soc* 37:173–183.

Rush D. 1993. Evaluating the nutrition screening initiative. *Am J Public Health* 83:944–945.

Sahyoun NR, Jacques PF, Dallal GE, Russell RM. 1997. Nutrition screening initiative checklist may be a better awareness/educational tool than a screening one. *J Am Diet Assoc* 97:760–764.

Sarkisian CA, Lachs MS. 1996. Failure to thrive in older adults. *Ann Intern Med* 124:1072–1078.

Schwartz RS. 1997. Obesity in the elderly. Pp. 103–114 in: Bray GA, Bouchard C, James WPT, eds. *Handbook of Obesity*. New York: Marcel Dekker, Inc.

Stevens J, Cai J, Pamuk ER, Williamson DF, Thun MJ, Wood JL. 1998. The effect of age on the association between body-mass index and mortality. *N Engl J Med* 338:1–7.

Sullivan DH, Walls RC. 1995. The risk of life-threatening complications in a select population of geriatric patients: The impact of nutritional status. *J Am Coll Nutr* 14:29–36.

Sullivan DH, Patch GA, Walls RC, Lipschitz DA. 1990. Impact of nutrition status on morbidity and mortality in a select population of geriatric rehabilitation patients. *Am J Clin Nutr* 51:749–758.

Sullivan DH, Walls RC, Lipschitz DA. 1991. Protein–energy undernutrition and the risk of mortality within 1 y of hospital discharge in a select population of geriatric rehabilitation patients. *Am J Clin Nutr* 53:599–605.

Sullivan DH, Sun S, Walls RC. 1999. Protein–energy undernutrition among elderly hospitalized patients: A prospective study. *J Am Med Assoc* 281:2013–2019.

Thompson FE, Byers T. 1994. Dietary Assessment Resource Manual. *J Nutr* 124:2245S–2317S.

USDHHS (U.S. Department of Health and Human Services). 2000. *Healthy People 2010*. Washington, D.C.: USDHHS.

Van Itallie TB. 1985. Health implications of overweight and obesity in the United States. *Ann Intern Med* 103:983–1008.

VA TPN (Veterans Affairs Total Parenteral Nutrition) Cooperative Study Group. 1991. Perioperative total nutrition in surgical patients. *N Engl J Med* 325:525–32.

Vellas B, Garvey J, Guigoz Y, eds. 1999. *Mini Nutritional Assessment (MNA) Research and Practice in the Elderly, Nestle Nutrition Workshop Series and Clinical Performance Programme,* Vol. 1. Basel: S. Karger AG.

Vita AJ, Terry RB, Hubert HB, Fries JF. 1998. Aging, health risks, and cumulative disability. *N Engl J Med* 338:1035–1041.

Volkert D, Kruse W, Oster P, Schlierf G. 1992. Malnutrition in geriatric patients: Diagnostic and prognostic significance of nutritional parameters. *Ann Nutr Metab* 36:97–112.

Wallace JI, Schwartz RS, LaCroix AZ, Uhlmann RF, Pearlman RA. 1995. Involuntary weight loss in older outpatients: Incidence and clinical significance. *J Am Geriatr Soc* 43:329–337.

3

Methods

For this report, the committee reviewed the published medical literature to determine whether nutrition-based therapies have a beneficial
impact in preventing or treating diseases among Medicare beneficiaries
(i.e., predominantly older-aged persons). The fundamental question was
one of efficacy: For the disease or condition under study, does manipulation of diet in older persons have beneficial effects? To answer this question, the committee reviewed the published medical literature with a focus on original research and systematic reviews. To identify relevant
literature, systematic searches of online databases were conducted and
key references were elicited from committee members, other experts (invited speakers and consultants), and the reference lists of publications.

Early in the course of this study, the committee developed and agreed
upon the literature search strategy. The initial focus was a comprehensive
search of relevant online databases. The online database Medline was
selected because it offers an effective and efficient means of searching the
medical literature. Medline was accessed through Ovid, a commercial
database vendor, and through Grateful Med of the National Library of
Medicine (NLM). The search strategy was individualized by topic area or
disease state. Searches were limited to human subjects, age ≥65 and/or
the entire population, the English language, and 1976–present. Searching
also incorporated standardized terminology found in NLM's Medical
Subject Headings (MeSH) and the MeSH tree structures.

All retrieved citations were reviewed to determine whether the cita-
tion was relevant to this report and if relevant, whether to obtain the full

paper. All citations were entered into the study's bibliographic database, which at the conclusion of the study contained approximately 850 references to abstracts, journal articles, books, congressional reports, and conference proceedings.

EVIDENCE AVAILABLE

Description

The evidence reviewed was heterogeneous (i.e., the types of nutrition-based therapies varied as did the types of outcomes reported). The latter included both "clinical" outcome variables (e.g., number of hip fractures, hospital admissions) and "intermediate" outcome variables (e.g., bone mineral density, blood pressure). The vast majority of studies report the effects of nutrition-based therapy on intermediate outcomes. The committee also evaluated the full spectrum of nutrition-based therapies. For example, for common outpatient conditions such as hypertension, the therapies included behavioral interventions that involved counseling, feeding studies that controlled food intake, and trials of dietary supplements. Multidisciplinary interventions were also evaluated as long as there was a nutritional component to the program. The type of individuals who conducted the study interventions and thus provided the nutrition therapy was not uniform: whereas a registered dietitian provided the nutrition-based therapy in most instances, there were several studies in which other personnel (e.g., nurses) administered the intervention. The setting for interventions varied as well (e.g., outpatient versus home-based, group versus individual counseling).

Although research conducted among the elderly was of primary interest, evidence from studies in non-elderly population groups, as well as evidence from studies that covered a broad age range of individuals—both non-elderly and elderly—was also considered. In many instances, fewer studies were conducted in elderly population groups than in the non-elderly. In this setting, the committee considered studies in non-elderly populations as relevant to its deliberations as long as the evidence appeared consistent across the adult lifespan.

Quality

In preparing this report, the committee evaluated and then classified the type and quality of available evidence for each of the diseases or conditions under study. Several classification schemes are available (NIH, 1998; USPSTF, 1995; Yusuf et al., 1998). For this report, the committee adapted the approach used by the National Institutes of Health (NIH) task force on the identification, evaluation and treatment of overweight and obesity (NIH, 1998). The only substantive difference between the approach in this report and that of the NIH task force is in the committee's classification of systematic reviews. In addition to meta-analyses, other types of systematic reviews were considered as long as the review involved a comprehensive search of the medical literature. A separate category, "systematic review," was also created—rather than having to combine these reports with randomized trials. The classification scheme, ordered from lowest to highest quality of evidence, is summarized below:

- *Consensus reports and guidelines.* In many instances, expert panels convened by professional societies or government agencies evaluated and synthesized the available evidence. In addition to describing the available data, these reports have the advantage of proposing clinical management strategies, which integrate nutrition-based therapy in the overall management of patients.
- *Observational studies.* In contrast to consensus reports and guidelines, this category pertains to original research and includes both observational studies (i.e., case series, case-control studies, cohort studies) and nonrandomized trials of nutrition-based therapies. Because individuals were not randomly allocated to the treatment under study, the potential for bias exists. Hence, this grade of evidence is less persuasive than randomized, controlled trials.
- *Systematic reviews.* In recent years, systematic approaches have been used to identify, evaluate, and synthesize evidence. This report includes meta-analyses of clinical trials as well as other systematic reviews as long as these reviews performed a comprehensive search of the medical literature. Systematic reviews are considered more complete and less subject to bias than expert opinion and previous types of reviews.
- *Some evidence from randomized, controlled trials.* For several conditions, clinical trials were conducted; however, the number or size of the trials was small and/or the data were somewhat inconsistent.
- *Extensive evidence from randomized, controlled trials.* This category applies to those nutrition-based therapies for which there are several clinical trials documenting a clinically meaningful health benefit from the therapy. Furthermore, the data from these trials had to be generally consistent. Overall, this is the strongest category of evidence supporting nutrition-based therapy.

COMMITTEE DELIBERATIONS

At its initial meeting, the committee identified common medical conditions for which nutrition-based therapy was generally recommended, as well as other conditions for which the evidence appeared much less persuasive. The committee then assigned working groups to review and summarize the published medical literature. The committee also sought expert advice from people who were not committee members, primarily through presentations at subsequent committee meetings. At several points, the working groups presented their assessments to the entire committee. These presentations included an overall assessment of the efficacy of nutrition-based therapy in the elderly, as well as practical aspects of implementation (e.g. Who is qualified to implement the therapy—a highly skilled professional or a variety of general health professionals? What is the appropriate setting? What number of contacts is required; and so forth). The committee then considered the costs of nutrition-based therapy and identified potential cost offsets. Methods pertaining to the cost analyses are presented separately in chapter 14.

REFERENCES

NIH (National Institutes of Health). 1998. Clinical guidelines on the identification, evaluation, and treatment of overweight and obesity in adults—The evidence report. *Obes Res* 2:51S–209S.

USPSTF (U.S. Preventive Services Task Force). 1995. *Guide to Clinical Preventive Services, 2nd ed. Report of the U.S. Preventive Services Task Force*. Washington, D.C.: U.S. Department of Health and Human Services, Office of Public Health, Office of Health Promotion and Disease Prevention.

Yusuf S, Cairns JA, Cann AJ, Fallen EL, Gerch BJ. 1998. *Evidence-Based Cardiology*. London: BMJ Publishing Group.

Section II

The Role of Nutrition in the Management of Disease

4

Undernutrition

As new markers of poor nutritional status have been identified, the definition of undernutrition has been considerably refined. Most notably, better methods of measuring body composition and biochemical measures of inflammation and nutritional health have led to refined classification systems of undernutrition. Concurrently, there has been increasing recognition of clinical syndromes that appear to have a major nutritional component (e.g., failure to thrive). This report considers several aspects of undernutrition including the following:

1. Markers of Undernutrition
   - Weight loss and morphometric measures of undernutrition
   - Poor nutritional intake
   - Biochemical markers of malnutrition (albumin, transferrin, retinol binding protein)

2. Syndromes of Undernutrition
   - Body composition changes with aging or sarcopenia
   - Cachexia
   - Wasting
   - Protein–energy undernutrition
   - Failure to thrive

None of these markers or syndromes (except poor nutritional intake) are specific for malnutrition, and it must be recognized that the interfaces between nutrition, energy requirements, and disease are complex. Moreover, approaches to diagnosis and management usually have not followed these definitions. Finally, despite global research efforts, there are still many gaps in the understanding of undernutrition in older persons.

For each of these markers and syndromes, the following topics are addressed where information is available:

- commonly used definitions,
- clinical importance in different settings (e.g., frequency, increased risk for adverse events),
- potentially treatable contributing factors and assessment methods (including current practice and a more optimal approach), and
- approaches to treatment and treatment outcomes.

There is considerable overlap across conditions with respect to assessment, contributing factors, and treatments. Although this chapter focuses on markers and syndromes of undernutrition, it must be recognized that undernutrition may affect the course of specific acute (e.g., pneumonia [Riquelme et al., 1996]) and chronic diseases (e.g., congestive heart failure, chronic obstructive pulmonary disease, pressure sores). In some instances, the treatment of these diseases (e.g., congestive heart failure) may lead to dietary restrictions that compromise nutritional status (Reuben et al., 1997). In others, the burden of the disorder may lead to increased energy requirements. Finally, some disorders (e.g., stroke with dysphagia, malabsorption) may precipitate undernutrition because of the inability to ingest or absorb nutrients. Although the recognition of these potential influences is important and may guide management, undernutrition accompanying specific diseases will eventually be expressed through the markers and syndromes described below.

MARKERS OF UNDERNUTRITION

Weight Loss

Several definitions of clinically important weight loss have been described. These vary according to the amount of weight lost and the duration of the weight loss. In outpatient settings, commonly employed definitions include more than 10 pounds in 6 months, 4 to 5 percent of body weight in 1 year, or 7.5 percent in 6 months.

In the nursing home, the definition of weight loss has usually followed that included in the Omnibus Budget Reconciliation Act (OBRA) regulations of 1987. This legislation mandated implementation of the

Minimum Data Set (MDS) and Resident Assessment Protocols (RAPs) in Medicare-certified nursing homes to ensure prompt identification and response to problems in nursing home residents. (The MDS is a functionally based assessment tool; RAPs utilize MDS assessment information to flag potential problem and risk areas in nursing home residents.) The OBRA MDS considers weight loss as greater than or equal to 5 percent of body weight in the past month or greater than or equal to 10 percent in the last 6 months.

Clinical Importance

A 4-year cohort study determined that the annual incidence of involuntary weight loss (defined as loss of more than 4 percent of body weight) among veterans followed in an outpatient setting was 13.1 percent. Over a 2-year follow-up period, those with involuntary weight loss had an increased risk of mortality (relative risk [RR] = 2.4, 95 percent confidence interval [CI] = 1.3–4.4), which was 28 percent among those who lost weight and 11 percent among those who did not. Individuals with voluntary weight loss had a 36 percent mortality rate during this time (Wallace et al., 1995). In a study of Alzheimer's patients followed for up to 6 years, greater than or equal to 5 percent weight loss in any year before death predicted mortality (RR 1.5, 95 percent CI = 1.09–2.07); 22 percent of Alzheimer's patients experienced such weight loss (White et al., 1998).

Two longitudinal studies also suggest that weight loss in later life predicts mortality. In the Established Populations for Epidemiologic Studies of the Elderly (EPESE) cohort, older persons who lost 10 percent of their body weight or more between ages 50 and 70 years had higher adjusted risks of mortality (men: RR = 1.69, 95 percent CI = 1.19–1.65; women: RR = 1.62, 95 percent CI = 1.45–1.97) (Losonczy et al., 1995). The Iowa Women's Health Study demonstrated that women greater than or equal to 55 years of age who had an episode of unintentional weight loss (19 percent of the study participants) had an adjusted OR of 1.45 (95 percent CI = 1.24–1.70) for all-cause 5-year mortality (French et al., 1999). Although the time spans utilized in these latter definitions are impractical for clinical purposes, they do provide evidence of an association between weight loss and subsequent mortality.

For the nursing home population, there are fewer prevalence data. One study found that 5 percent of residents at one nursing home met these criteria (Blaum et al., 1997). Weight loss may be an insensitive measure of malnutrition because nursing home residents may stop eating for several weeks between weight measurements.

Potentially Treatable Contributing Factors and Assessment Methods

Many of the causes of weight loss (e.g., depression, type 2 diabetes, hyperthyroidism, gastrointestinal diseases, cancer) are treatable with effective therapies supported by randomized clinical trials (Blaum et al., 1995; Morley and Kraenzle, 1994; Wilson et al., 1998).

Among nursing home residents, reversible factors such as poor oral intake, feeding dependency, chewing problems, depressive symptoms or behavior, medications, and swallowing disorders were related to observed weight loss in two cross-sectional studies (Blaum et al., 1995; Morley and Kraenzle, 1994).

In hospital settings (defined here as short-stay, acute care hospitals), the current approach to assessment of causes of weight loss and undernutrition is generally haphazard. Although many nursing intake forms include questions on weight loss, functional status related to nutrition, and special dietary needs, staff complete these forms in an inconsistent manner. At many institutions, dietary technicians spend significant amounts of time collecting data, which may have little clinical value, in order to meet the Joint Commission for Accreditation of Healthcare Organizations (JCAHO) mandate of nutritional assessment data collection of all hospitalized persons.

Usually nursing home residents are weighed once a month. When the RAP for malnutrition is triggered by any of the MDS nutrition criteria, there must be documentation of responses by the health care team, including an assessment of feeding as well as investigation, when appropriate, for medical disorders that can cause weight loss.

The assessment of weight loss is guided by other associated symptoms (e.g., gastrointestinal, cancer-related, depression, diabetes) if they are present. In addition, other potential contributors to weight loss or any of the other undernutrition disorders are evaluated for potentially remediable conditions. This assessment may include some or all of the following:

• assessment of food security, if the older person is community dwelling (e.g., specific questions about financial status, referral to social worker);
• assessment of food-related functional status (e.g., specific questions about shopping, meal preparation, and feeding);
• assessment of appetite and documentation of dietary intake (e.g., dietitian referral, 72-hour calorie count);
• assessment of depressive symptoms (e.g., dietitian referral, 72-hour calorie count);

- assessment of dental and chewing status (e.g., documented oral examination or referral to a dentist);
- assessment of swallowing ability (e.g., bedside swallowing study, referral for swallowing study, or videofluoroscopy);
- assessment of medications that might be associated with decreased appetite (e.g., digoxin, fluoxetine, anticholinergics);
- assessment of cognitive impairment (e.g., screening for dementia with the Mini-Mental State Examination); and
- assessment of disease-related dietary restrictions (e.g., low salt, low protein).

Approaches to Treatment and Treatment Outcomes

Treatment of specific identified causes of weight loss such as cancer or thyroid disease is supported by clinical trials. However, to date, no randomized clinical trial data have evaluated the ability of consultation by a dietitian or the use of nutritional supplements to provide clinical or health utilization benefits for older persons other than in situations following recovery from pneumonia or hip fracture (Schürch et al., 1998; Woo et al., 1994).

Among homebound elderly with involuntary weight loss or baseline low body mass index (BMI), a case series of 12 weeks of dietary supplements (500 kcal per day) demonstrated increases in weight, total lymphocyte count, and general well-being score (Gray-Donald et al., 1994). A subsequent randomized clinical trial using the same intervention demonstrated increases in weight (2.1 kg in the supplemented group compared to 0.6 kg in the control group, $p < 0.01$) but no changes in functional status (Gray-Donald et al., 1995). A case-series of persons who had lost at least 20 percent of their body weight or at least 10 percent in 3 months demonstrated improvement in nutritional parameters, including serum albumin, after being hospitalized in a nutritional support unit and receiving enteral nutrition via a nasogastric tube which provided approximately three times the measured energy expenditure for 4 weeks (Hébuterne et al., 1995).

In nursing home settings, many residents who sustain weight loss do so because they are not adequately fed, in part due to limitations of nursing resources (see discussion of "poor nutritional intake" below) (Kayser-Jones and Schell, 1997). Although no studies are available to suggest that nursing home staffing or behavioral changes can improve dietary intake, these problems are potentially correctable. A case-control study of nursing home residents who were receiving oral supplements at least twice daily for weight loss or poor appetite demonstrated that most of these residents regained weight back to their admission weight over a period of 9 to 10 months (Johnson et al., 1993). In a nonrandomized study that provided increased nutritional support to nursing home residents, undernourished residents (defined by BMI, weight loss, and anthropometric measurements) who gained weight over 10 months had fewer recurring infections and were less likely to die. They had a 17 percent mortality rate, compared to a 45 percent mortality rate among those who were undernourished but lost weight during the follow-up period, and a 35 percent mortality rate among those who were undernourished and maintained their weight (Keller, 1995).

Anthropometric Measurements

Anthropometric measures are used in research and in some clinical settings to identify older persons with malnutrition. Some of the more common measurements include: triceps skinfold thickness (TSF), which is measured on the upper arm, halfway between the inferior border of the acromion process and the tip of the olecranon process, and mid-arm muscle circumference (MAMC) (Bienia et al., 1982; Shenkin et al., 1996). The MAMC is calculated using the mid upper-arm circumference (AC) and the standard formula: MAMC = AC − 3.14 (TSF) (Bienia et al., 1982).

Clinical Importance

Because TSF thickness spans a wide range among normal individuals, sequential changes in the same individual may be more valuable than one-time measurements (Shenkin et al., 1996). However, measurement error increases with size of skinfold, and inter- and intraobserver variation may be large (Fuller et al., 1991). Moreover, these anthropometric measurements suffer from poorer reliability in elderly compared to younger subjects, in part because of difficulties in accurately locating anatomic landmarks (Sullivan et al., 1989) and because of age-related changes in skin elasticity. For example, a TSF measurement taken at the level of the midarm may vary by as much as 150 percent from a measurement taken only 1 to 2 centimeters above or below this point (Sullivan et al., 1989). With aging, a smaller proportion of total body fat is subcutaneous; therefore, skinfold thickness is less likely to indicate total body fat in older compared to younger persons.

Nevertheless, in community-dwelling older persons, low corrected arm muscle area and low TSF predict subsequent 40- to 46-month age-adjusted mortality. For example, in a prospective cohort study, having a corrected arm muscle area below the 5th percentile was associated with a RR of 3.5 (95 percent CI = 1.6–8.2), and having a corrected arm muscle area between the 5th and 10th percentiles was associated with a RR of 2.2 (95 percent CI = 1.0–4.9). In the same study, having a TSF below the 5th percentile was associated with a RR of 4.9 (95 percent CI = 2.1–11.1). BMI did not remain in the logistic model and the authors noted that BMI determinations can be inaccurate in the elderly due to difficulties in obtaining accurate heights and the effects of edema or dehydration on weight (Campbell et al., 1990).

Potentially Treatable Contributing Factors and Assessment Methods

The contributors to anthropometric abnormalities have not been formally studied but are not likely to differ substantially from those contributing to weight loss or low BMI. Assessment methods for abnormal anthropometric measures are similar to those used for weight loss.

Approaches to Treatment and Treatment Outcomes

Anthropometric measures have been used as entry criteria in some clinical trials of nutritional supplementation in hospitalized older persons (Bastow et al., 1983; Gariballa et al., 1998). A randomized clinical trial studied the administration of a 600 kcal and 20 g protein supplementation twice daily to patients who had sustained a stroke and who had anthropometric evidence of undernutrition by TSF and MAMC. Subjects in the supplemented group demonstrated a smaller decrease in serum albumin than those in the control group (mean decrease 1.5 g/L compared to 4.4 g/L, $p = 0.025$) and a nonsignificant reduction in 3-month mortality (10 percent in the supplemented group versus 35 percent in the control group, $p = 0.12$) (Gariballa et al., 1998). Another clinical trial of women hospitalized for hip fracture who were classified as thin or very thin based on arm circumference and TSF studied the effect of overnight supplementary nasogastric tube feedings of 1,000 calories, which were continued until discharge or death. Rehabilitation time to independent mobility (median 16 days in the treated group compared to 23 days in the control group, $p = 0.02$) and hospital stay were shortened (median 29 days in the treated group compared to 38 days in the control group, $p = 0.04$), particularly among the very thin (Bastow et al., 1983).

Low Body Mass Index

Low BMI (weight [kg] versus height [m^2]) is considered definitive for chronic protein–energy undernutrition (PEU) if less than 17 and for being consistent with but not diagnostic of PEU if between 17 to 20 (Shenkin et al., 1996).

Clinical Importance

Among community-dwelling older persons, BMI has been shown to demonstrate a U-shaped relationship to functional impairment, with increased risk among those at the lowest and highest BMIs (Galanos et al., 1994). However, change in BMI may be more important than actual value. In the EPESE study, persons who were in the lowest quintile of BMI at age 50 were not at increased risk of mortality during old age (Losonczy et al., 1995).

Potentially Treatable Contributing Factors and Assessment Methods

There are two population groups of older persons who have low BMI: those who have always been thin and those whose BMI has declined. Among the latter group, the causes of low BMI are not likely to differ substantially from the causes of weight loss. Assessment methods for low BMI are similar to those used for weight loss.

Approaches to Treatment and Treatment Outcomes

A randomized clinical trial of nutritional supplements for demented patients with low BMI (15.1–19.9) who were admitted to a psychiatric hospital and who received a 600 kcal oral supplement demonstrated significant increases in weight (3.7 versus 0.6 kg), MAMC (0.5 cm versus no change), and TSF (1.5 versus 0.5 mm) at 12 weeks compared to the placebo group (Carver and Dobson, 1995).

Other studies have included low BMI, in addition to weight loss or abnormal anthropometric measurements, as an entry criterion (see discussion of weight loss above).

Poor Nutritional Intake

Generally, poor nutritional intake has been defined as average or usual intake of servings of food groups, nutrients, or energy below recommended amounts. Estimates for energy needs may be obtained from published references (WHO/FAO/UNU, 1985) or calculated using regression equations (e.g., Harris-Benedict). Many of the regression equations in use take into account age, height, and/or body weight. The energy needs are then adjusted for the estimates of activity level and the effects of disease and treatment.

A threshold percentage used to define poor nutritional intake has been 66 or 75 percent of the Recommended Dietary Allowance (RDA) (IOM, 1994). This is not an appropriate use of the RDA as the numbers are derived in multiple ways from available data (IOM, 1997; NRC, 1986).

While some of these recommended intakes are based on the minimum average amount most individuals are thought to need to prevent deficiency, plus additional amounts to account for decreased absorption or bioavailability of the nutrient and for individual variation in requirements, others are based on what appear to be average intakes of healthy groups of people (IOM, 1994).

Newer methodology indicates that a more appropriate reference intake for use in assessing adequacy for a specific nutrient in a group of people is the Estimated Average Requirement (IOM, 1994, 1997). However, these reference intakes are not yet available for all nutrients of interest (IOM, 1997, 1998). Some recent studies conducted in hospital settings have used less than or equal to 30 and 50 percent of estimated energy requirements as a threshold (Incalzi et al., 1998; Sullivan et al., 1999). The MDS uses less than 75 percent of food provided as the threshold to trigger the malnutrition resident assessment protocol. These are subjective assessments frequently conducted by nursing staff.

Prior to implementation of the MDS, the RDA was used as a goal for monitoring nutritional intake and is still used as a standard by many dietitians working in nursing home settings. Subsequent to OBRA implementation in 1987, the specific MDS items for poor nutritional intake are the following:

- The resident complains about the taste of many foods.
- The resident regularly or repeatedly complains of hunger.
- The resident leaves 25 percent or more of his or her food uneaten at most meals.

The unreliability and subjective nature of accurately assessing these measures have been raised. Two studies have documented that nursing home staff significantly overestimate nutritional intake of nursing home residents (Kayser-Jones et al., 1997; Pokrywka et al., 1997).

In summary, efforts to develop assessment tools for use with elderly have not yet been able to identify aspects of health and status that can be monitored and evaluated objectively in older individuals with varying stages of functional capability that will accurately discriminate between those at risk and those not.

Clinical Importance

Although older persons under-report energy intake (Goran and Poehlman, 1992; Sawaya et al., 1996; Tomoyasu et al., 1999), community surveys estimate that between 37 to 40 percent of elderly men and women (those age 65 and over) report energy intakes less than two-thirds of the

RDA (Ryan et al., 1992). A recent study identified poor nutrient intake (less than 50 percent of calculated maintenance energy requirements) in 21 percent of hospitalized older persons (Sullivan et al., 1999). These persons had higher rates of in-hospital (RR = 8.0, 95 percent CI = 2.8–22.6) and 90-day mortality (RR = 2.9, 95 percent CI = 1.4–6.1). Another prospective observational study demonstrated that low caloric intake (less than 30 percent of estimated need) during the first 3 days of hospitalization could predict in-hospital mortality independently of serum albumin, lymphocytopenia, and activities of daily living impairment on admission (Incalzi et al., 1998).

A review of 14 surveys of nutritional status conducted among chronically institutionalized older persons concluded that 5 to 18 percent of nursing home residents had energy intakes below their recommended average energy expenditure (Rudman and Feller, 1989). In one study, 26 percent of nursing home residents met the MDS criterion for poor oral intake and 9 percent met the criterion for hunger (Blaum et al., 1997).

Potentially Treatable Contributing Factors and Assessment Methods

In hospitalized older persons, diagnostic testing and other reasons for a "nothing by mouth" restriction may contribute to poor nutritional intake beyond the burden of their acute illness. However, in hospital settings, nurses and aides can routinely observe dietary intake and thus offer the potential for inexpensive detection of potential nutritional disorders among hospitalized older persons. In addition, dietetic staff also frequently monitor nutritional intake of older hospitalized patients to meet JCAHO requirements. In general though, the methods for communicating poor dietary intake observed by nursing staff and dietary technicians to physicians have been informal and haphazard. Whether formal calorie counts obtained by food records provide additional value beyond nurse and aide observations has not been established. One report documented that among hospitalized patients, a 1-day calorie count corresponded very closely to the values obtained by a 3-day calorie count for energy and protein intake (Breslow and Sorkin, 1993).

In a qualitative study at two community nursing homes, the following problems with nursing home feeding were identified, largely due to an inadequate number of qualified staff (Kayser-Jones and Schell, 1997):

- lack of personal care,
- residents being served their meals in bed,
- residents being poorly positioned at mealtimes,
- trays being poorly positioned at mealtimes,
- poor quality of care at mealtimes,

- staff-enhanced dependency,
- residents being fed quickly and forcibly,
- solid food being mixed with liquids,
- dysphagia being undiagnosed and unrecognized, and
- some residents receiving little or no food.

In addition, many of the medical contributing factors mentioned above (see weight loss) are also applicable to poor intake in the nursing home.

Approaches to Treatment and Treatment Outcomes

There is a large body of literature supporting the value of providing inpatient parenteral and enteral nutrition to older persons who have inadequate intake in the hospital. In addition, there is anecdotal evidence of appetite stimulation and resulting increased energy intake among older persons following administration of large doses of megesterol acetate, an appetite stimulant (Castle et al., 1995). Although evidence supports the use of this appetite stimulant in acquired immune deficiency syndrome (AIDS) and cancer patients (Loprinzi et al., 1994; Oster et al., 1994; Von Roenn et al., 1994), randomized clinical trials indicating benefit in older persons have not been published and toxicity in older persons remains a concern.

Biochemical Markers of Malnutrition

Visceral Proteins

Although the relationship between serum albumin and nutritional intake is not well established, hypoalbuminemia is commonly considered a sign of malnutrition. However, low serum albumin levels may be a better measure of inflammation and associated decrease in albumin synthesis, increase in albumin degradation, and transcapillary leakage than of malnutrition (Rothschild et al., 1988). Thus, the relationship between hypoalbuminemia and adverse outcomes may not necessarily be directly related to nutrition. Hypoalbuminemia is considered in greater detail below in the discussion of PEU. Other proteins, particularly prealbumin and transferrin, are also considered nutritional markers. These proteins have shorter half-lives (prealbumin's half-life is 48 hours; transferrin's is 7 to 10 days). Accordingly, they may reflect more recent intake and may be valuable in monitoring response to treatment and like serum albumin, are also affected by inflammation. They are also considered in greater detail below in the discussion of PEU.

Other Biochemical Markers of Undernutrition

Several biological markers of nutritional disorders are being actively investigated in research protocols. They are mentioned only briefly here because many of these are nonspecific markers of inflammation (e.g., C-reactive protein [CRP] and cytokines) and because research on these markers, especially with respect to assessment and treatment, is limited. Cytokines are discussed briefly below under "cachexia." Low or falling serum cholesterol has been explored as another nutritional marker. In a case-control study of older persons with normal cholesterol levels on admission to the hospital (≥160 mg/dL), those whose cholesterol levels fell to less than or equal to 120 mg/dL during hospitalization (9 percent of admissions among persons ≥65 years) had more infectious and noninfectious complications, and their length of stay was nearly three times as long as those who maintained normal cholesterol levels. Inpatient mortality rates were higher in the acquired hypocholesterolemia group, although not significantly so (Noel et al., 1991). Another study indicated that at their hospital discharge nutritional assessment, 26 percent of hospitalized older persons had serum cholesterol less than 150 mg/dL (Sullivan et al., 1995). However, acquired hypocholesterolemia may not be nutritionally mediated. Ongoing inflammation and proinflammatory cytokines, particularly interleukin-6 (IL-6), may be responsible for acquired hypocholesterolemia (Ettinger et al., 1995).

A variety of demographic and nutrition-related variables were considered as potential predictors of 1-year mortality in a prospective cohort study at a Department of Veterans Affairs nursing home (Rudman and Feller, 1989). In multivariate analysis, only serum cholesterol and hematocrit remained statistically significant. The authors reported a "mortality risk index" (MRI) using the equation: 0.1 (serum cholesterol in mg/dl) + (hematocrit in %) = MRI. When MRI was less than 60, patients were classified as at high risk of dying (when MRI = 60, specificity was 85 percent and sensitivity was 90 percent). Another study found that total cholesterol was predictive of pressure ulcers among tube-fed residents of a long-term care facility (Henderson et al., 1992).

SYNDROMES OF UNDERNUTRITION

Body Composition Changes with Aging

The aging process affects multiple organ system functions that may impact on nutritional assessment and intervention. For example, changes in the skin may alter anthropometric measures. Changes in cardiac and/or renal functions may necessitate fluid restrictions that alter feeding pre-

---

BOX 4.1 Factors Affecting Changes in Body Composition

• Reduced physical activity or sedentary lifestyle
• Changes in trophic hormonal or neurologic functions
• Chronic disease
• Medications
• Diet
• Genetics

---

scriptions. The degree of change observed in organ function varies considerably among older individuals. Individualized assessment and intervention are therefore necessary.

The aging process is associated with notable changes in body composition. Therefore, well-standardized nutrient requirements for younger or middle-aged adults may not be applicable to older persons. With aging, a gradual decline in lean body mass (LBM) and an increase in body fat occur (Baumgartner et al., 1995) (see Box 4.1). A reduction in LBM results in a lower basal metabolic rate, thus reducing the energy needs of older persons. Novak (1972) studied 500 men and women, aged 18 to 85 years, and observed that body fat was increased, respectively, from 18 to 36 percent in younger versus older men and from 33 to 44 percent in younger versus older women. As total body fat increases with aging, intra-abdominal fat stores often increase. Abdominal adiposity has been linked to the development of insulin resistance, coronary artery disease, dyslipidemia, hypertension, and type 2 diabetes mellitus (Poehlman et al., 1995).

Sarcopenia

Age-related loss of skeletal muscle mass is referred to as sarcopenia (Rosenberg, 1989). Biopsy studies reveal a reduction in the number and size of type II muscle fibers with aging, while type I fibers are spared (Lexell, 1995).

Clinical Importance

There has been considerable interest in studying sarcopenia because of its possible relationship to loss of strength and functional decline (Evans and Campbell, 1993). Two recent major symposia have summarized current knowledge regarding sarcopenia and have highlighted limitations in understanding it (Kehayias and Heymsfield, 1997; Lexell and Dutta, 1997).

The prevalence of clinically relevant sarcopenia is unknown (Baumgartner et al., 1998); moreover, the relationship between sarcopenia and undernutrition has not been established. It is not clear whether sarcopenia is an inexorable part of aging, or is more a reflection of sedentary lifestyle or as yet unrecognized factors. The role, if any, of nutritional intervention awaits further clarification. It is clear, however, that assessment of energy needs for many older persons must take into consideration a decline in lean body mass and reduced physical activity.

Potentially Treatable Contributing Factors and Assessment Methods

Possible causal factors for sarcopenia include age-related accelerated muscle loss or changes in muscle accretion or responsiveness to trophic hormonal or neurologic factors. Decline in endogenous growth hormone production, altered cytokine regulation, decreased androgen and estrogen production, and loss of alpha motor neurons in the spinal column have been suggested as factors (Roubenoff et al., 1997). Changes in dietary intake, protein metabolism, or disuse atrophy resulting from a sedentary lifestyle may also be contributors (Bortz, 1982; Dutta and Hadley, 1995; Evans and Campbell, 1993).

Major difficulties in the study of sarcopenia include the lack of valid methods for routine assessment of skeletal muscle mass and function in humans. Current high-technology standards for the measurement of muscle mass include total body counting of the naturally occurring potassium isotope (^{40}K), dual-energy x-ray absorptiometry, computed tomography, and magnetic resonance imaging (Chumlea et al., 1995; Heymsfield et al., 1990; Selberg et al., 1993; Sjostrom, 1991).

Approaches to Treatment and Treatment Outcomes

Potential approaches to treatment of sarcopenia include administration or modulation of trophic factors (Rudman et al., 1990) or resistance strength training (Evans and Cyr-Campbell, 1997). Growth hormone (GH) levels may be 29 to 70 percent lower in elderly compared with younger men (Corpas et al., 1993). Papadakis and coworkers (1996) randomized 52 men to 6 months of GH replacement versus placebo, and found that LBM increased by an average of 4.3 percent in men who received GH, in comparison to a decrease of 0.1 percent in those receiving placebo. Fat mass also declined in the treatment group (down 13.1 percent with therapy versus 0.1 percent with placebo). Despite favorable improvements in body composition, there were no statistically significant improvements in muscle strength, systemic endurance, or functional status. Insulin-like growth factor I (IGF-I), which is released by the liver in response to GH, also declines with age. Rudman et al. (1990) randomized 21 healthy men aged 61 to 81 with low plasma IGF-I levels into GH treatment for 6 months or a no-treatment group. At follow-up, the treatment group exhibited an 8.8 percent increase in LBM, a 14.4 percent decrease in total body fat, a 7.1 percent increase in skin thickness, and a recovery of IGF-I to levels usually observed in younger people. The no-treatment group exhibited little change in outcome variables.

Testosterone also declines in aging men. When six elderly men with reduced testosterone concentrations were administered testosterone by injection for 4 weeks to achieve serum concentrations comparable to younger men, increased fractional synthetic rate of muscle protein and increased muscle strength (hamstring and quadriceps) were observed (Urban et al., 1995). Since increased mRNA concentrations of IGF-I were detected, it was suggested that IGF-I might mediate the observed response to testosterone. A prospective, randomized trial of testosterone versus placebo injection in 32 older men over a 12-month period found significant improvement in hand-grip strength and increased hemoglobin and lowered leptin levels in the treatment group in comparison to placebo (Sih et al., 1997). A more recent prospective, randomized trial of testosterone versus placebo by cutaneous patch in 108 older men over a 36-month period found a significant increase in LBM and a decrease in total body fat, but no increase in strength of knee flexion and extension in the treatment group in comparison to placebo (Snyder et al., 1999). Serum IGF-I concentrations fell significantly in both groups during study, but significantly less in the treatment group.

Skeletal muscle mass is responsive to changes in physical activity. Fiatarone and colleagues (1994) conducted a randomized, placebo-controlled trial of resistance exercise and/or multinutrient supplementation for over 10 weeks in 100 frail nursing home residents. Participants who received resistance exercise training had significant improvements in muscle strength, gait velocity, and stair-climbing power. Cross-sectional thigh muscle area increased in exercisers but declined in nonexercisers. Nutrient supplementation alone or as a supplement to exercise had no beneficial effect on primary outcome measures.

Cachexia

Cachexia and wasting, in which body cell mass is diminished, occur in illness, injury, or disease and are not part of the normal aging process. Because these are newly defined conditions, research on their clinical importance, assessment, and treatment is limited. Although the terms "cachexia" and "wasting" have often been used interchangeably in the clinical setting to describe patients with severe weight loss and compromised nutrition intake, Roubenoff and coworkers (1997) have recently suggested distinct syndrome definitions based on the presence or absence of cytokine-mediated response to injury or disease. Although patients may exhibit components of both inflammatory or injury response and semistarvation, this framework serves as a useful conceptual approach. Patients with components of both cachexia (cytokine-mediated inflammatory/injury response) and wasting (semi-starvation) are particularly challenging to treat successfully.

Cachexia is characterized by increased cytokine production as a result of underlying inflammatory disease or critical illness or injury. The inflammatory cytokines (tumor necrosis factor [TNF], IL-1, and IL-6) may mediate changes in metabolism indirectly by altering the secretion of hormones and directly by affecting target organs (Roubenoff, 1997). The resulting hormonal milieu favors a catabolic state. It is noteworthy that TNF was originally called "cachectin" because of its suspected role in cachexia (Beutler et al., 1985). These three cytokines are believed to play key roles in triggering the acute-phase metabolic response to inflammation or injury. Manifestations of this response may include elevation in resting energy expenditure, a net export of amino acids from muscle to liver, an increase in gluconeogenesis, a shift toward the production of acute-phase proteins, and a decline in the synthesis of albumin (Kushner, 1993). Despite the loss of body cell mass, observable weight loss may be modest or nonexistent because of an increase in the extracellular fluid compartment.

Clinical Importance

Although the acute-phase metabolic response may be an appropriate adaptive response for acute injury or inflammation, it can be associated with increased complications and mortality if severe or protracted. Life is not sustainable when body cell mass falls below 60 percent of usual levels (Kotler et al., 1989; Winick, 1979).

Potentially Treatable Contributing Factors

Diseases or injury states in which cachexia is present at varying degrees include rheumatoid arthritis, congestive heart failure, chronic obstructive pulmonary disease, human immunodeficiency virus (HIV) infection without serious opportunistic infection, and critical injury with adequate nutrition support (Roubenoff et al., 1997). Patients with rheumatoid arthritis who had adequate nutritional intakes evidenced reduced body cell mass in comparison to weight-matched controls (Roubenoff et al., 1992, 1994). Rheumatoid patients with the highest levels of catabolic cytokines had the lowest lean body mass (Roubenoff et al., 1992). Congestive heart failure patients may suffer appreciable loss of body cell mass with concomitant increase in extracellular water, resulting in net weight gain. Elevated levels of TNF and its soluble receptors have been detected in patients with heart failure (Anker et al., 1997). Decline of body cell mass in HIV patients without severe weight loss was found to identify individuals with subsequent risk of mortality (Kotler et al., 1989). Severe burn injury can elicit a profound cytokine-mediated catabolic response that may result in negative nitrogen balance even in the face of aggressive nutrition support (Cannon et al., 1992; Wolfe, 1996).

Approaches to Treatment and Treatment Outcomes

Anticytokine agents and anabolic hormones offer potential to modulate response to inflammation or injury, but have been applied in limited settings (e.g., rheumatic diseases) to date. Adjunctive nutrition support may serve to blunt semistarvation and associated wasting.

Wasting

Wasting has been differentiated from cachexia by its loss of body cell mass without increased cytokine production (Roubenoff et al., 1997). Semi-starvation results in obvious nonvolitional weight loss without manifestations of the acute-phase metabolic response. In pure wasting syndrome, resting energy expenditure may well be reduced and visceral proteins preserved. Increased extracellular fluid is not observed. The common feature of wasting conditions is poor dietary intake that results in weight loss.

Potentially Treatable Contributing Factors

Disorders in which wasting is a clinically observable component include marasmus, cancer, advanced AIDS with opportunistic infection, critical illness without nutrition support, and chronic organ failure syndromes (i.e., renal, hepatic, lung) (Roubenoff et al., 1997). Many patients with these disorders may have evidence of inflammation as measured by cytokine and CRP stimulation. Thus, the distinction between wasting and cachexia may not be as clear as previously thought. Marasmus is the classic syndrome of semistarvation with loss of subcutaneous fat and skeletal muscle that may be readily detected by change in body weight and upper-arm anthropometry. Among cancer, AIDS, and organ failure syndrome patients, observed weight loss determined to be due to wasting carries a poor prognosis.

Approaches to Treatment and Treatment Outcomes

Interventions for wasting syndromes have generally focused on increasing nutrient intake through nutritional supplementation and appetite stimulation via drug therapy. However, outcome and ability to accrue lean body mass appear largely to be determined by the underlying disease process.

Protein–Energy Undernutrition

PEU is defined by the presence of both clinical (physical signs such as wasting, low BMI) and biochemical (albumin or other protein) evidence of insufficient intake. The most commonly used threshold to define PEU, albumin less than 3.5 g/dL, was derived in hospitalized patients (Bistrian et al., 1974). More recently, this threshold has been questioned as increased risk of adverse outcomes has been identified among hospitalized patients with higher levels of serum albumin (Del Savio et al., 1996).

Clinical Importance

The prevalence of PEU varies widely across settings. Using a threshold of less than or equal to 3.5 g/dL, 25 to 53 percent of elderly patients meet this criteria among hospitalized older persons (Bienia et al., 1982; Constans et al., 1992), as do 35 percent of geriatric rehabilitation unit patients (Sullivan et al., 1995). Among community-dwelling older persons sampled in the first National Health and Nutrition Examination Survey (NHANES), 1 percent of persons 55 to 74 years of age had albumin levels less than 3.5 g/dL, but 8 percent had values of less than or equal to 3.8 g/dL (Reuben et al., 1997). The prevalence of hypoalbuminemia rises with age as a result of the increased burden of diseases and probably a slight physiological decrease in albumin level with aging. Among those 90 years of age or older in the EPESE cohort, 10 percent had values less than 3.5 g/dL (Salive et al., 1992). Community-dwelling older persons who are homebound appear to be at particular risk for hypoalbuminemia; 19 percent had serum albumin levels less than 3.5 g/dL in one survey (Ritchie et al., 1997). In the nursing home setting, approximately 28 percent of residents have albumin levels less than 3.5 g/dL (Abbasi and Rudman, 1993).

Numerous studies have associated low serum albumin in hospitalized older persons (measured at various times during hospitalization) with in-hospital complications, longer hospital stays, more frequent readmissions, in-hospital mortality, and increased mortality at 90 days and at 1 year (Agarwal et al., 1988; Anderson et al., 1984; Burness et al., 1996; Cederholm et al., 1995; D'Erasmo et al., 1997; Ferguson et al., 1993;

Friedmann et al., 1997; Harvey et al., 1981; Herrmann et al., 1992; Incalzi et al., 1998; Marinella and Markert, 1998; McClave et al., 1992; Patterson et al., 1992; Sullivan and Walls 1995; Sullivan et al., 1995; Volkert et al., 1992). When considering mortality, the lower the albumin level, the higher the risk of death. Among nursing home residents who were hospitalized, one prospective cohort study found that severe hypoalbuminemia predicted mortality (Ferguson et al., 1993).

Low serum albumin has been predictive of 1-year mortality in male nursing home residents (Rudman et al., 1987). Similarly, a prospective cohort study found that hypoalbuminemia predicted 3-month mortality among long-term care residents receiving tube feedings (Henderson et al., 1992).

In community-dwelling populations, hypoalbuminemia predicts higher mortality rates at 3, 5, and 9 to 10 years (Agarwal et al., 1988; Corti et al., 1994; Klonoff-Cohen et al., 1992; Sahyoun et al., 1996) and in healthier older persons (Reuben et al., 1999). The magnitude of this risk is most pronounced in those who meet the classic hypoalbuminemic criterion of less than 3.5 g/dL. In the EPESE cohort, the adjusted RR of mortality over 5 years for those who met this criterion was 1.9 for men and 3.7 for women. That study also noted significantly increased RR (1.9 for men and 2.5 for women) among persons with more modest hypoalbuminemia (≤3.8 g/dL). In the MacArthur Studies of Successful Aging, which enrolled older persons who had little or no functional impairment at the study's onset, those with albumin levels less than 3.8 g/dL had an adjusted RR of 3-year mortality of 1.8 (Reuben et al., 1999).

Prealbumin has also been shown to provide long-term prognostic value of mortality for patients admitted to a geriatric assessment unit (Mühlethaler et al., 1995). Low prealbumin and transferrin levels predicted short-term (3 month) mortality among nursing home residents (Woo et al., 1989).

Potentially Treatable Contributing Factors and Assessment Methods

Using data from the first NHANES, 14 risk factors for hypoalbuminemia were identified (Reuben et al., 1997). These included age greater than or equal to 65 years; receipt of welfare; having a condition that interferes with eating; vomiting greater than or equal to 3 days per month; prior surgery for gastrointestinal tumor; having heart failure; having recurring cough attacks; feeling tired, worn out, or exhausted; loss of teeth or having poor dentition; getting little or no exercise; being prescribed a low salt diet; currently smoking cigarettes; trouble chewing firm meats; and having albuminuria, glycosuria, or hematuria. Those who had between three and five of these conditions had an odds ratio of 2.73 for having an albumin level less than or equal to 3.8 g/dL, and those with six or more risk factors had an odds ratio of 6.44. Many of these risk factors are modifiable; however, the link between modifying risk factors and reduction of hypoalbuminemia and subsequent consequences has not yet been established.

The assessment of hypoalbuminemia includes tests of liver and renal function to exclude cirrhosis and nephrotic syndrome. Other assessment methods are similar to those used to evaluate weight loss and are described above.

Approaches to Treatment and Treatment Outcomes

Among hospitalized older persons, the most relevant research has been that aimed at poor nutritional intake (summarized above and in chapter 2). There have been no randomized clinical trials of specific treatments for PEU or hypoalbuminemia in community-dwelling older persons, but a small case-series indicated that a nurse-administered, in-home assessment may uncover remediable problems that contribute to hypoalbuminemia (Reuben et al., 1999).

Failure to Thrive

This term was originally coined to describe infants who failed to achieve height, weight, or behavioral milestones consistent with population-based normative data. It was later adapted to describe older persons who lose weight, decline in physical and/or cognitive function, and demonstrate signs of hopelessness and helplessness (Braun et al., 1988). In 1991, the National Institute on Aging described failure to thrive as "a syndrome of weight loss, decreased appetite and poor nutrition, and inactivity, often accompanied by dehydration, depressive symptoms, impaired immune function, and low cholesterol" (Lonergan, 1991). Some people have advocated abandoning this term as a disease construct in favor of four treatable contributing domains: (1) impaired physical functioning, (2) malnutrition, (3) depression, and (4) cognitive impairment (Sarkisian and Lachs, 1996). Because failure to thrive has not been approached systematically, prevalence data are not available. Specific treatments have not been developed or tested. Accordingly, the approach to failure to thrive is not considered separately.

LIMITATIONS OF CURRENT EVIDENCE

The detection of undernutrition in older persons in all settings is limited by the lack of valid and reliable detection methods. Other than in specific situations (e.g., after hip fracture), the treatment of undernutrition is more empirical than evidence based.

SUMMARY

Undernutrition is exceedingly common among hospitalized older persons. Some are undernourished at the time of admission; others become undernourished during the hospitalization as a result of poor nutritional intake and high energy requirements. The treatment for undernutrition depends on the underlying cause. Although there are limited data supporting nutritional intervention in this setting, efforts to assess dietary intake and intervene should be encouraged. The JCAHO has designated the geriatric population as being at high risk and has required screening within 24 hours. Although the details of this screening are not specified, in practice, substantial amounts of dietitian and dietary technician time are spent in attempting to meet JCAHO requirements with little evidence that this actually benefits the care of patients.

Undernutrition among nursing home residents is also common. Inadequate numbers of qualified staff and resulting feeding problems are major contributors. Treatable acute and chronic medical problems may also be important contributing factors.

Most markers (i.e., weight loss, body composition, and biochemical) that are used to indicate undernutrition are not specific for this disorder and may be affected by both acute and chronic illness. Nevertheless, all convey valuable prognostic information.

Newly defined syndromes, such as sarcopenia, cachexia, and wasting, may occur singly or in combination. The contributions of nutritional components as well as age-related changes and disease must be considered. The role(s) for nutritional therapy in the treatment of these syndromes awaits clarification.

There is a pressing need for research on undernutrition in older persons. In many instances, key issues have not been formally studied. In other instances, the research previously conducted does not provide definitive answers.

RECOMMENDATIONS

• **Although the optimal method for identifying undernutrition in hospitalized older persons has not been determined, the currently employed methods are time consuming and insufficient. The current standards for screening for risk of malnutrition in hospitalized Medicare beneficiaries must be revised and standardized. While additional research is being conducted, it is rational to focus on assessments that** have prognostic value (e.g., weight loss, serum proteins) or which indicate that patients are not receiving adequate intake in the hospital, particularly patients whose hospitalization exceeds 72 hours. If potential undernutrition is identified, it is imperative that this information be communicated formally to the physician responsible for the patient's care.

• Community-dwelling older persons and nursing home residents who have experienced weight loss should be evaluated by a dietitian for potentially reversible causes as part of their Medicare benefits. This evaluation should include some or all of the following:

— food security
— food-related functional status
— appetite and dietary intake
— depressive symptoms
— swallowing ability
— medications that might be associated with decreased appetite
— cognitive impairment
— disease-related dietary restrictions.

• Adequacy of feeding assistance in nursing home and hospital settings should be a performance standard for licensing.

• The federal government, through agencies such as the National Institute on Aging, the Agency for Healthcare Research and Quality, and the Health Care Financing Administration, should support clinical research on nutrition in older persons. Some of the most important research questions include the following:

— Which body composition and biochemical measures are most specific for undernutrition?
— What are the best methods for identifying older persons with undernutrition in hospital settings?
— What are the benefits of provision of nutritional supplements among older persons who have experienced decreased appetite during hospitalization?
— What are the benefits of provision of nutritional supplements among older persons who have lost weight for which an identifiable cause has not been found?
— What are the most appropriate methods for providing nutritional intake for older persons who will not or cannot safely ingest sufficient nutritional intake?

— What are the best methods to ensure that nursing home residents are adequately fed?

— What are the most effective combinations of nutrition therapy, exercise, trophic factors, and appetite stimulants that lead to optimal outcomes among those with undernutrition?

— What is the role of nutrition therapy among older persons who have evidence of sarcopenia, cachexia, or wasting syndromes?

REFERENCES

Abbasi AA, Rudman D. 1993. Observations on the prevalence of protein–calorie undernutrition in VA nursing homes. *J Am Geriatr Soc* 41:117–121.

Agarwal N, Acevedo F, Leighton LS, Cayten CG, Pitchumoni CS. 1988. Predictive ability of various nutritional variables for mortality in elderly people. *Am J Clin Nutr* 48:1173–1178.

Anderson CF, Moxness K, Meister J, Burritt MF. 1984. The sensitivity and specificity of nutrition-related variables in relationship to the duration of hospital stay and the rate of complications. *Mayo Clin Proc* 59:477–483.

Anker SD, Clark AL, Kemp M, Salsbury C, Teixeira MM, Hellewell PG, Coats AJS. 1997. Tumor necrosis factor and steroid metabolism in chronic heart failure: Possible relation to muscle wasting. *J Am Coll Cardiol* 30:997–1001.

Bastow MD, Rawlings J, Allison SP. 1983. Benefits of supplementary tube feeding after fractured neck of femur: A randomised controlled trial. *Br Med J* 287:1589–1592.

Baumgartner RN, Stauber PM, McHugh D, Koehler KM, Garry PJ. 1995. Cross-sectional age differences in body composition in persons 60+ years of age. *J Gerontol* 50A:M307–M316.

Baumgartner RN, Koehler KM, Gallagher D, Romero L, Heymsfield SB, Ross RR, Garry PJ, Lindeman RD. 1998. Epidemiology of sarcopenia among the elderly in New Mexico. *Am J Epidemiol* 147:755–763.

Beutler B, Mahoney J, Le Trang N, Pekala P, Cerami A. 1985. Purification of cachectin, a lipoprotein lipase-suppressing hormone secreted by endotoxin-induced RAW 264.7 cells. *J Exp Med* 161:984–995.

Bienia R, Ratcliff S, Barbour GL, Kummer M. 1982. Malnutrition in the hospitalized geriatric patient. *J Am Geriatr Soc* 30:433–436.

Bistrian BR, Blackburn GL, Hallowell E, Heddle R. 1974. Protein status of general surgical patients. *J Am Med Assoc* 230:858–860.

Blaum CS, Fries BE, Fiatarone MA. 1995. Factors associated with low body mass index and weight loss in nursing home residents. *J Gerontol* 50A:M162–M168.

Blaum CS, O'Neill EF, Clements KM, Fries BE, Fiatarone MA. 1997. Validity of the Minimum Data Set for assessing nutritional status in nursing home residents. *Am J Clin Nutr* 66:787–794.

Bortz WM II. 1982. Disuse and aging. *J Am Med Assoc* 248:1203–1208.

Braun JV, Wykle MH, Cowling WR III. 1988. Failure to thrive in older persons: A concept derived. *Gerontologist* 28:809–812.

Breslow RA, Sorkin JD. 1993. Comparison of one-day and three-day calorie counts in hospitalized patients: A pilot study. *J Am Geriatr Soc* 41:923–927.

Burness R, Horne G, Purdie G. 1996. Albumin levels and mortality in patients with hip fractures. *N Z Med J* 109:56–57.

Campbell AJ, Spears GFS, Brown JS, Busby WJ, Borrie MJ. 1990. Anthropometric measurements as predictors of mortality in a community population aged 70 years and over. *Age Ageing* 19:131–135.

Cannon JG, Friedberg JS, Gelfand JA, Tompkins RG, Burke JF, Dinarello CA. 1992. Circulating interleukin-1 beta and tumor necrosis factor-alpha concentrations after burn injury in humans. *Crit Care Med* 20:1414–1419.

Carver AD, Dobson AM. 1995. Effects of dietary supplementation of elderly demented hospital residents. *J Hum Nutr Dietetics* 8:389–394.

Castle S, Nguyen C, Joaquin A, Coyne B, Heuston C, Chan A, Percy L, Ohmen J. 1995. Megestrol acetate suspension therapy in the treatment of geriatric anorexia/cachexia in nursing home patients. *J Am Geriatr Soc* 43:835–836.

Cederholm T, Jägrén C, Hellström K. 1995. Outcome of protein–energy malnutrition in elderly medical patients. *Am J Med* 98:67–74.

Chumlea WC, Guo SS, Vellas B, Guigoz Y. 1995. Techniques of assessing muscle mass and function (sarcopenia) for epidemiological studies of the elderly. *J Gerontol* 50A:45–51.

Constans T, Bacq Y, Bréchot J-F, Guilmot J-L, Choutet P, Lamisse F. 1992. Protein-energy malnutrition in elderly medical patients. *J Am Geriatr Soc* 40:263–268.

Corpas E, Harman SM, Blackman MR. 1993. Human growth hormone and human aging. *Endocr Rev* 14:20–39.

Corti MC, Guralnik JM, Salive ME, Sorkin JD. 1994. Serum albumin level and physical disability as predictors of mortality in older persons. *J Am Med Assoc* 272:1036–1042.

Del Savio GC, Zelicof SB, Wexler LM, Byrne DW, Fish D, Ende KA. 1996. Preoperative nutritional status and outcome of elective total hip replacement. *Clin Orthop* 326:153–161.

D'Erasmo E, Pisani D, Ragno A, Romagnoli S, Spagna G, Acca M. 1997. Serum albumin level at admission: Mortality and clinical outcome in geriatric patients. *Am J Med Sci* 314:17–20.

Dutta C, Hadley EC. 1995. The significance of sarcopenia in old age. *J Gerontol A Biol Sci Med Sci* 50S:1–4.

Ettinger WH Jr, Harris T, Verdery RB, Tracy R, Kouba E. 1995. Evidence for inflammation as a cause of hypocholesterolemia in older people. *J Am Geriatr Soc* 43:264–266.

Evans WJ, Campbell WW. 1993. Sarcopenia and age-related changes in body composition and functional capacity. *J Nutr* 123:465–468.

Evans WJ, Cyr-Campbell D. 1997. Nutrition, exercise, and healthy aging. *J Am Diet Assoc* 97:632–638.

Ferguson RP, O'Connor P, Crabtree B, Batchelor A, Mitchell J, Coppola D. 1993. Serum albumin and prealbumin as predictors of clinical outcomes of hospitalized elderly nursing home residents. *J Am Geriatr Soc* 41:545–549.

Fiatarone MA, O'Neill EF, Ryan ND, Clements KM, Solares GR, Nelson ME, Roberts SB, Kehayias JJ, Lipsitz LA, Evans WJ. 1994. Exercise training and nutritional supplementation for physical frailty in very elderly people. *N Engl J Med* 330:1769–1775.

French SA, Folsom AR, Jeffery RW, Williamson DF. 1999. Prospective study of intentionality of weight loss and mortality in older women: The Iowa Women's Health Study. *Am J Epidemiol* 149:504–514.

Friedmann JM, Jensen GL, Smiciklas-Wright H, McCamish MA. 1997. Predicting early nonelective hospital readmission in nutritionally compromised older adults. *Am J Clin Nutr* 65:1714–1720.

Fuller NJ, Jebb SA, Goldberg GR, Pullicino E, Adams C, Cole TJ, Elia M. 1991. Inter-observer variability in the measurement of body composition. *Eur J Clin Nutr* 45:43–49.

Galanos AN, Pieper CF, Cornoni-Huntley JC, Bales CW, Fillenbaum GG. 1994. Nutrition and function: Is there a relationship between body mass index and the functional capabilities of community-dwelling elderly? *J Am Geriatr Soc* 42:368–373.

Gariballa SE, Parker SG, Taub N, Castleden CM. 1998. A randomized, controlled, single-blind trial of nutritional supplementation after acute stroke. *J Parenter Enteral Nutr* 22:315–319.

Goran MI, Poehlman ET. 1992. Total energy expenditure and energy requirements in healthy elderly persons. *Metabolism* 41:744–753.

Gray-Donald K, Payette H, Boutier V, Page S. 1994. Evaluation of the dietary intake of homebound elderly and the feasibility of dietary supplementation. *J Am Coll Nutr* 13:277–284.

Gray-Donald K, Payette H, Boutier V. 1995. Randomized clinical trial of nutritional supplementation shows little effect on functional status among free-living frail elderly. *J Nutr* 125:2965–2971.

Harvey KB, Moldawer LL, Bistrian BR, Blackburn GL. 1981. Biological measures for the formulation of a hospital prognostic index. *Am J Clin Nutr* 34:2013–2022.

Hébuterne X, Broussard J-F, Rampal P. 1995. Acute renutrition by cyclic enteral nutrition in elderly and younger patients. *J Am Med Assoc* 273:638–643.

Henderson CT, Trumbore LS, Mobarhan S, Benya R, Miles TP. 1992. Prolonged tube feeding in long-term care: Nutritional status and clinical outcomes. *J Am Coll Nutr* 11:309–325.

Herrmann FR, Safran C, Levkoff SE, Minaker KL. 1992. Serum albumin level on admission as a predictor of death, length of stay, and readmission. *Arch Intern Med* 152:125–130.

Heymsfield SB, Smith R, Aulet M, Bensen B, Lichtman S, Wang J, Pierson RN Jr. 1990. Appendicular skeletal muscle mass: Measurement by dual-photon absorptiometry. *Am J Clin Nutr* 52:214–218.

Incalzi RA, Capparella O, Gemma A, Landi F, Pagano F, Cipriani L, Carbonin P. 1998. Inadequate caloric intake: A risk factor for mortality of geriatric patients in the acute-care hospital. *Age Ageing* 27:303–310.

IOM (Institute of Medicine). 1994. *How Should the Recommended Dietary Allowances Be Revised?* Washington, D.C.: National Academy Press.

IOM (Institute of Medicine). 1997. *Dietary Reference Intakes for Calcium, Phosphorus, Magnesium, Vitamin D, and Fluoride.* Washington, D.C.: National Academy Press.

IOM (Institute of Medicine). 1998. *Dietary Reference Intakes for Thiamin, Riboflavin, Niacin, Vitamin B_6, Folate, Vitamin B_{12}, Pantothenic Acid, Biotin, and Choline.* Washington, D.C.: National Academy Press.

Johnson LE, Dooley PA, Gleick JB. 1993. Oral nutritional supplement use in elderly nursing home patients. *J Am Geriatr Soc* 41:947–952.

Kayser-Jones J, Schell E. 1997. The effect of staffing on the quality of care at mealtime. *Nurs Outlook* 45:64–72.

Kayser-Jones J, Schell E, Porter C, Paul S. 1997. Reliability of percentage figures used to record the dietary intake of nursing home residents. *Nurs Home Med* 5:69–76.

Kehayias J, Heymsfield S, eds. 1997. Symposium: Sarcopenia: Diagnosis and mechanisms. *J Nutr* 127:989S–1016S.

Keller HH. 1995. Weight gain impacts morbidity and mortality in institutionalized older persons. *J Am Geriatr Soc* 43:165–169.

Klonoff-Cohen H, Barrett-Connor EL, Edelstein SL. 1992. Albumin levels as a predictor of mortality in the healthy elderly. *J Clin Epidemiol* 45:207–212.

Kotler DP, Tierney AR, Wang J, Pierson RN Jr. 1989. Magnitude of body-cell-mass depletion and the timing of death from wasting in AIDS. *Am J Clin Nutr* 50:444–447.

Kushner I. 1993. Regulation of the acute phase response by cytokines. *Perspect Biol Med* 36:611–622.

Lexell J. 1995. Human aging, muscle mass, and fiber type composition. *J Gerontol* 50A:11–16.

Lexell JL, Dutta C, eds. 1997. Sarcopenia and physical performance in old age. Proceedings of a workshop. *Muscle Nerve* 5:S1–S120.

Lonergan ET, ed. 1991. *Extending Life, Enhancing Life: A National Research Agenda on Aging.* Washington, D.C.: National Academy Press.

Loprinzi CL, Bernath AM, Schaid DJ, Malliard JA, Athmann LM, Michalak JC, Tschetter KL, Hatfield AK, Morton RF. 1994. Phase III evaluation of 4 doses of megestrol acetate as therapy for patients with cancer anorexia and/or cachexia. *Oncology* 51:S2–S7.

Losonczy KG, Harris TB, Cornoni-Huntley J, Simonsick EM, Wallace RB, Cook NR, Ostfeld AM, Blazer DG. 1995. Does weight loss from middle age to old age explain the inverse weight mortality relation in old age? *Am J Epidemiol* 14:312–321.

Marinella MA, Markert RJ. 1998. Admission serum albumin level and length of hospitalization in elderly patients. *S Med J* 91:851–854.

McClave SA, Mitoraj TE, Thielmeier KA, Greenburg RA. 1992. Differentiating subtypes (hypoalbuminemic vs marasmic) of protein–calorie malnutrition: Incidence and clinical significance in a university hospital setting. *Parenter Enteral Nutr* 16:337–342.

Morley JE, Kraenzle D. 1994. Causes of weight loss in a community nursing home. *J Am Geriatr Soc* 42:583–585.

Mühlethaler R, Stuck AE, Minder CE, Frey BM. 1995. The prognostic significance of protein-energy malnutrition in geriatric patients. *Age Ageing* 24:193–197.

Noel MA, Smith TK, Ettinger WH. 1991. Characteristics and outcomes of hospitalized older patients who develop hypocholesterolemia. *J Am Geriatr Soc* 39:455–461.

Novak LP. 1972. Aging, total body potassium, fat-free mass, and cell mass in males and females between ages 18 and 85 years. *J Gerontol* 27:438–443.

NRC (National Research Council). 1986. *Nutrient Adequacy. Assessment Using Food Consumption Surveys.* Washington, D.C.: National Academy Press

Oster MH, Enders SR, Samuels SJ, Cone, LA, Hooton, TM, Browder HP, Flynn NM. 1994. Megestrol acetate in patients with AIDS and cachexia. *Ann Intern Med* 121:400–408.

Papadakis MA, Grady D, Black D, Tierney MJ, Gooding GAW, Schambelan M, Grunfeld C. 1996. Growth hormone replacement in healthy older men improves body composition but not functional ability. *Ann Intern Med* 124:708–716.

Patterson BM, Cornell CN, Carbone B, Levine B, Chapman D. 1992. Protein depletion and metabolic stress in elderly patients who have a fracture of the hip. *Am J Bone Joint Surg* 74:251–260.

Poehlman ET, Toth MJ, Bunyard LB, Gardner AW, Donaldson KE, Colman E, Fonong T, Ades PA. 1995. Physiological predictors of increasing total and central adiposity in aging men and women. *Arch Intern Med* 155:2443–2448.

Pokrywka HS, Koffler KH, Remsburg R, Bennett RG, Roth J, Tayback M, Wright JE. 1997. Accuracy of patient care staff in estimating and documenting meal intake of nursing home residents. *J Am Geriatr Soc* 45:1223–1227.

Reuben DB, Moore AA, Damesyn M, Keeler E, Harrison GG, Greendale GA. 1997. Correlates of hypoalbuminemia in community-dwelling older persons. *Am J Clin Nutr* 66:38–45.

Reuben DB, Effros RB, Hirsch SH, Zhu X, Greendale GA. 1999. An in-home nurse-administered geriatric assessment for hypoalbuminemic older persons: Development and preliminary experience. *J Am Geriatr Soc* 47:1244–1248.

Riquelme R, Torres A, El-Ebiary M, de la Bellacasa JP, Estruch R, Mensa J, Fernandez-Sola J, Hernandez C, Rodriguez-Roisin R. 1996. Community-acquired pneumonia in the elderly: A multivariate analysis of risk and prognostic factors. *Am J Respir Crit Care Med* 154:1450–1455.

Ritchie CS, Burgio KL, Locher JL, Cornwell A, Thomas D, Hardin M, Redden D. 1997. Nutritional status of urban homebound older adults. *Am J Clin Nutr* 66:815–818.

Rosenberg IH. 1989. Summary comments. *Am J Clin Nutr* 50:1231S–1233S.

Rothschild MA, Oratz M, Schreiber SS. 1988. Serum albumin. *Hepatology* 8:385–401.

Roubenoff R. 1997. Inflammatory and hormonal mediators of cachexia. *J Nutr* 127:1014S–1016S.

Roubenoff R, Roubenoff RA, Ward LM, Holland SM, Hellmann DB. 1992. Rheumatoid cachexia: Depletion of lean body mass in rheumatoid arthritis. Possible association with tumor necrosis factor. *J Rheumatol* 19:1505–1510.

Roubenoff R, Roubenoff RA, Cannon JG, Kehayias JJ, Zhuang H, Dawson-Hughes B, Dinarello CA, Rosenberg IH. 1994. Rheumatoid cachexia: Cytokine-driven hypermetabolism accompanying reduced body cell mass in chronic inflammation. *J Clin Invest* 93:2379–2386.

Roubenoff R, Heymsfield SB, Kehayias JJ, Cannon JG, Rosenberg IH. 1997. Standardization of nomenclature of body composition in weight loss. *Am J Clin Nutr* 66:192–196.

Rudman D, Feller AG. 1989. Protein-calorie undernutrition in the nursing home. *J Am Geriatr Soc* 37:173–183.

Rudman D, Feller AG, Nagraj HS, Jackson DL, Rudman IW, Mattson DE. 1987. Relation of serum albumin concentration to death rate in nursing home men. *J Parenter Enteral Nutr* 11:360–363.

Rudman D, Feller AG, Nagraj HS, Gergans GA, Lalitha PY, Goldberg AF, Schlenker RA, Cohn L, Rudman IW, Mattson DE. 1990. Effects of human growth hormone in men over 60 years old. *N Engl J Med* 323:1–6.

Ryan AS, Craig LD, Finn SC. 1992. Nutrient intakes and dietary patterns of older Americans: A national study. *J Gerontol* 47:M145–M150.

Sahyoun NR, Jacques PF, Dallal G, Russell RM. 1996. Use of albumin as a predictor of mortality in community-dwelling and institutionalized elderly populations. *J Clin Epidemiol* 49:981–988.

Salive, ME, Cornoni-Huntley J, Phillips C, Guralinik JM, Cohen HJ, Ostfeld AM, Wallace RB. 1992. Serum albumin in older persons: Relationship with age and health status. *J Clin Epidemiol* 45:213–221.

Sarkisian CA, Lachs MS. 1996. "Failure to thrive" in older adults. *Ann Intern Med* 124:1072–1078.

Sawaya AL, Tucker K, Tsay R, Saltzman E, Dallal GE, Roberts SB. 1996. Evaluation of four methods for determining energy intake in young and older women: Comparison with doubly-labeled water measurements of total energy expenditure. *Am J Clin Nutr* 63:491–499.

Schürch M-A, Rizzoli R, Slosman D, Vadas L, Vergnaud P, Bonjour J-P. 1998. Protein supplements increase serum insulin-like growth factor-I levels and attenuate proximal femur bone loss in patients with recent hip fracture. A randomized, double-blind, placebo-controlled trial. *Ann Intern Med* 128:801–809.

Selberg O, Burchert W, Graubner G, Wenner C, Ehrenheim C, Muller MJ. 1993. Determination of anatomical skeletal muscle mass by whole body nuclear magnetic resonance. *Basic Life Sci* 60:95–97

Shenkin A, Cederblad G, Elia M, Isaksson B. 1996. Laboratory assessment of protein–energy status. *Clin Chim Acta* 253:S5–S59.

Sih R, Morley JE, Kaiser FE, Perry HM 3rd, Patrick P, Ross C. 1997. Testosterone replacement in older hypogonadal men: A 12-month randomized controlled trial. *J Clin Endocrinol Metab* 82:1661–1667.

Sjostrom L. 1991. A computer-tomography based multicompartment body composition technique and anthropometric predictions of lean body mass, total and subcutaneous adipose tissue. *Int J Obes* 15:S19–S30.

Snyder PJ, Peachey H, Hannoush P, Berlin JA, Loh L, Lenrow DA, Holmes JH, Dlewati A, Santanna J, Rosen CJ, Strom BL. 1999. Effect of testosterone treatment on body composition and muscle strength in men over 65 years of age. *J Clin Endocrinol Metab* 84:2647–2653.

Sullivan DH, Walls RC. 1995. The risk of life-threatening complications in a select population of geriatric patients: The impact of nutritional status. *J Am Coll Nutr* 14:29–36.

Sullivan DH, Patch GA, Baden AL, Lipschitz DA. 1989. An approach to assessing the reliability of anthropometrics in elderly patients. *J Am Geriatr Soc* 37:607–613.

Sullivan DH, Walls RC, Bopp MM. 1995. Protein–energy undernutrition and the risk of mortality within one year of hospital discharge: A follow-up study. *J Am Geriatr Soc* 43:507–512.

Sullivan DH, Sun S, Walls RC. 1999. Protein–energy undernutrition among elderly hospitalized patients: A prospective study. *J Am Med Assoc* 281:2013–2019.

Tomoyasu NJ, Toth MJ, Poehlman ET. 1999. Misreporting of total energy intake in older men and women. *J Am Geriatr Soc* 47:710–715.

Urban RJ, Bodenburg YH, Foxworth J, Coggan AR, Wolfe RR, Ferrando A. 1995. Testosterone administration to elderly men increases skeletal muscle strength and protein synthesis. *Am J Physiol* 269:E820–E826.

Volkert D, Kruse W, Oster P, Schlierf G. 1992. Malnutrition in geriatric patients: Diagnostic and prognostic significance of nutritional parameters. *Ann Nutr Metab* 36:97–112.

Von Roenn JH, Armstrong D, Kotler DP, Cohn DL, Klimas NG, Tchekmedyian NS, Cone L, Brennan PJ, Weitzman SA. 1994. Megestrol acetate in patients with AIDS-related cachexia. *Ann Intern Med* 121:393–399.

Wallace JI, Schwartz RS, LaCroix AZ, Uhlmann RF, Pearlman RA. 1995. Involuntary weight loss in older outpatients: Incidence and clinical significance. *J Am Geriatr Soc* 43:329–337.

White H, Pieper C, Schmader K. 1998. The association of weight change in Alzheimer's disease with severity of disease and mortality: A longitudinal analysis. *J Am Geriatr Soc* 46:1223–1227.

WHO/FAO/UNU (World Health Organization, Food and Agriculture Organization, United Nations University). 1985. *Energy and Protein Requirements*. Geneva: WHO.

Wilson M-MG, Vaswani S, Liu D, Morley JE, Miller DK. 1998. Prevalence and causes of undernutrition in medical outpatients. *Am J Med* 104:56–63.

Winick M. 1979. *Hunger Disease—Studies by Jewish Physicians in the Warsaw Ghetto*. New York: John Wiley & Sons.

Wolfe RR. 1996. Herman Award Lecture, 1996: Relation of metabolic studies to clinical nutrition—the example of burn injury. *Am J Clin Nutr* 64:800–808.

Woo J, Chan SM, Mak YT, Swaminathan R. 1989. Biochemical predictors of short term mortality in elderly residents of chronic care institutions. *J Clin Pathol* 42:1241–1245.

Woo J, Ho SC, Mak YT, Law LK, Cheung A. 1994. Nutritional status of elderly patients during recovery from chest infection and the role of nutritional supplementation assessed by a prospective randomized single-blind trial. *Age Ageing* 23:40–48.

5

Cardiovascular Disease

Cardiovascular diseases are the leading cause of death and major contributors to medical utilization and disability (Havlik et al., 1987). In 1996, a total of 959,227 deaths occurred from cardiovascular diseases (CVD)[1], including 476,227 deaths from coronary heart disease (CHD)[2] and 159,942 from stroke (AHA, 1998). Table 5.1 displays mortality rates for heart disease by age, gender, and race or ethnicity from 1989 to 1991. It is evident from this table that heart disease afflicts both men and women, independent of race or ethnicity. Furthermore, there is a striking age-related rise in mortality from heart disease such that the vast majority of deaths due to heart disease occur in persons age 65 and older.

The costs associated with CVD are enormous. According to data compiled by the American Heart Association (AHA, 1998), the estimated direct costs of health care for CVDs in 1999 will be $178.2 billion. An additional $108 billion in costs will occur as a result of indirect expenses. In view of the high prevalence and incidence of CVDs in the elderly, a substantial fraction of Medicare expenditures are related to these conditions. For instance, in 1995, Medicare spent $24.6 billion for hospital expenses

---

[1]CVD refers to stroke and any disease pertaining to the heart and/or blood vessels.

[2]CHD refers to conditions such as myocardial infarction and angina which result from an insufficient blood supply to the heart, typically from atherosclerotic changes in coronary arteries.

TABLE 5.1 Death Rate due to Heart Disease per 100,000 Population, 1989 to 1991

Age (years)	Men			Women		
	White	Black	Hispanic	White	Black	Hispanic
15–24	3	7	—	2	4	—
24–44	25	58	—	8	2	28
45–54	171	340	111	50	156	58
55–64	518	838	346	193	445	149
65–74	1,234	1,645	840	584	1,023	435
75–84	2,959	3,115	1,988	1,877	2,289	1,294
>85	7,515	6,343	4,861	6,550	5,767	4,488

SOURCE: Adapted from Srinath et al. (1995). Data for the age groups between 15 and 44 years were obtained from NCHS (1993). Data for the groups over age 45 were obtained from NCHS (1994).

related to CVDs, an amount that corresponds to 33 percent of its hospitalization expenditures.

Through well-accepted risk factors (i.e., dyslipidemia, hypertension), dietary factors have a prominent role in the genesis of athersclerotic CVDs (i.e., CHD, stroke, heart failure[3]). Although atherosclerosis is a chronic process beginning in youth, there is abundant evidence that therapies initiated in older-aged persons can prevent or delay clinical events. Furthermore, because of the high incidence of CVD events in older age, even relatively small improvements in risk factors (i.e., small reductions in blood pressure and low-density lipoprotein [LDL] cholesterol through diet), should be of substantial benefit to the general population. However, there is a lag period, likely 2 or more years, between the onset of therapy and a reduced risk of clinical events, such as CHD and stroke. The situation is quite different for heart failure, in which case adherence to dietary and medication therapies can lead to early benefits, such as reduced rate of hospitalization and reduced length of stay.

The following sections discuss the role of diet as a means to improve cardiovascular risk factors (dyslipidemia and hypertension) and as a means to treat heart failure.

DYSLIPIDEMIA

Dyslipidemia is a powerful risk factor for atherosclerotic diseases, particularly CHD. The term dyslipidemia applies to a high blood level of

---

[3]Heart failure refers to a clinical condition in which the heart becomes weakened or stiff and pumps blood inefficiently.

total cholesterol, as well as other abnormalities in blood lipid levels including an elevated LDL cholesterol level, a decreased high-density lipoprotein (HDL) cholesterol level, and an elevated triglyceride level. Each of these conditions increases the risk of atherosclerotic disease. Still, the primary focus of treatment has been on reducing total and LDL cholesterol (NCEP, 1994), each of which is amenable to nutrition therapy.

Dyslipidemia is commonplace among the elderly. According to the Third National Health and Nutrition Examination Survey (NHANES III) (NCHS, 1997), approximately 28 percent of men and 43 percent of women, ages 65 to 74, have elevated total cholesterol defined as a total cholesterol greater than or equal to 240 mg/dL. A somewhat lower percentage of persons, ages 75 and older, have an elevated total cholesterol level (i.e., 19 percent of men and 39 percent of women). Such data underestimate the prevalence of dyslipidemia, which would include persons with an elevated LDL cholesterol level, a low HDL cholesterol level, or a high triglyceride level despite a total cholesterol level of less than 240 mg/dL. Furthermore, the actual prevalence is also underestimated by the number in these age groups under treatment for dyslipidemia. Current treatment guidelines advocate aggressive treatment of persons with less severe lipid abnormalities who have other risk factors for atherosclerotic disease or who have had prior CVD (NCEP, 1994).

The relationship of blood levels of total and LDL cholesterol to subsequent CHD events has been documented in several major observational studies (e.g., Kahn et al., 1984; Martin et al., 1986; MRFIT, 1996; Shekelle et al., 1981) and in pooled analyses across 20 or more cohorts (Jacobs et al., 1992; Manolio et al., 1992). In general, the risk of CHD increases progressively as the blood levels of serum total and LDL cholesterol rise. The association of total mortality with total serum cholesterol is similar, except that total mortality may increase in the group of persons with the lowest levels of total cholesterol, perhaps as a result of the association of very low total cholesterol with serious noncardiovascular illnesses (Jacobs et al., 1992). Although it is generally recognized that LDL and total cholesterol are directly related to CHD risk, it is noteworthy that an increasing body of evidence has linked dyslipidemias to the occurrence of stroke (Ross et al., 1999). Also, a large body of evidence indicates that an elevated triglyceride level is at least a marker, if not an independent risk factor, for heart disease (Hokanson and Austin, 1996).

In the elderly, the risk of CHD also increases with increasing blood levels of total and LDL cholesterol (Grundy et al., 1999; Manolio et al., 1992). Previous studies have questioned the importance of elevated cholesterol as a risk factor for CHD in the elderly. In part, such uncertainties resulted from the presentation of risk estimates (i.e., the ratio of CHD risk in high versus low cholesterol groups [risk ratio] conveys a different impression than the absolute difference in CHD risk between groups with high and low cholesterol). Because CHD is commonplace in the elderly, even among persons with lower levels of serum cholesterol, the ratio of risks in high- versus low-cholesterol groups among the elderly is typically less than that observed in middle-aged persons. In fact, because of the high risk of CHD in the elderly, a reduction in blood cholesterol levels should prevent more CHD events than a comparable reduction in blood cholesterol in younger persons.

Evidence that a Change in Risk Factors Affects Morbidity and Mortality

Reduction of plasma cholesterol levels by dietary and/or pharmacological means has been shown to prevent CHD events both in persons with and without prior CHD. Effective interventions include several types of medications (bile acid sequestrants, niacin, and statin medications as prescribed by physicians) and dietary intervention. As a result of the inherent difficulties of conducting long-term dietary intervention trials, evidence tends to be stronger for drug therapies than for diet therapy (Muldoon et al., 1990). The health benefits from cholesterol reduction therapies occur without evidence of deleterious effects on noncardiovascular mortality. The magnitude of the reduction in CHD has been defined for people with initial serum cholesterol levels in the 250 to 300 mg/dL range. For each 1 percent reduction in the serum cholesterol level, a 2 percent reduction in the incidence of CHD is expected (Lipid Research Clinics Program, 1984).

The benefits of cholesterol-reducing therapy extend to the elderly (Grundy et al., 1999). Both dietary therapies and pharmacologic therapies favorably affect lipid levels in the elderly (LaRosa et al., 1994) and can prevent CVD events. Of particular interest is the Los Angeles Veterans Administration domiciliary study that involved older men, average age 66 years, who were free of signs of definite CHD (Dayton et al., 1969). In this dietary intervention trial, moderate cholesterol reduction was achieved and sustained in the active intervention group by institutional feeding of a fat-modified diet, low in saturated fat and cholesterol and high in polyunsaturated fat. A significant 31 percent reduction in the incidence of severe atherosclerotic events (coronary, cerebral, peripheral) occurred over 8.5 years of follow-up. These findings lend strong support to the judgment that risk factor modification in the elderly can prevent CVD.

In large-scale trials that enrolled persons without prior atherosclerotic cardiovascular disease (ASCVD) (Downs et al., 1998; Shepherd et al., 1995) and in other trials that enrolled persons with prior ASCVD (Sacks et al., 1996; Scandinavian Simvastatin Survival Study Group, 1994), cholesterol lowering medication significantly reduced cardiovascular morbidity and mortality, and in several instances reduced total mortality. Additional aspects of these trials are noteworthy. First, in subgroup analyses restricted to older-aged enrollees, significant reductions in cardiovascular end points were documented. Second, in each trial, the effects of the medications were tested in individuals who were also being given nutrition therapy.

Modifying Risk Factors Through Nutrition Therapy

The mainstays of dietary counseling for dyslipidemia have been advice to reduce saturated fat and dietary cholesterol intake and to increase polyunsaturated fat intake (NCEP, 1994). Such approaches reflect observational studies that have linked these aspects of diet with lipid levels as well as clinical trials that tested the effects of modifying these nutritional factors on CHD. Although reductions in total fat have also been recommended, particularly for weight reduction or weight control, the emphasis of nutrition therapy for dyslipidemia has been a reduction in saturated fat. In general, diets high in unsaturated fat have been considered more successful than low-fat diets in lowering serum cholesterol levels and decreasing the risk of coronary artery disease (Sacks, 1998).

Preliminary evidence suggests that other dietary strategies may also be effective. For instance, a diet rich in alpha-linolenic acid led to a significant reduction in the risk of subsequent coronary events in patients with previous CVD, even though cholesterol levels did not change (de Lorgeril et al., 1994, 1999). Also, Burr et al. (1989) demonstrated that advice to eat two fish meals weekly significantly decreased the risk of total mortality and coronary mortality in patients with previous myocardial infarction.

To date, the impact of vitamin supplementation (i.e., either antioxidant vitamins or those given to reduce homocysteinemia) on CHD is uncertain. Evidence primarily from observational studies suggests that certain vitamin supplements, particularly folate and vitamin E, may decrease the risk of ASCVD in some population groups. For vitamin E, a few clinical trials have been completed. One trial demonstrated a reduction in ASCVD morbidity but not mortality from supplemental vitamin E among persons with preexisting CHD (Stephens et al., 1996). In another trial, a comparatively low dose of vitamin E had no benefit on ASCVD outcomes in approximately 20,000 Finnish male smokers (Alpha-Tocopherol, Beta Carotene Cancer Prevention Study Group, 1994). In a large secondary prevention trial, vitamin E had no significant benefit in preventing ASCVD (GISSI-Prevenzione Investigators, 1999). Overall, data are insufficient for recommendations pertaining to vitamin E as a means to prevent ASCVD. For folate supplements, evidence predominantly from retrospective observational studies (Boushey et al., 1995) indirectly suggests that an increased dietary intake of folate may prevent ASCVD; however, no clinical trials of supplemental folate have been completed. Hence, available evidence is insufficient to recommend either vitamin E or folate supplements as a means for preventing ASCVD.

The Step I diet proposed by the National Cholesterol Education Program (NCEP, 1994) has been shown to decrease plasma total cholesterol by 7 to 9 percent compared with the average American diet (Stone et al., 1996). A Step II diet has been shown to decrease total cholesterol and LDL cholesterol by 10 to 20 percent (Stone et al., 1996). Short-term studies typically demonstrate greater effects than long-term studies, and feeding or metabolic studies achieve greater reductions than studies conducted in free-living persons (Kris-Etherton and Dietschy, 1997).

Thirty-seven intervention studies published between 1981 and 1997 were analyzed by Yu-Poth et al. (1999). Some were sequential studies, but most were randomized, parallel-arm studies. The dietary interventions ranged from vegetarian diets providing less than 10 percent of energy as fat, less than 6 percent of energy as saturated fat, and less than 100 mg cholesterol to a Step I diet providing less than or equal to 30 percent of energy as fat, less than 10 percent of energy as saturated fat, and less than or equal to 300 mg cholesterol per day. Average reductions in LDL cholesterol were 12 percent with a Step I diet and 16 percent with a Step II diet. Changes in plasma total cholesterol, LDL cholesterol, and HDL cholesterol were significantly correlated with changes in dietary total fat and saturated fatty acids.

Several studies utilized registered dietitians in their intervention programs. In a study of patients aged 22 to 79 with hypercholesterolemia (>5.20 mmol/L [>201 mg/dL]), assignment to a dietitian for nutrition therapy led to a mean reduction in serum cholesterol level of 9 percent. In a study by Katzel et al. (1995), a Step I isocaloric diet was sequentially compared to a Step I hypocaloric diet for 3 months in elderly men with silent myocardial ischemia. The sequential interventions decreased triglyceride levels by 44 percent, LDL cholesterol by 18 percent, and the LDL to HDL ratio by 19 percent. Reduction in total serum cholesterol levels correlated with increased time spent with a dietitian.

A group of hypercholesterolemic patients (mean age 61) took part in an 8-week nutrition intervention program provided by registered dietitians before initiating treatment with a cholesterol-lowering medication (Sikand et al., 1998). The nutrition part of the intervention lowered total cholesterol by 13 percent ($p > 0.001$), LDL cholesterol by 15 percent ($p >$

0.0001), triglyceride by 11 percent ($p = 0.05$), and HDL cholesterol by 4 percent ($p = 0.05$). After dietary counseling, 34 of 67 (51 percent) subjects were no longer candidates for drug therapy (per NCEP guidelines). The magnitude of LDL cholesterol reduction increased with greater time spent with the dietitian. A similar finding was also reported by McGehee and colleagues (1995), whose research documented that a minimum of two visits was required.

HMG-CoA Reductase Inhibitors (Statins)

β-Hydroxy-β-methylglutaryl-coenzyme A (HMG-CoA) reductase inhibitors (statins) are medications that have potent effects on blood lipid levels. Through such effects (i.e., reductions in LDL cholesterol of 17–54 percent and total cholesterol of 6–21 percent), these medications have been shown to reduce total mortality by 24 percent, fatal heart attacks by 39 percent, nonfatal heart attacks by 31 percent, fatal stroke by 23 percent, and nonfatal stroke by 31 percent (Ross et al., 1999). The populations studied have included persons with prior heart attacks, persons without prior heart attacks but at high risk for CVD, and older-aged persons. The impressive impact of statin medications on lipid levels and clinical cardiovascular events has led some to reconsider the role of nutrition therapy in the management of persons with dyslipidemia.

Still, there is a strong rationale to advocate nutrition therapy as initial therapy in persons not on statins and as adjunctive therapy in persons on medication. First, it is important to emphasize that the reductions in lipid levels and CVDs documented in trials of statin therapy were achieved in the context of concomitantly administered nutrition therapy. Second, through nutrition therapy, many persons can reduce their lipid levels to the point that they do not need or no longer require medication. A report from the National Cholesterol Education Adult Treatment Panel suggests that if all patients who are eligible for nutrition therapy experienced a 15 percent drop in LDL cholesterol, the number of patients who need drug therapy could be cut in half (Carleton et al., 1991). Third, as documented by Hunninghake et al. (1993) and others, the effects of medication and dietary therapies appear additive. Finally, dietary changes may provide additional benefits beyond that of lipid-lowering alone.

Dyslipidemia: Summary and Recommendations

Substantial evidence from observational studies and from randomized trials supports the use of nutrition therapy as a means for improving lipid profiles and thereby preventing or delaying CVD in the elderly. Furthermore, numerous professional organizations including the American Heart Association, the National Cholesterol Education Program of the National Heart, Lung, and Blood Institute, and the Second Joint Task Force of European and Other Societies on Coronary Prevention (Wood et al., 1998) advocate nutrition therapy as an integral part of routine medical therapy for persons with dyslipidemia. Recommendations for nutrition therapy extend to those individuals not on cholesterol-lowering therapy as well as persons on medications such as statins. Although the number and frequency of visits with a nutrition professional is uncertain, data suggest that at least two visits would be required. Additional research is needed to identify behavioral strategies that can accomplish and sustain long-term changes in dietary intake, the impact of different health care providers on lipid levels, and continued research on the optimal dietary pattern that reduces cardiovascular risk.

Summary of Evidence—Nutrition Therapy for Dyslipidemia

Consensus statements: Recommended as part of the standard of care in guidelines prepared by the American Heart Association (Krauss et al., 1996) and the National Heart, Lung and Blood Institute (LaRosa et al., 1990; NCEP, 1994)

Observational studies: Strong evidence (e.g., Martin et al., 1986; Shekelle et al., 1981)

Randomized trials: Strong evidence (e.g., Dayton et al., 1969; Downs et al., 1998; Lipid Research Clinic Program, 1984; Sacks et al., 1996; Shepherd et al., 1995)

Systematic reviews: Several (e.g., Grundy et al., 1999; Jacobs et al., 1992; Ross et al., 1999; Stone et al., 1996; Yu-Poth et al., 1999)

HYPERTENSION

Elevated blood pressure is among the most common and important risk factors for ASCVD in the general population and among older-aged persons. According to NHANES III data, approximately 50 percent of the more than 30 million persons age 65 or older have hypertension (defined as a systolic blood pressure ≥140 mm Hg, a diastolic blood pressure ≥90 mm Hg, and/or the use of antihypertensive medication) (Burt et al., 1995). In certain groups, the prevalence of hypertension is almost ubiquitous; for example, nearly 80 percent of black women age 60 and older have hypertension (Burt et al., 1995).

The evidence that elevated blood pressure is causally related to

ASCVD (both CHD and stroke) and to kidney disease is strong and consistent. Such data include the results of numerous longitudinal studies that assessed the occurrence of clinical ASCVD outcomes by blood pressure level. These studies were summarized in an analysis in which the relationship between blood pressure and both stroke and CHD was direct, progressive, and graded throughout the range of blood pressure (MacMahon et al., 1990). The relationship of end-stage renal disease to blood pressure is likewise direct and progressive (Klag et al., 1996). Although both systolic and diastolic blood pressure predict risk, systolic blood pressure tends to be a stronger predictor than diastolic blood pressure.

More than 20 major clinical trials have assessed the impact of blood pressure-reducing pharmacologic therapy on clinical ASCVD events, including several studies conducted exclusively in older-aged persons (MRC Working Party, 1992; SHEP Cooperative Research Group, 1991; Staessen et al., 1997). The totality of evidence suggests that a typical diastolic blood pressure reduction of 5 to 6 mm Hg prevents approximately 40 percent of strokes and 15 percent of CHD events (Hebert et al., 1993). It is assumed that blood pressure reductions from nonpharmacologic interventions would likewise prevent ASCVD events, although direct evidence from clinical trials is unavailable, primarily because of the difficulty in conducting such trials.

The contemporary approach to preventing blood pressure-related ASCVD includes nonpharmacologic blood pressure-reducing therapy (also termed lifestyle modification), as well as pharmacologic approaches. In individuals with hypertension, nonpharmacologic therapies can serve as initial therapy in Stage 1 hypertension[4] before the addition of medication and as an adjunct to medication in persons already on drug therapy. In hypertensive patients with controlled blood pressure, nonpharmacologic therapies can facilitate medication stepdown or even withdrawal in certain individuals. In nonhypertensive individuals, nonpharmacologic interventions have the potential to prevent the onset of hypertension and, more broadly, to reduce blood pressure and thereby lower the risk of ASCVD in the general population (National High Blood Pressure Education Program Working Group, 1993).

The Sixth Report of the Joint National Committee on the Detection, Evaluation and Treatment of High Blood Pressure (JNC VI, 1997) concluded that several dietary approaches effectively lower blood pressure (i.e., reduced sodium intake, weight loss, reduced alcohol consumption, increased potassium intake, and adoption of an overall healthy diet, such

---

[4] Stage 1 hypertension refers to either a systolic blood pressure of 140 to 159 mm Hg or a diastolic blood pressure of 90 to 99 mm Hg.

as the Dietary Approaches to Stop Hypertension Trial [DASH] diet). The evidence supporting these recommendations comes from observational studies as well as controlled clinical trials.

Reduced Sodium Intake

The preponderance of available evidence indicates that a high intake of salt (sodium chloride) adversely affects blood pressure. Such data include results from observational studies of diet and blood pressure (Intersalt Cooperative Research Group, 1988; Khaw and Barrett-Connor, 1990) and clinical trials of reduced salt intake. In three meta-analyses of randomized trials (Cutler et al., 1997; Graudal et al., 1998; Midgley et al., 1996), a reduced sodium intake lowered both systolic and diastolic blood pressure in hypertensive patients (range of pooled effects, 3.9–5.9 mm Hg for systolic blood pressure and 1.9–3.8 mm Hg for diastolic blood pressure); lesser reductions occurred in normotensive individuals. Many older-aged persons and African-Americans of all age groups appear particularly sensitive to the effects of salt on blood pressure. Recent trials show that behavior change interventions can reduce intake by approximately 30 to 50 mmol per day in the elderly (Whelton et al., 1998) and in other population groups (Neaton et al., 1993; TOHP Collaborative Research Group, 1992, 1997).

Weight Loss

A persuasive and consistent body of evidence from both observational and experimental studies indicates that weight is positively (directly) associated with blood pressure and hypertension (Stamler, 1991). The importance of this relationship is reinforced by the high and increasing prevalence of overweight in the United States (Kuczmarski et al., 1994). According to NHANES III data, the combined prevalence of overweight and obesity (a body mass index of >25 kg/m^2) is 59 percent in men and 51 percent in women (NIH, 1998). All but one of the 16 clinical trials that examined the influence of weight loss on blood pressure in hypertensive individuals have documented a substantial and significant reduction in blood pressure from weight loss interventions (NIH, 1998). Reductions in blood pressure occur before (and without) attainment of desirable body weight. In one study that aggregated results across 11 weight loss trials, the average systolic and diastolic blood pressure reduction per kilogram of weight loss was 1.6/1.1 mm Hg (Staessen et al., 1989). Recent lifestyle intervention trials have uniformly achieved short-term weight loss. In several instances (Neaton et al., 1993; Whelton et al., 1998), substantial weight loss has also been sustained over the long term (3 or more years).

Reduced Alcohol Intake

The relationship between high alcohol intake (typically three or more drinks per day) and elevated blood pressure has been reported in a large number of observational studies (Klatsky et al., 1977; MacMahon, 1987). A few trials have also demonstrated that reductions in alcohol intake among heavy drinkers can lower blood pressure in normotensive and hypertensive men (Puddey et al., 1985, 1987). In the Prevention and Treatment of Hypertension Study, a reduction in alcohol intake among non-dependent moderate to heavy drinkers also reduced blood pressure to a small, nonsignificant, extent (Cushman et al., 1998).

Increased Potassium Intake

In contrast to the direct relationship of sodium intake with blood pressure, the relationship between potassium intake and blood pressure is inverse (i.e., high levels of potassium are associated with low blood pressure). Whereas observational data have been reasonably consistent, the data from clinical trials have been less consistent and persuasive. However, a recent meta-analysis has documented a significant impact of potassium supplements on blood pressure (Whelton et al., 1997). On average, supplementation of the diet with a typical dose of 60 to 120 mmol of potassium per day reduced systolic and diastolic blood pressure, respectively, by 4 4 and 2.5 mm Hg in hypertensives and by 1.8 and 1.0 mm Hg in normotensives. This analysis also documented greater blood pressure reduction from potassium supplementation at higher levels of salt intake Because a high intake of potassium can easily be achieved through diet and because potassium derived from foods also comes with a variety of other nutrients, the preferred strategy for increasing potassium intake is via foods rather than supplements.

Healthy Dietary Pattern

Certain dietary patterns have been associated with low blood pressure. For instance, in observational studies, vegetarian diets have been associated with lower blood pressure even after controlling for other factors known to affect blood pressure (Sacks et al., 1974). In clinical trials, vegetarian diets also reduced blood pressure (Margetts et al., 1986; Rouse et al., 1983). Such findings spawned efforts to identify the nutrients responsible for blood pressure reduction, especially since vegetarian diets are not widely followed in the general population.

The nutrients responsible for the blood pressure-lowering effects of these diets have remained elusive. Attention has focused on macronutrients (particularly the type and amount of fat), potassium, magnesium, calcium, and fiber. Modification of fat intake, particularly saturated and total fat intake, has been tested in several trials, but the results have generally been disappointing (Morris, 1994). Trials of other nutrients have likewise been inconclusive. For instance, trials of magnesium supplementation have been inconsistent. The effects of calcium on blood pressure have likewise been equivocal. In a meta-analysis of 23 observational studies, Cappuccio et al. (1995) documented an inverse association between blood pressure and dietary calcium intake (as measured by 24-hour dietary recalls or food frequency questionnaires). However, the effect size was relatively small, and there was evidence of publication bias and heterogeneity across studies. Subsequently, meta-analyses of randomized trials have determined that calcium supplementation (typically 1–1.5 g per day) may reduce systolic blood pressure by approximately 1 mm Hg but not diastolic blood pressure (Allender et al., 1996). A high intake of potassium, as discussed above, may be partially responsible for the blood pressure-lowering effects of vegetarian diets.

In view of these perplexing data, the Dietary Approaches to Stop Hypertension (DASH) study was designed to test the impact of modifying whole dietary patterns (Appel et al., 1997). DASH was a controlled feeding study demonstrating that a healthy dietary pattern can substantially reduce blood pressure. This dietary pattern emphasized fruits, vegetables, and low-fat dairy products. It included whole grains, poultry, fish, and nuts, and reduced fat red meat, sweets, and sugar-containing beverages. Among 326 nonhypertensive individuals, this dietary pattern reduced systolic and diastolic blood pressure by 3.5 and 2.1 mm Hg, respectively. The corresponding blood pressure reductions in 133 hypertensive patients were 11.4 and 5.5. African Americans had greater blood pressure reductions than non-African Americans (Svetkey et al., 1999). The blood pressure reductions observed in hypertensive patients have obvious clinical significance and are similar in magnitude to the blood pressure reductions from drug monotherapy. Still, because DASH was a feeding study, additional research in free-living persons is clearly warranted.

Effects of Lifestyle Modification on Blood Pressure in the Elderly

Although most trials of lifestyle interventions were conducted in middle-age persons, several have been conducted in older-age people. The Trials of Nonpharmacologic Interventions in the Elderly (TONE) was a randomized, controlled trial that tested the effects of three lifestyle interventions (sodium reduction, weight loss, and combined weight loss and sodium reduction) on blood pressure control in the elderly over 18 to

30 months (Whelton et al., 1998). Participants were 975 adults, ages 60 to 80 years, with a systolic blood pressure less than 145 mm Hg and a diastolic blood pressure less than 85 mm Hg on one medication. Medication withdrawal was attempted 3 months after the start of interventions. The primary outcome variable was the need to resume drug therapy. Registered dietitians conducted the interventions, which consisted primarily of group sessions (weekly for 3 months, then biweekly for another 3 months, then monthly) supplemented by individual counseling. Over 2.5 years, those assigned to a sodium reduction intervention achieved and sustained an average reduction in sodium intake of nearly 40 mmol per day. Likewise, those assigned to a weight loss intervention achieved and sustained an average reduction in weight of nearly 10 pounds. Mean net reductions in systolic and diastolic blood pressure, prior to medication withdrawal, were 2.6/1.1 mm Hg from sodium reduction, 3.2/0.3 mm Hg from weight loss, and 4.5/2.6 mm Hg from the combination of reduced sodium and weight loss (each $p < 0.001$). Compared to controls, among the 585 obese participants, there was a 40 percent reduction in the need for medication from reduced sodium intake alone, 36 percent from weight loss alone, and 53 percent from the combination of reduced sodium and weight loss (each $p < 0.05$). Among the 390 nonobese participants, there was a 25 percent reduction in the need for medication from a reduced sodium intake. Results from this trial indicate that reduced sodium intake and weight loss are feasible, effective, and safe nonpharmacologic interventions in older persons.

In a pilot study that preceded the TONE trial, Applegate et al. (1992) tested the effects of a multifactorial lifestyle intervention of sodium reduction, weight loss, and physical activity on blood pressure control in 56 individuals with a mean systolic blood pressure of 144 and a diastolic blood pressure 87 mm Hg. After 6 months, the intervention group achieved a net reduction in systolic blood pressure/diastolic blood pressure of 4.2/4.9 (each $p < 0.05$). In a separate trial of 47 elderly persons (18 who were normotensive and 29 hypertensive), a reduction in salt intake of 83 mmol/day was associated with significant reductions in supine systolic blood pressure/diastolic blood pressure of 7.2/3.2 (each $p < 0.05$) (Cappuccio et al., 1997). The results of these trials, each of which included sodium reduction, are consistent with observational studies indicating that the blood pressure of older-aged persons is particularly sensitive to changes in salt intake (Law et al., 1991).

Although the above trials document the feasibility and efficacy of lifestyle modification in the elderly, the available data are limited in other respects. First, none of these trials compared different providers, settings, and intensities of intervention. Most interventions consisted of a combination of group and individual sessions, and most were implemented by skilled interventionists, typically registered dietitians. A corollary issue is that none of the trials explicitly tested a dietitian-based intervention similar to what would be provided in routine clinical practice. Also, no trial has tested the impact of reduced alcohol intake, increased potassium intake, or adoption of the DASH diet in the elderly. Finally, no trial has tested the feasibility and efficacy of an intervention that simultaneously implements all lifestyle modifications.

Nonetheless, the results of above trials, as well as numerous studies conducted in younger adults, provides the basis for clinical algorithms that incorporate lifestyle modifications as part of routine standard of care of hypertensive patients. According to JNC VI (1997), lifestyle modification (salt reduction, weight loss, exercise, reduced alcohol intake, and desirable dietary pattern) should be the initial therapy for 6 to 12 months in persons with uncomplicated hypertension and an adjunctive therapy in other individuals.

Hypertension: Summary and Recommendations

Available evidence from several trials conducted in the elderly and from numerous studies conducted in other populations strongly supports nutrition-based therapy as an effective means to reduce blood pressure in older-aged persons with hypertension. At a minimum, such therapy can be an adjuvant to medication. In selected individuals, medication stepdown and potentially medication withdrawal are feasible. Although available data are insufficient to determine the qualifications of persons who should provide nutrition-based therapy, as well as the intensity of such therapy, the complexity of dietary changes suggests that providers skilled in behavioral change should implement nutrition-based therapies. The intensity of therapy required to affect life-style changes is also unknown. Despite these uncertainties, the reductions in blood pressure from nutrition-based therapies should lower blood pressure and thereby have a substantial benefit in reducing the occurrence of blood pressure-related complications (CHD, stroke, and renal failure) in the elderly.

Summary of Evidence—Nutrition Therapy for Hypertension

Consensus of opinion:　　　Recommended as part of standard of care (JNC VI, 1997) and the Working Group Report on Hypertension in the Elderly (National High Blood Pressure Education Program Working Group, 1994)

Observational studies: Strong evidence (e.g., Intersalt Cooperative Research Group, 1988; Khaw and Barrett-Connor, 1990)

Randomized trials: Several consistent trials in the elderly (Applegate et al., 1992; Cappuccio et al., 1997; Whelton et al., 1998) as well as numerous trials in other populations

Systematic reviews: Several (Cutler et al., 1997; Graudal et al., 1998; Midgley et al., 1996; NIH, 1998)

HEART FAILURE

Heart failure is a major public health problem. According to the National Heart, Lung, and Blood Institute, more than 2 million Americans have heart failure, about 400,000 new cases occur annually, and about 200,000 people die each year of this disease. Heart failure is the most frequent cause of hospitalization among Medicare beneficiaries, accounting for more than 1 million hospitalizations per year. Heart failure is now considered the most costly cardiovascular illness in the United States (Rich and Nease, 1999).

Heart failure is a clinical syndrome resulting from several conditions that damage the heart (e.g., uncontrolled hypertension; myocardial infarction; viral, alcohol-related, or idiopathic cardiomyopathies). In these instances, the heart becomes weakened or stiff and pumps blood ineffectively. Although heart failure can occur at any age, the vast majority of heart failure patients are elderly. The symptoms and signs of heart failure reflect volume or fluid overload (fluid in the lungs, abdomen, or legs [edema]) and/or inadequate perfusion of tissues, resulting in fatigue and poor exercise tolerance. Clinically, it is characterized by intermittent, acute exacerbations of symptoms. Between these acute episodes, patients are either in a state of well-compensated heart failure, which is virtually asymptomatic, or in a clinical state characterized by chronic symptoms of leg swelling (edema), fatigue, and/or shortness of breath. During the acute exacerbations, severe shortness of breath from accumulation of fluid in the lungs and/or excessive edema are the typical symptoms that prompt hospitalization.

In addition to pharmacologic therapy for heart failure, nonpharmacologic therapies are commonly recommended as standards of care. The goals of therapy, both pharmacologic and nonpharmacologic, are to control symptoms, improve the quality of life, prolong survival, and prevent acute exacerbations that prompt hospitalization. Previously, digoxin and diuretics had been the mainstay of drug therapy. Recently, medical therapy has improved considerably. Specifically, angiotensin-converting enzyme inhibitors and beta-blockers have been shown to increase survival and improve quality of life (Garg and Yusuf, 1995; Rich and Nease, 1999). The primary, diet-related nonpharmacologic therapy is sodium restriction, which should reduce the extent of fluid overload and potentially lower the dose of diuretic therapy. Water restriction is also recommended for patients with severe heart failure, who are at risk of hyponatremia.

Interestingly, no trial has specifically tested the effects of dietary recommendations alone in the management of heart failure. The absence of such data does not reflect uncertainty over this aspect of heart failure treatment. Rather, sodium restriction has been and remains a widely accepted component of standard medical care for heart failure patients. Presently, joint guidelines from the American College of Cardiology and the American Heart Association (Packer and Cohn, 1999) and guidelines from the Agency for Healthcare Research and Quality (formerly the Agency for Health Care Policy and Research (AHCPR, 1994) recommend diet therapy as a component of the standard management of patients with heart failure.

The factors leading to exacerbations of heart failure include nonadherence to medication or diet, inadequate therapy, social or environmental issues, abnormal heart rhythms, and intercurrent noncardiac conditions. In one case series from an urban medical center, the most common factor associated with hospital admissions for heart failure was noncompliance with the medical regimen (diet and/or drugs), and was present in 64 percent of patients admitted with heart failure (Ghali et al., 1988). Other common factors were cardiac arrhythmias (29 percent), social or environmental issues (26 percent), inadequate therapy (17 percent), and pulmonary infections (12 percent) (many persons had several problems simultaneously). In view of the diversity of these precipitating factors, subsequent studies have evaluated the effects of multidisciplinary programs designed to improve several aspects of care, rather than unidimensional programs (e.g., nutrition therapy alone).

In a comprehensive review of the medical literature on nonpharmacologic treatments for heart failure, Dracup et al. (1994) concluded that counseling and education can improve medical outcomes and decrease hospitalizations. At the time of that publication, only one study had demonstrated reduced numbers of hospitalizations from such interventions. Specifically, in a nonrandomized trial (Rosenberg, 1971), a group-based, behavioral intervention program designed to improve compliance with diet and medications reduced hospital admissions compared to the previous year (46 versus 12 percent) and compared to patients at another hospital (31 versus 17 percent).

Subsequent studies that used stronger research methods have corroborated the above findings. As part of a larger trial examining the effects of a single, postdischarge home intervention visit across a broad population of hospitalized patients in Australia, Stewart et al. (1999) reported the effects of this visit on 97 heart failure patients. The post-discharge visit included measures to optimize medication management, identify early clinical deterioration, and intensify medical follow-up and caregiver vigilance. In comparison to the control group, the group that received the postdischarge visit (by a nurse and pharmacist) had fewer unplanned readmissions (64 versus 125, $p = 0.02$) and outpatient deaths (2 versus 9, $p = 0.02$) over 18 months.

In another randomized controlled trial, Rich et al. (1995) tested the effects of an intensive intervention (with both inpatient and home care components) in older-aged patients (aged 70+) who were hospitalized for heart failure and were at risk for readmission. The intervention team included a cardiovascular research nurse, registered dietitian, social worker, and cardiologist. During the inpatient phase of the intervention, the dietitian completed a dietary assessment and provided individualized instruction on sodium reduction that subsequently was reinforced by the study nurse. Over a follow-up period of 90 days, the intensive intervention compared to control led to fewer patients who were readmitted (29 versus 42 percent of patients, $p = 0.03$), fewer days of hospitalization (556 versus 865, $p = 0.04$), and fewer readmissions for heart failure (24 versus 54, $p = 0.04$).

In a randomized, controlled clinical trial conducted in Sweden, Cline et al. (1998) evaluated the effects of a nurse-directed intervention that provided patient education and promoted adherence and self-monitoring to patients hospitalized for heart failure. The nurse provided the counseling during the hospitalization and in an outpatient clinic. Compared to control participants at 1 year, patients assigned to the intervention group had a longer mean time to readmission (141 versus 106 days, $p < 0.05$), trends toward fewer hospitalizations (0.7 versus 1.1, $p = 0.08$) and readmissions per patient (39 versus 54 percent, $p = 0.08$), a shorter length of hospital stay (4.2 versus 8.2 days, $p = 0.07$), and lower mean annual health costs (U.S. \$2,294 versus \$3,594 per patient, $p = 0.07$). One-year mortality rates and quality of life did not differ between the two groups.

Kostis et al. (1994) tested the effects of a multidimensional, intensive nonpharmacologic approach (a 12-week outpatient program of diet, exercise, and cognitive-behavioral therapy, presented in a group format) in comparison to two other treatments (digoxin alone and placebo). The dietary component of the program, which focused on reducing salt intake and reducing weight (among overweight participants), was conducted by a dietitian who led weekly meetings. The study population consisted of 20 outpatients (mean age 65 years) with moderate heart failure. In the digoxin group, the ejection fraction improved (as measured by echocardiography) but without corresponding changes in exercise tolerance or quality-of-life. In contrast, the nonpharmacologic approach improved exercise tolerance, improved mood, and reduced weight.

In response to such studies, multidisciplinary "heart failure teams" have been established at many medical centers as a means to reduce morbidity and mortality from heart failure, as well as prevent hospitalizations and their attendant costs. Typically, the team is overseen by a cardiologist and directed by a nurse experienced in the management of patients with heart failure. Dietitians and exercise counselors are often members of such teams. The structure, content and setting of the programs also vary. Component activities include education about heart failure and its treatment; medication adjustment; efforts to improve adherence to diet and medication and to increase physical activity; discharge planning in the setting of hospitalizations; telephone follow-up; and self-monitoring. In a recent review by Rich and Nease (1999), such multidisciplinary programs are cost-effective and potentially cost saving.

Some heart failure programs have reported their experience. At the University of Nebraska, a multidisciplinary team has reduced hospital days by 42 percent, hospital admissions by 30 percent, and length of stay by 17 percent (Chapman and Torpy, 1997). Pezzella et al. (1997) reported on an ambulatory program designed to reduce readmissions in high-risk heart failure patients. Each patient received comprehensive education provided by a primary care nurse in collaboration with a registered dietitian. The nutrition component consisted of a 45–60 minute group session in which the nutrition professional used participatory, problem-solving strategies to implement dietary recommendations, and individual counseling sessions as needed on referral by the primary care nurse. Preliminary data indicate a 1-day reduction in length of stay and a decrease of 60-day readmission rate by 1.1 percent (using historical utilization data).

Heart Failure: Summary and Recommendations

Available evidence from several small clinical trials and a few observational studies supports the use of nutrition therapy in the context of multidisciplinary programs. Such programs can prevent readmissions for heart failure, reduce subsequent length of stay, and improve functional status and quality-of-life. The programs often include both inpatient predischarge counseling and outpatient components that may even be home based. Evidence is unavailable to separate the effects of nutrition therapy from other aspects of these programs and to compare the effectiveness of different types of counselors (dietitians versus nurses). In view of the high costs of managing heart failure, particularly admissions for heart failure exacerbations, and the rapid response to therapies, there is a real potential for cost savings from multidisciplinary heart failure programs that include nutrition therapy. The high morbidity, mortality, and costs associated with heart failure and the paucity of data on the effects of nutritional therapies in this condition provide a strong rationale for additional research.

Summary of Evidence—Nutrition Therapy for Heart Failure

Consensus statements:	Recommended as part of standard of care in guidelines prepared by the American College of Cardiology (Packer and Cohn, 1999), American Heart Association (AHA, 1999), and by the Agency for Health Care Policy and Research (AHCPR, 1994)
Observational studies:	Consistent evidence from diverse types of studies (Chapman and Torpy, 1997; Ghali et al., 1988; Rosenberg, 1971)
Randomized trials:	Consistent evidence from a few small clinical trials (Kostis et al., 1994; Rich et al., 1995; Stewart et al., 1999) that tested the effects of programs that included nutrition therapy
Systematic review:	Dracup et al. (1994); Rich and Nease (1999)

RESEARCH RECOMMENDATIONS

Available evidence strongly supports the efficacy of nutrition therapy as a means to improve lipid profiles, reduce blood pressure and, in the context of multidisciplinary programs, treat heart failure. Still, there are numerous unresolved issues that include the following:

• What is the optimal diet that reduces cardiovascular risk? For instance, although there is a broad consensus that the diet should be low in saturated fat, it is unclear what type of nutrient (protein, carbohydrate, or unsaturated fat) should replace saturated fat as the source of calories.

• Does supplementation of diet with specific nutrients have a cardioprotective role? For instance, preliminary studies suggest that certain nutrients (e.g., folate or other B vitamins) may reduce the risk of CVD. However, clinical trials are needed to confirm the efficacy and safety of diet supplementation with any nutrient.

• What are the optimal public health strategies that accomplish favorable dietary changes? In view of the high prevalence of hypertension and dyslipidemia, efficient and effective strategies need to be developed and tested in a rigorous fashion.

• What is the optimal intervention strategy for use in the clinic setting? Corollary issues are to determine the number of provider contacts required to accomplish dietary change, the impact of different types of nutrition providers, and the impact of individual-based versus group-based interventions.

• What dietary changes other than sodium reduction (e.g., weight loss, DASH diet) favorably affect the course of congestive heart failure?

REFERENCES

AHA (American Heart Association). 1999. *1999 Heart and Stroke Statistical Update*. Dallas, Tex.: American Heart Association.

AHCPR (Agency for Health Care Quality and Research). 1994. *Heart Failure: Management of Patients With Left-Ventricular Systolic Dysfunction. Quick Reference Guide for Clinicians, No. 11*. Rockville, Md.: AHCPR.

Allender PS, Cutler JA, Follmann D, Cappuccio FP, Pryer J, Elliott P. 1996. Dietary calcium and blood pressure: A meta-analysis of randomized clinical trials. *Ann Intern Med* 124:825–831.

Alpha-Tocopheral, Beta Carotene Cancer Prevention Study Group. 1994. The effect of vitamin E and beta carotene on the incidence of lung cancer and other cancers in male smokers. *N Eng J Med* 330:1029–1035.

Appel LJ, Moore TJ, Obarzanek E, Vollmer WM, Svetkey LP, Sacks FM, Bray GA, Vogt TM, Cutler JA, Windhauser MM, Lin P-H, Karanja N. 1997. A clinical trial of the effects of dietary patterns on blood pressure. *N Engl J Med* 336:1117–1124.

Applegate WB, Miller ST, Elam JT, Cushman WC, El Derwi D, Brewer A, Graney MJ. 1992. Nonpharmacologic intervention to reduce blood pressure in older patients with mild hypertension. *Arch Intern Med* 152:1162–1166.

Boushey CJ, Beresford SAA, Omenn GS, Motulsky AG. 1995. A quantitative assessment of plasma homocysteine as a risk factor for vascular disease. Probable benefits of increasing folic acid intakes. *J Am Med Assoc* 274:1049–1057.

Burr ML, Fehily AM, Gilbert JF, Rogers S, Holliday RM, Sweetnam PM, Elwood PC, Deadman NM. 1989. Effects of changes in fat, fish, and fibre intakes on death and myocardial reinfarction: Diet and Reinfarction Trial. *Lancet* 2:757–761.

Burt VL, Whelton P, Roccella EJ, Brown C, Cutler JA, Higgins M, Horan MJ, Labarthe D. 1995. Prevalence of hypertension in the U.S. adult population. Results from the Third National Health and Nutrition Examination Survey, 1988–1991. *Hypertension* 25:305–313.

Cappuccio FP, Elliott P, Allender PS, Pryer J, Follman DA, Cutler JA. 1995. Epidemiologic association between dietary calcium intake and blood pressure: A meta-analysis of published data. *Am J Epidemiol* 142:935–945.

Cappuccio FP, Markandu ND, Carney C, Sagnella GA, MacGregor GA. 1997. Double-blind randomised trial of modest salt restriction in older people. *Lancet* 350:850–854.

Carleton RA, Dwyer J, Finberg L, Flora J, Goodman, DS, Grundy SM, Havas S, Hunter GT, Kritchevsky D, Lauer RM, Luepker RV, Ramirez AG, Van Horn L, Stason WB, Stokes J III. 1991. Report of the Expert Panel on Population Strategies for Blood Cholesterol Reduction. A statement from the National Cholesterol Education Program, National Heart, Lung, and Blood Institute, National Institutes of Health. *Circulation* 83:2154–2232.

Chapman DB, Torpy J. 1997. Development of a heart failure center: A medical center and cardiology practice join forces to improve care and reduce costs. *Am J Manag Care* 3:431–437.

Cline CM, Israelsson BY, Willenheimer RB, Broms K, Erhardt LR. 1998. Cost effective management programme for heart failure reduces hospitalisation. *Heart* 80:442–446.

Cushman WC, Cutler JA, Hanna E, Bingham SF, Follmann D, Harford T, Dubbert P, Allender PS, Dufour M, Collings JF, Walsh SM, Kirk GF, Burg M, Felicetta JV, Hamilton BP, Katz LA, Perry HM Jr, Willenbring ML, Lakshman R, Hamburger RJ. 1998. Prevention and treatment of hypertension study (PATHS): Effects of an alcohol treatment program on blood pressure. *Arch Intern Med* 158:1197–1207.

Cutler JA, Follmann D, Allender PS. 1997. Randomized trials of sodium reduction: An overview. *Am J Clin Nutr* 65:643S–651S.

Dayton S, Pearce ML, Hashimoto S, Dixon WJ, Tomiyasu U. 1969. A controlled clinical trial of a diet high in unsaturated fat in preventing complications of atherosclerosis. *Circulation* 39–40:1–63.

de Lorgeril M, Renaud S, Mamelle N, Salen P, Martin J-L, Monjaud I, Guidollet J, Touboul P, Delaye J. 1994. Mediterranean alpha-linolenic acid-rich diet in secondary prevention of coronary heart disease. *Lancet* 343:1454–1459.

de Lorgeril M, Salen P, Martin JL, Monjaud I, Delaye I, Mamelle N. 1999. Mediterranean diet, traditional risk factors, and the rate of cardiovascular complications after myocardial infarction: Final report of the Lyon Diet Heart Study. *Circulation* 99:779–785.

Downs JR, Clearfield M, Weis S, Whitney E, Shapiro DR, Beere PA, Langendorfer A, Stein EA, Kruyer W, Gotto AM Jr. 1998. Primary prevention of acute coronary events with lovastatin in men and women with average cholesterol levels: Results of AFCAPS/TexCAPS. Air Force/Texas Coronary Atherosclerosis Prevention Study. *J Am Med Assoc* 279:1615–1622.

Dracup K, Baker DW, Dunbar SB, Dacey RA, Brooks NH, Johnson JC, Oken C, Massie BM. 1994. Management of heart failure. II. Counseling, education, and lifestyle modifications. *J Am Med Assoc* 272:1442–1446.

Garg R, Yusuf S. 1995. Overview of randomized trials of angiotensin-converting enzyme inhibitors on mortality and morbidity in patients with heart failure. *J Am Med Assoc* 273:1450–1456.

Ghali JK, Kadakia S, Cooper R, Ferlinz J. 1988. Precipitating factors leading to decompensation of heart failure. Traits among urban blacks. *Arch Intern Med* 148:2013–2016.

GISSI-Prevenzione Investigators. 1999. Dietary supplementation with n-3 polyunsaturated fatty acids and vitamin E after myocardial infarction: Results of the GISSI-Prevenzione trial. *Lancet* 354:447–455.

Graudal NA, Galløe AM, Garred P. 1998. Effects of sodium restriction on blood pressure, renin, aldosterone, catecholamines, cholesterols, and triglyceride. A meta-analysis. *J Am Med Assoc* 279:1383–1391.

Grundy SM, Cleeman JI, Rifkind BM, Kuller LH. 1999. Cholesterol lowering in the elderly population. *Arch Intern Med* 159:1670–1678.

Havlik RJ, Liu BM, Kovar MG, Suzman R, Feldman JJ, Harris T, Van Nostrand J. 1987. *Health Statistics on Older Persons, United States 1966*. Vital and Health Statistics, Series 3, No. 25. Washington, D.C.: National Center for Health Statistics.

Hebert PR, Moser M, Mayer J, Glynn RJ, Hennekens CH. 1993. Recent evidence on drug therapy of mild to moderate hypertension and decreased risk of coronary heart disease. *Arch Intern Med* 153:578–581.

Hokanson JE, Austin MA. 1996. Plasma triglyceride level is a risk factor for cardiovascular disease independent of high-density lipoprotein cholesterol level: A meta-analysis of population-based prospective studies. *J Cardiovasc Risk* 3:213–219.

Hunninghake DB, Stein EA, Dujovne CA Harris WS, Feldman EB, Miller VT, Tobert JA, Laskarzewski PM, Wuiter E, Held J, Taylor AM, Hopper S, Leonard SB, Brewer BK. 1993. The efficacy of intensive dietary therapy alone or combined with lovastatin in outpatients with hypercholesterolemia. *N Engl J Med* 328:1213–1219.

Intersalt Cooperative Research Group. 1988. Intersalt: An international study of electrolyte excretion and blood pressure. Results for 24 hour urinary sodium and potassium excretion. *Br Med J* 297:319–328.

Jacobs D, Blackburn H, Higgins M, Reed D, Iso H, McMillan G, Neaton J, Nelson J, Potter J, Rifkind B. 1992. Report of the Conference on Low Blood Cholesterol: Mortality associations. *Circulation* 86:1046–1060.

JNC VI (Joint National Committee on Prevention, Detection, Evaluation, and Treatment of High Blood Pressure). 1997. The sixth report of the Joint National Committee on Prevention, Detection, Evaluation, and Treatment of High Blood Pressure. *Arch Intern Med* 157:2413–2446.

Kahn HA, Phillips RL, Snowdon DA, Choi W. 1984. Association between reported diet and all-cause mortality. Twenty-one-year follow-up on 27,530 adult Seventh-Day Adventists. *Am J Epidemiol* 119:775–787.

Katzel LI, Coon PJ, Dengel J, Goldberg AP. 1995. Effects of an American Heart Association Step I Diet and weight loss on lipoprotein lipid levels in obese men with silent myocardial ischemia and reduced high-density lipoprotein cholesterol. *Metabolism* 44:307–314.

Khaw KT, Barrett-Connor E. 1990. Increasing sensitivity of blood pressure to dietary sodium and potassium with increasing age. A population study using casual urine specimens. *Am J Hypertens* 3:505–511.

Klag MJ, Whelton PK, Randall BL, Neaton JD, Brancati FL, Ford CE, Shulman NB, Stamler J. 1996. Blood pressure and end-stage renal disease in men. *N Engl J Med* 334:13–18.

Klatsky AL, Friedman GD, Siegelaub AB, Gerard MJ. 1977. Alcohol consumption and blood pressure. Kaiser-Permanente Multiphasic Health Examination data. *N Engl J Med* 296:1194–1200.

Kostis JB, Rosen RC, Cosgrove NM, Shindler DM, Wilson AC. 1994. Nonpharmacologic therapy improves functional and emotional status in congestive heart failure. *Chest* 106:996–1001.

Krauss RM, Deckelbaum RJ, Ernst N, Fisher E, Howard BV, Knopp RH, Kotchen T, Lichtenstein AH, McGill HC, Pearson TA, Prewitt TE, Stone NJ, Van Horn L, Weinberg R. 1996. Dietary guidelines for healthy American adults. A statement for health professionals from the Nutrition Committee, American Heart Association. *Circulation* 94:1795–1800.

Kris-Etherton PM, Dietschy J. 1997. Design criteria for studies examining individual fatty acid effects on cardiovascular disease risk factors: Human and animal studies. *Am J Clin Nutr* 65:1590S–1596S.

Kuczmarski RJ, Flegal KM, Campbell SM, Johnson CL. 1994. Increasing prevalence of overweight among U.S. adults. The National Health and Nutrition Examination Surveys, 1960 to 1991. *J Am Med Assoc* 272:205–211.

LaRosa JC, Hunninghake D, Bush D, Criqui MH, Getz GS, Gotto AM Jr., Grundy SM, Rakita L, Robertson RM, Weisfeldt ML. 1990. The cholesterol facts. A summary of the evidence relating dietary fats, serum cholesterol, and coronary heart disease. A joint statement by the American Heart Association and the National Heart, Lung, and Blood Institute. *Circulation* 81:1721–1733.

LaRosa JC, Applegate W, Crouse JR III, Hunninghake DB, Grimm R, Knopp R, Eckfeldt JH, Davis CE, Gordon DJ. 1994. Cholesterol lowering in the elderly. Results of the Cholesterol Reduction in Seniors Program (CRISP) pilot study. *Arch Intern Med* 154:529–539.

Law MR, Frost CD, Wald NJ. 1991. By how much does dietary salt reduction lower blood pressure? I—Analysis of observational data among populations. *Br Med J* 302:811–815.

Lipid Research Clinics Program. 1984. The Lipid Research Clinic's Coronary Primary Prevention Trial Results, II: The relationship of reduction in incidence of coronary heart disease to cholesterol lowering. *J Am Med Assoc* 251:365.

MacMahon S. 1987. Alcohol consumption and hypertension. *Hypertension* 9:111–121.

MacMahon S, Peto R, Cutler J, Collins R, Sorlie P, Neaton J, Abbott R, Godwin J, Dyer A, Stamler J. 1990. Blood pressure, stroke, and coronary heart disease. Part 1, Prolonged differences in blood pressure: Prospective observational studies corrected for the regression dilution bias. *Lancet* 335:765–774.

Manolio TA, Pearson TA, Wenger NK, Barrett-Connor E, Payne GH, Harlan WR. 1992. Cholesterol and heart disease in older persons and women: Review of an NHLBI workshop. *Ann Epidemiol* 2:161–176.

Margetts BM, Beilin LJ, Vandongen R, Armstrong BK. 1986. Vegetarian diet in mild hypertension: A randomized controlled trial. *Br Med J* 293:1468–1471.

Martin MJ, Hulley SB, Browner WS, Kuller LH, Wentworth D. 1986. Serum cholesterol, blood pressure and mortality: Implications from a cohort of 361,662 men. *Lancet* 2: 933–936.

McGehee MM, Johnson EQ, Rasmussen HM, Sahyoun N, Lynch MM, Carey M. 1995. Benefits and costs of medical nutrition therapy by registered dietitians for patients with hypercholesterolemia. *J Am Diet Assoc* 95:1041–1043.

Midgley JP, Matthew AG, Greenwood CMT, Logan AG. 1996. Effect of reduced dietary sodium on blood pressure. A meta-analysis of randomized controlled trials. *J Am Med Assoc* 275:1590–1597.

Morris MC. 1994. Dietary fats and blood pressure. *J Cardiovasc Risk* 1:21–30.

MRC (Medical Research Council) Working Party. 1992. Medical Research Council trial of treatment of hypertension in older adults: Principal results. *Br Med J* 304:405–412.

MRFIT (Multiple Risk Factor Intervention Trial). 1996. Mortality after 16 years for participants randomized to the Multiple Risk Factor Intervention Trial. *Circulation* 94:946–951.

Muldoon MF, Manuck SB, Matthews KA. 1990. Lowering cholesterol concentrations and mortality: A quantitative review of primary prevention trials. *Br Med J* 301:309–314.

National High Blood Pressure Education Program Working Group. 1993. National High Blood Pressure Education Program Working Group Report on primary prevention of hypertension. *Arch Intern Med* 1993;153:186–208.

National High Blood Pressure Education Program Working Group. 1994. National High Blood Pressure Education Program Working Group report on hypertension in the elderly. *Hypertension* 23:275–285.

NCEP (National Cholesterol Education Program) 1994. Second report of the Expert Panel on the Detection, Evaluation, and Treatment of High Blood Cholesterol in Adults (Adult Treatment Panel II). *Circulation* 89:1329–1445.

NCHS (National Center for Health Statistics). 1993. Advance report on final mortality statistics, 1991. *Mon Vital Stat Rep* 42:1–64.

NCHS (National Center for Health Statistics). 1994. *Health United States, 1993*. Hyattsville, Md.: Public Health Service.

NCHS (National Center for Health Statistics). 1997. *Third National Health and Nutrition Examination Survey* (Series 11, No. 1, SETS version 1.22a). [CD-ROM]. Washington, D.C.: U.S. Government Printing Office.

Neaton JD, Grimm RH Jr, Prineas RJ, Stamler J, Grandits GA, Elmrt PJ, Cutler JA, Flack JM, Schoenberger JA, McDonald R, Lewis CE, Liebson PR. 1993. Treatment of mild hypertension study. Final results. *J Am Med Assoc* 270:713–724.

NIH (National Institutes of Health), National Heart, Lung, and Blood Institute. 1998. Clinical guidelines on the identification, evaluation, and treatment of overweight and obesity in adults—the evidence report. *Obes Res* 6:51S–209S.

Packer M, Cohn JN, eds. 1999. Consensus recommendations for the management of chronic heart failure. *Am J Cardiol* 83:1A–38A.

Pezzella SM, O'Mara P, Donahue JN. 1997. An ambulatory care program for managing high-risk congestive heart failure patients. *J Clin Outcomes Mgmt* 4:27–35.

Puddey IB, Beilin LJ, Vandongen R, Rouse IL, Rogers P. 1985. Evidence for a direct effect of alcohol consumption on blood pressure in normotensive men. A randomized controlled trial. *Hypertension* 7:707–713.

Puddey IB, Beilin LJ, Vandongen R. 1987. Regular alcohol use raises blood pressure in treated hypertensive subjects. A randomized controlled trial. *Lancet* 1:647–651.

Rich MW, Nease RF. 1999. Cost-effectiveness analysis in clinical practice. The case of heart failure. *Arch Intern Med* 159:1690–1700.

Rich MW, Beckham V, Wittenberg C, Leven CL, Freedland KE, Carney RM. 1995. A multidisciplinary intervention to prevent the readmission of elderly patients with congestive heart failure. *N Engl J Med* 333:1190–1195.

Rosenberg SG. 1971. Patient education leads to better care for heart patients. *HSMHA Health Rep* 86:793–802.

Ross SD, Allen IA, Connelly JE, Korenblat BM, Smith ME, Bishop D, Luo D. 1999. Clinical outcomes in statin treatment trials: A meta-analysis. *Arch Intern Med* 159:1793–1802.

Rouse IL, Beilin LJ, Armstrong BK, Vandongen R. 1983. Blood-pressure-lowering effect of a vegetarian diet: Controlled trial in normotensive subjects. *Lancet* 1:5–10.

Sacks FM. 1998. Why cholesterol as a central theme in coronary artery disease? *Am J Cardiol* 82:14T–17T.

Sacks FM, Rosner B, Kass EH. 1974. Blood pressure in vegetarians. *Am J Epidemiol* 100:390–398.

Sacks FM Sacks FM, Pfeffer MA, Moye LA, Rouleau JL, Rutherford JD, Cole TG, Brown L, Warnica JW, Arnold JM, Wun CC, Davis BR, Braunwald E. 1996. The effect of Pravastatin on coronary events after myocardial infarction in patients with average cholesterol levels. *N Engl J Med* 335:1001–1009.

Scandinavian Simvastatin Survival Study Group. 1994. Randomized trial of cholesterol lowering in 4444 patients with coronary heart disease: The Scandinavian Simvastatin Survival Study (4S). *Lancet* 344:1383–1389.

Shekelle RB, Shryock AM, Paul O, Lepper M, Stamler J, Liu S, Raynor WJ Jr. 1981. Diet, serum cholesterol, and death from coronary heart disease. The Western Electric study. *N Engl J Med* 304:65–70.

SHEP Cooperative Research Group. 1991. Prevention of stroke by antihypertensive drug treatment in older persons with isolated systolic hypertension. Final results of the Systolic Hypertension in the Elderly Program (SHEP). *J Am Med Assoc* 265:3255–3264.

Shepherd J, Cobbe SM, Ford I, Isles CG, Lorimer AR, Macfarlane PW, McKillop JH, Packard CJ. 1995. Prevention of coronary heart disease with Pravastatin in men with hypercholesterolemia. West of Scotland Coronary Prevention Study Group. *N Engl J Med* 333:1301–1307.

Sikand G, Kashyap ML, Yang I. 1998. Medical nutrition therapy lowers serum cholesterol and saves medication costs in men with hypercholesterolemia. *J Am Diet Assoc* 98:889–894.

Srinath U, Jonnalagadda SS, Naglak MC, Champagne C, Kris-Etherton PM. 1995. Diet in the prevention and treatment of atherosclerosis. A perspective for the elderly. *Clin Geriatr Med* 11:591–611.

Staessen J, Fagard R, Lijnen P, Amery A. 1989. Body weight, sodium intake and blood pressure. *J Hypertens* 7:S19–S23.

Staessen JA, Fagard R, Thijs L Celis H, Arabidze GG, Birkenhäger WH, Bulpitt CJ, de Leeuw PW, Dollery CT, Fletcher AE, Forette F, Leonetti G, Nachev C, O'Brien ET, Rosenfeld J, Rodicio JL, Tuomilehto J, Zanchetti A. 1997. Randomized double-blind comparison of placebo and active treatment for older patients with isolated systolic hypertension. *Lancet* 350:757–764.

Stamler J. 1991. Epidemiologic findings on body mass and blood pressure in adults. *Ann Epidemiol* 1:347–362.

Stephens, NG, Parsons A, Schofield PM, Kelly F, Cheeseman K, Mitchinson MJ, Brown MJ. 1996. Randomised controlled trial of vitamin E in patients with coronary disease: Cambridge Heart Antioxidant Study (CHAOS). *Lancet* 347:781–786.

Stewart S, Vandenbroek AJ, Pearson S, Horowitz JD. 1999. Prolonged beneficial effects of a home-based intervention on unplanned readmissions and mortality among patients with congestive heart failure. *Arch Intern Med* 159:257–261.

Stone NJ, Nicolosi RJ, Kris-Etherton P, Ernst ND, Krauss RM, Winston M. 1996. AHA conference proceedings. Summary of the Scientific Conference on the Efficacy of Hypocholesterolemic Dietary Interventions. *Circulation* 94:3388–3391.

Svetkey LP, Simons-Morton D, Vollmer WM, Appel LJ, Conlin PR, Ryan DH, Ard J, Kennedy BM. 1999. Effects of dietary patterns on blood pressure: Subgroup analysis of the Dietary Approaches to Stop Hypertension (DASH) randomized clinical trial. *Arch Intern Med* 159:285–293.

The TOHP (Trials of Hypertension Prevention) Collaborative Research Group. 1992. The effects of non-pharmacological interventions on blood pressure of persons with high normal levels. *J Am Med Assoc* 267:1213–1220.

The TOPH (Trials of Hypertension Prevention) Collaborative Research Group. 1997. Effects of weight loss and sodium reduction intervention on blood pressure and hypertension incidence in overweight people with high-normal blood pressure. The Trials of Hypertension Prevention, Phase II. *Arch Intern Med* 157:657–667.

Whelton PK, He J, Cutler JA Brancati FL, Appel L, Follmann D, Klag MJ. 1997. Effects of oral potassium on blood pressure. Meta-analysis of randomized controlled clinical trials. *J Am Med Assoc* 277:1624–1632.

Whelton PK, Appel LJ, Espeland MA, Applegate WB, Ettinger WH Jr, Kostis JB, Kumanyika S, Lacy CR, Johnson KC, Folmar S, Cutler JA. 1998. Sodium reduction and weight loss in the treatment of hypertension in older persons. A randomized controlled trial of nonpharmacologic interventions in the elderly (TONE). *J Am Med Assoc* 279:839–846.

Wood D, De Backer G, Faergeman O, Graham I, Mancia G, Pyörälä K, Second Joint Task Force of European and Other Societies on Coronary Prevention. 1998. Prevention of coronary heart disease in clinical practice. Recommendations of the Second Joint Task Force of European and other Societies on Coronary Prevention. *Eur Heart J* 19:1434–1503.

Yu-Poth S, Zhao G, Etherton T, Naglak M, Jonnalagadda S, Kris-Etherton PM. 1999. Effects of the National Cholesterol Education Program's Step I and Step II dietary intervention programs on cardiovascular disease risk factors: A meta-analysis. *Am J Clin Nutr* 69:632–646.

6

Diabetes Mellitus

Diabetes mellitus type 1 is an autoimmune disease that destroys the beta cells of the pancreas, leading to insulin deficiency. The resulting hyperglycemia can lead to microvascular and macrovascular disease. The microvascular complications include retinopathy, nephropathy, and neuropathy. The macrovascular complications include coronary artery disease, peripheral vascular disease with amputation, stroke, and renal disease. The disease usually manifests early in life, although it can also occur in adulthood.

Diabetes mellitus type 2 is a familial hyperglycemia that occurs primarily in adults but can also occur in children and adolescents. It is caused by an insulin resistance whose etiology is multiple and not totally understood. The net result of the insulin resistance is to initially cause a compensatory hyperinsulinemia. Subsequently, the beta cells of the pancreas fail to meet the compensatory need, less insulin secretion occurs than is required for the adequate elimination and utilization of glucose, and hyperglycemia results. Dyslipidemia and hypertension are common in patients with type 2 diabetes, and about 80 percent of patients with type 2 diabetes are obese (LaPorte et al., 1995). The complications arising from this condition are the same as those described for type 1 diabetes mellitus. Because of the later age of onset in persons with type 2 compared to type 1 diabetes, evidence of clinically significant microvascular complications is less.

Estimates of prevalence have increased over the years in part due to more stringent diagnostic criteria as well as the continued rise in obesity.

In 1997, the diagnostic criterion for a diagnosis of diabetes was lowered from a fasting glucose tolerance test result of 140 mg/dL to 126 mg/dL (American Diabetes Association, 1997). Based on the diagnostic criteria of a fasting glucose tolerance test of 110 to 126 mg/dL as impaired glucose tolerance and greater than or equal to 126 mg/dL as diabetes, 18.4 percent or 6.3 million people age 65 or older have diabetes. Approximately 40 to 45 percent of persons age 65 years or older have either type 2 diabetes or impaired glucose tolerance. Diabetes is the seventh leading cause of death in the United States, and more than 187,000 persons died from the disease and its complications in 1995 (HCFA, 1999).

Individuals with diabetes mellitus, regardless of type, typically have several risk factors associated with increased morbidity and mortality. The risk factors include abnormal fasting glucose, postprandial glucose, hemoglobin A_{1c} (HbA$_{1c}$), low-density lipoprotein cholesterol, high-density lipoprotein cholesterol, triglycerides, microalbuminuria, blood pressure, a procoagulant state, and abdominal obesity.

EVIDENCE THAT A CHANGE IN RISK FACTORS CHANGES MORBIDITY AND MORTALITY

A series of long-term, randomized, controlled trials shows the effect of tight glucose and HbA$_{1c}$ control on complications of the disease and are described below.

Diabetes Control and Complications Trial

Investigators in the Diabetes Control and Complications Trial (DCCT), a randomized controlled trial, followed 1,400 patients with type 1 diabetes, between the ages of 15 and 39 years, for 7 years to determine what effect normalizing blood glucose and HbA$_{1c}$ had on chronic complications of the disease (DCCT Research Group, 1993). The study showed a sustained difference in the levels of glucose and HbA$_{1c}$ between the conventionally treated group and the tightly controlled experimental group. The trial was stopped after 7 years because of the significant lowering of microvascular complication rates in the experimental group compared to the conventionally treated control group. Microvascular disease was defined as retinopathy, neuropathy, and urinary albumin excretion. All three end points showed a significant difference. Macrovascular disease events in diabetes usually include myocardial infarction, sudden death, stroke, and peripheral vascular disease. While the DCCT study lacked the statistical power to detect a difference in macrovascular disease in this relatively young population with type 1 diabetes, a trend toward a lower incidence of macrovascular end points was suggested in the tightly controlled group.

Stockholm Diabetes Intervention Study

This small randomized clinical trial of 102 patients with type 1 diabetes included a group that was treated intensively and a group with usual care (Reichard et al., 1993). The patients' age at baseline was 30 ± 8 years in the intensive group and 32 ± 7 years in the standard group. The intensive group had extensive educational intervention, including blood glucose monitoring, and most of the patients (82 percent) took at least three insulin injections daily. The standard treatment group continued with routine diabetes care. The patients were followed for 7.5 years. As in the DCCT, intensive glucose control led to a decreased incidence of microvascular complications (retinopathy, nephropathy, and neuropathy). Macrovascular end points were not assessed.

Kumamoto Study

This randomized controlled trial in Japan (Ohkubo et al., 1995) studied the effect of multiple insulin injections versus conventional insulin injections in 110 middle-aged patients with type 2 diabetes. The appearance and progression of retinopathy, nephropathy, and neuropathy were evaluated every 6 months over a 6-year period. The group with the tight control had significantly lower HbA_{1c} values and developed fewer microvascular complications. Although the study lacked the statistical power to measure the effect on macrovascular disease, the trend was for fewer events in the tightly controlled group.

Veterans Affairs Diabetes Feasibility Trial

Investigators in this pilot study randomized 153 men with type 2 diabetes to either conventional or intensive insulin therapy (Abraira et al., 1997). The mean age was 60 ± 6 years and the length of diagnosis of non-insulin-dependent diabetes mellitus was 7.8 ± 4.0 years. While the standard treatment was one injection each morning, intensive insulin therapy was a stepped plan with up to multiple insulin injections as necessary to attain near normal glycemia. Despite a 2 percent absolute HbA_{1c} difference in glycemic control between the two groups, which were followed for an average of 27 months, the trial reported no significant difference in cardiovascular events (when adjusted for baseline characteristics). Cardiovascular events were defined as myocardial infarction, stroke, and sudden death. This pilot study did not have the statistical power to come to a definite conclusion concerning macrovascular end points.

United Kingdom Prospective Diabetes Study

The United Kingdom Prospective Diabetes Study (UKPDS) was a large, multicenter randomized control trial in which 3,867 patients with type 2 diabetes were followed for 10 years (UKPDS Group, 1998). The median age of patients was 54 years at baseline, with a range of 48 to 60 years. The study compared the effects of intensive blood glucose control with either sulfonylureas, insulin, or conventional treatment on both microvascular and macrovascular complications. Treatment for all groups included a standard diet, exercise prescription, and/or drugs as needed to attain the designated level of blood glucose control for each group. The aim in the intensive group was a fasting plasma glucose (FPG) of less than 108 mg/dL. The aim in the conventional group was the best achievable FPG with diet or exercise alone. Drugs were added in the conventional group only if there were hyperglycemic symptoms or FPG of at least 270 mg/dL. To assess differences between conventional and intensive treatment the study focused on three aggregate end points:

1. any diabetes-related end point (sudden death, death from hyperglycemia or hypoglycemia, fatal or nonfatal myocardial infarction, angina, heart failure, stroke, renal failure, amputation, vitreous hemorrhage, retinopathy requiring photocoagulation, blindness in one eye, or cataract extraction);
2. diabetes-related death (defined as death from myocardial infarction, stroke, peripheral vascular disease, renal disease, hyperglycemia or hypoglycemia, and/or sudden death); and
3. all-cause mortality.

All analyses included the intention-to-treat model, where all patients assigned to a particular protocol are followed to the end as part of that group, whether they carry out the intervention or not. Over 10 years, HbA_{1c} was 7.0 percent in the intensive group and 7.9 percent in the conventional group. Compared to the conventional group, the risk in the intensive group was 12 percent lower for any diabetes-related end point, 10 percent lower for any diabetes-related death, and 6 percent lower for all-cause mortality. There was a 25 percent reduction in microvascular end points in the intensive compared to the conventional group ($p = 0.0099$). Tighter control significantly reduced the development of retinopathy and nephropathy, and was borderline with regard to neuropathy. Epidemiological analysis of the UKPDS data showed a continuous relationship between the risk of microvascular complications and glycemia. For every percentage point decrement in HbA_{1c} (e.g., 9 to 8 percent), a 35 percent reduction in the risk of microvascular complications occurred. The effect of tighter control on macrovascular disease resulted in a nonsignificant trend, with a 16 percent reduction in the risk of combined fatal or nonfatal myocardial infarction and sudden death in the intensively treated group. Tight control of blood pressure (<134/82 mm Hg) had a profound effect on both micro- and macrovascular complications in both the intensive and the conventional treatment groups, significantly reducing strokes, diabetes-related deaths, heart failure, microvascular complications, and visual loss. This landmark study confirms that for inpatients with type 2 diabetes, lowering blood glucose is definitely beneficial in reducing macrovascular complications and reemphasizes the importance of blood pressure control in patients with diabetes mellitus.

THE ROLE OF NUTRITION INTERVENTION IN THE MANAGEMENT OF DIABETES

Nutrition intervention is considered an essential component in the management of diabetes. For this reason, it has been provided to participants in both control and intervention groups of studies designed to evaluate the impact of improved glycemic control on the development of diabetic complications in both patients with type 1 and 2 diabetes (DCCT Research Group, 1993; UKPDS Group, 1998). While there are few studies in which nutrition intervention is the only variable (Bitzen et al., 1988; Franz et al., 1995; Kulkarni et al., 1998), many studies have demonstrated the effectiveness of multidisciplinary patient education which includes a nutrition component on glycemic control (Agurs-Collins et al., 1997; García and Suárez, 1996; Gilden et al., 1989; Glasgow et al., 1992).

While these studies demonstrate improved outcomes, it is difficult to tease out benefits specifically attributable to the nutritional component of the education. Researchers have studied diabetes patient education extensively. Three meta-analyses have shown that patient education is effective in improving knowledge, skills, psychosocial adjustment, and metabolic control (Brown, 1988, 1990; Padgett et al., 1988). Overall, evidence from many types of studies involving nutrition therapy in the management of diabetes is supportive of nutrition intervention. The American Diabetes Association has recognized the value of medical nutrition therapy and considers it an essential component of diabetes management (American Diabetes Association, 1999b).

Nutrition Intervention in Trials of Intensive Management

In the DCCT study, the control and intervention groups both received counseling by a dietitian. However, while the control group received nutrition counseling every 6 months, the intensive management group received nutrition counseling every month. In the DCCT, several behaviors were shown to be associated with lower HbA_{1c} levels among patients with type 1 diabetes randomized to intensive insulin therapy (Delahanty and Halford, 1993). Within the intensively managed group, those who reported following their prescribed diets had average HbA_{1c} levels 0.9 percent lower than those who did not follow their meal plan. Adjusting food and/or insulin resulted in significantly lower HbA_{1c} levels. This substudy on 687 patients provides evidence that dietary behaviors positively alters indicators of glycemic control when used in combination with appropriate insulin management (Delahanty and Halford, 1993).

In the UKPDS study, all treatment and control groups received nutritional advice from a dietitian every 3 months. Initial monthly clinic visits resulted in an average weight loss of 5 kg after 3 months (UKPDS Group, 1995).

Nutrition Intervention as a Component of Diabetes Education

García and Suárez (1996) described a continuing interactive educational model for elderly patients with diabetes. Elderly individuals who had previously attended the Diabetes Basic Information Course at the National Institute of Endocrinology in Havana, Cuba were invited to participate in small interactive groups (≤ 15 participants) with no more than two health professionals over a period of 5 years. The health professionals included an endocrinologist, health educator, teaching nurse, dietitian, podiatrist, and social worker. A total of 148 elderly individuals (mean age 72 years) along with many spouses attended the monthly sessions. Data showed a significant increase in diabetes self management knowledge and skills ($p < 0.001$), a reduction in body weight ($p < 0.01$), and a reduction in the need for medication ($p < 0.05$). Overall, mean levels of HbA_{1c} declined from 12.4 percent to 7.9 percent after 5 years ($p < 0.02$). The need for emergency services declined from 97 percent in the year before the course to less than 2 percent after 5 years ($p = 0.000$). In addition, the social support and education received through this interactive model overall resulted in patients feeling "less sick, depressed and isolated" (García and Suárez, 1996).

Gilden and colleagues (1989) demonstrated improvement in quality of life outcomes for older patients and their spouses. They evaluated the outcomes of 45 older male patients who ranged in age from 65 to 82 years (mean age 70 years) following 6 weeks of diabetes education (one session per week). A multidisciplinary team including a diabetologist, nurse-educator, dietitian, psychologist, podiatrist, and social worker administered the program. Results indicated a reduction in stress that correlated with their increase in knowledge ($p < 0.05$) and their improved diet-related quality of life ($p < 0.02$). The decrease in stress level was still apparent 6 months later ($p < 0.01$). Their perceived quality of life with regard to lifestyle modifications such as diet and exercise increased ($p < 0.01$) and was still evident after 6 months (Gilden et al., 1989).

The Diabetes Care for Older Adults Project was a 3-year randomized clinical trial that compared an intensive team care program to conventional therapy in 103 participants with a mean age of 70 years. Diabetes education and social support were provided by an interdisciplinary team consisting of a clinical nurse specialist, a dietitian, both of whom were certified diabetes educators (CDE), and a social worker. Glycosylated hemoglobin dropped an average of 3.2 percentage points in the treatment group versus 1.0 percentage point in the control group after an 18-month intervention period in which groups met 12 times (Funnell et al., 1997; Halter et al., 1993).

Glasgow and colleagues (1992) studied 102 patients over the age of 60 with type 2 diabetes in a crossover intervention using a multidisciplinary team that included a registered dietitian. Results demonstrated a significantly greater reduction in caloric intake and percent of calories from fat in the intervention group compared to the control group who received delayed intervention. In this crossover study, the intervention resulted in a decline in HbA_{1c} from 6.8 percent to 6.3 percent. The HbA_{1c} rebounded to 6.7 percent during the subsequent control period. When control patients crossed over to the intervention, their HbA_{1c} declined from 7.4 percent to 6.4 percent (Glasgow et al., 1992).

In a randomized control trial, researchers randomly assigned 64 overweight African-American patients (55–79 years) with type 2 diabetes to one of two groups. Subjects participated in either one individual and eighteen group sessions given by a registered dietitian or in a "usual" care program, which included one group meeting and two follow-up mailings. Topics focused on nutrition and exercise interventions. The intensive intervention participants had significantly greater decreases in HbA_{1c} (–1.6 compared to –2.4 percent, $p < 0.01$) and an average of 2 to 2.5-kg reduction in weight ($p = 0.006$) compared to controls (Agurs-Collins et al., 1997).

Impact of the Intensity of Nutrition Intervention
on Glycemic Control

Franz and associates (1995) completed a randomized trial in 179 persons, 38 to 76 years of age, with type 2 diabetes, comparing the usual nutrition care of one visit to a more intensive nutrition intervention of at least three visits led by a dietitian. The results demonstrated that any nutrition intervention provided by dietitians resulted in significant improvements in medical and clinical outcomes, with FPG decreasing by 50 to 100 mg/dL and HbA_{1c} dropping by 1 to 2 percentage points. Both groups demonstrated improvement in diabetes control, with the more intensive nutrition intervention reducing FPG by 10.5 percent and the usual care by 5.3 percent. A similarly treated but nonrandomized control group who had no contact with a dietitian resulted in HbA_{1c} levels showing no improvement during the same 6-month period of study (8.2 versus 8.4 percent) (Franz et al., 1995). In a prospective randomized trial, Kulkarni et al. (1998) also compared the use of a more intensive nutrition intervention in patients with type 1 diabetes to a control group who received standard nutrition intervention. At 3 months, the HbA_{1c} improved in 88 percent of the participants who had received the more intensive nutrition intervention and in 53 percent of those receiving the standard nutrition intervention. The patients who received the more intensive nutrition intervention also achieved greater decrements in HbA_{1c} levels than the usual care patients (-1.00 versus -0.33, $p < 0.05$). Both of these studies demonstrate that regardless of the intensity of the nutrition intervention, improvements in blood glucose levels can be achieved with nutrition therapy. In addition, these studies indicate that when practice guidelines are used, increasing the intensity of the nutrition therapy by both time spent and the number of visits, greater improvements in glycemic control result.

Bitzen and colleagues (1988) studied the effect of dietary intervention in 38 hyperglycemic patients who had never been treated by diet or medication (insulin or oral hypoglycemic agents). The participants had a mean age of 63 years. Each received a standardized meal plan by a nurse and weight reduction was advocated for all participants who were above ideal body weight (36 of 38 participants). The education was reinforced at 2- to 3-week intervals over a 10-week period. Each participant also received at least one home visit during the study period. After 10 weeks, 82 percent of participants were found to have significantly reduced both fasting blood glucose (148 mg/dL to 117 mg/dL, $p < 0.001$) and HbA_{1c} (7.6 percent to 6.7 percent, $p < 0.001$).

PROVIDERS OF NUTRITION THERAPY FOR DIABETES

In the studies cited above, the formats for interventions varied from multiple individualized visits with dietitians to group sessions with an interdisciplinary team that included a nutrition professional. The DCCT clearly demonstrated the value of a multidisciplinary team in the care of patients with diabetes. Health professionals who contribute to the management of patients with diabetes include physicians, nurses, dietitians, pharmacists, podiatrists, exercise specialists, and social workers. In the management of care for elderly persons, the inclusion of a health professional with particular expertise in the care of elderly persons would be optimal (Fonseca and Wall, 1995).

Prior to results of the DCCT in 1992, data had been less clear regarding the impact of specific nutrition interventions. This, in part, was due to the role of the dietitian in diabetes management intensifying given the demonstrated need for dietary adherence in the DCCT. Since this landmark trial, dietitians have become more focused on individualizing nutrition therapy for patients with diabetes (Delahanty et al., 1993).

The individualized approach requires changes in the lifestyle and goals of each patient and can result in complex dietary interventions. Individualization involves a knowledge of food as it relates to culture, nutrient composition, and meal preparation. For this reason, the American Diabetes Association (1999b) has recommended that a registered dietitian, knowledgeable and skilled in implementing nutritional interventions, be the team member providing nutrition education. In addition, the American Diabetes Association (1999c) has also recommended that education be conducted in the outpatient or home setting because of less frequent and shorter acute care admissions for patients with diabetes.

MEDICARE REIMBURSEMENT FOR DIABETES SELF-MANAGEMENT TRAINING

Prior to July 1, 1998, Medicare Part B covered diabetes education only if provided to registered patients of hospital outpatient departments. These diabetes education programs were required to address diet, exercise, and blood glucose self-monitoring; establish treatment plans for insulin-dependent patients; and motivate patients to manage their conditions. Services could be provided in group or individual sessions. Like other hospital outpatient services, reimbursement was on a "reasonable cost" basis.

Section 4105(a) of the Balanced Budget Act of 1997 added a new benefit to the Medicare program for diabetes self-management training services. This legislation provided coverage for educational and training services furnished in an outpatient setting by qualified personnel to patients with diabetes, if a physician certifies that such services are needed as part of a comprehensive plan of care. The services are paid under the Medicare physician fee schedule in amounts determined by the Secretary of Health and Human Services. The law specifies that payment may be made to "certified providers" who meet quality standards as determined through regulation, and who also are eligible to receive payment for providing other services to Medicare beneficiaries.

The new benefit has been partially implemented since July 1, 1998. Final implementation is expected early in 2000. In the interim, diabetes self-management training programs that meet the *National Standards for Diabetes Self-Management Education Programs* and are recognized by the American Diabetes Association, or programs that were receiving reimbursement, are considered to meet the requirements for Medicare coverage. As of October 1999, nationwide there were a total of 978 diabetes self-management education programs sites recognized by the American Diabetes Association. There are, however, widespread rural areas in which access to approved diabetes self-management training is severely limited.

To be an approved provider of diabetes self-management training services, a program must meet certain quality standards. Standards proposed by the Health Care Financing Administration include, among other things, that training be conducted by a team consisting of at least a registered dietitian and a CDE (although for an initial 3-year period a nurse may substitute for the CDE) (HCFA, 1999). Training must address 15 subject areas, including nutrition and the relationships among nutrition, exercise, medication, and blood glucose levels.

The proposed regulations would allow reimbursement for 10 hours of training during a 12-month period and one follow-up training session in each subsequent year. In general, training is to be in group sessions, although individual sessions would be allowed under certain circumstances (e.g., when no group session is available) or with certification that the patient has special needs (e.g., physical impairments, severe language challenges). Patients eligible for the initial 10 training sessions would include those who, within a year before referral, (1) experienced new onset diabetes, (2) had poor glycemic control, (3) experienced a change in medication or use of insulin, (4) had high risk for complications from poor glycemic control, or (5) had experienced certain complications of the foot, eye, or kidney.

Under the proposed rule, entities eligible to provide diabetes self-management training programs include settings such as hospitals, renal dialysis facilities and clinics, and certain independent practitioners who by current law are eligible to receive Medicare reimbursement. These health professionals include physicians, advanced practice nurses, clinical social workers, psychologists, nurse midwives, and pharmacists. Ironically, at present, the current regulation does not allow the specific health professionals who are required to provide the service (dietitians and CDEs) to bill and receive reimbursement for their services.

Payment for diabetes self-management under the Medicare physician fee schedule is proposed to be $32.62 for group sessions and $55.41 for individual sessions in 1999 (adjusted for geographic variation according to Medicare fee schedule rules). Medicare deductible and coinsurance requirements would apply; thus beneficiaries would pay 20 percent of the proposed amounts, if they had satisfied the $100 annual Part B deductible.

There is a distinct need for repeated training throughout the life of a person with diabetes. The DCCT showed that the diet adherence of a patient occurs in peaks and valleys (DCCT Research Group, 1993). The ability to attain adequate control to prevent costly complications requires continued attention to changes in the severity of the disease, weight, life style, and age. Corrective nutritional education is often necessary.

LIMITATIONS OF DATA AND FUTURE RESEARCH NEEDS

Although a number of studies support the usefulness of nutrition therapy in helping patients attain better control of diabetes and improving outcomes, the number of randomized, controlled trials that specifically explore this question are few. In addition, most of these studies involve nutritional intervention as part of an overall team approach to diabetes education. Therefore, it is not possible to dissect out the specific benefit of the nutritional intervention as a single component of therapy. In addition, it is seldom clear from the studies what type of provider is needed to effect a positive nutritional intervention in patients with diabetes. It is important to extend these studies so that the best provider mix and intensity of intervention can be determined. Additional studies focusing on special populations, such as the elderly and cultural minorities, are also indicated. There is a need for more definitive research on group versus individual formats, the number of encounters and methods needed to achieve improved clinical outcomes in weight, HgA_{1c} levels, lipid levels, blood pressure, and patient satisfaction.

SUMMARY

Diabetes mellitus is one of the most prevalent diseases among the U.S. population. This is especially true in the elderly, where nearly 18.4 percent of persons older than 65 have diabetes (American Diabetes Association, 1997). There is reasonable evidence from randomized clinical trials that nutrition intervention as part of overall diabetes education improves blood glucose and HbA_{1c} levels in persons with diabetes, including data in substantial numbers of individuals over age 65. Although nutrition therapy is best carried out when a patient is first diagnosed, it appears to be effective at any time during the disease process and refresher therapy may be of value.

The American Diabetes Association, other national diabetes organizations, and the World Health Organization all support a recommendation for nutrition therapy in patients with diabetes mellitus.

RECOMMENDATIONS

The committee recommends that individualized nutrition therapy, provided by a registered dietitian, be a covered benefit as part of the multidisciplinary approach to the management of diabetes which includes diet, exercise, medications, and blood glucose monitoring. This recommendation is consistent with that of the American Diabetes Association (1999a).

Summary of Evidence:
Nutrition Therapy for Diabetes

Consensus statements:	Recommended as part of the standard of care by the American Diabetes Association (1999a) and the World Health Organization (1994)
Observational studies:	Supportive evidence (Agurs-Collins et al., 1997; Bitzen et al., 1988; Delahanty and Halford, 1993; Franz et al., 1995; García and Suárez, 1996; Gilden et al., 1989; Glasgow et al., 1992; Kulkarni et al., 1998)
Randomized trials:	Reasonable (DCCT Research Group, 1993; UKPDS Group, 1998)
Meta-analyses of trials:	Supportive evidence (Brown, 1988, 1990; Padgett et al., 1988)
Systematic reviews:	Several

REFERENCES

Abraira C, Colwell J, Nuttall F, Sawin CT, Henderson W, Comstock JP, Emanuele NV, Levin SR, Pacold I, Lee HS. 1997. Cardiovascular events and correlates in the Veterans Affairs Diabetes Feasibility Trial. Veterans Affairs Cooperative Study on Glycemic Control and Complications in Type II Diabetes. *Arch Intern Med* 157:181–188.

Agurs-Collins TD, Kumanyika SK, Ten Have TR, Adams-Campbell LL. 1997. A randomized controlled trial of weight reduction and exercise for diabetes management in older African-American subjects. *Diabetes Care* 20:1503–1511.

American Diabetes Association. 1997. Diabetes facts and figures. Available at: http://www.diabetes.org/ada/c20f.asp. Accessed September 8, 1999.

American Diabetes Association. 1999a. Clinical practice recommendations. *Diabetes Care* 22:S1–S114.

American Diabetes Association. 1999b. Nutrition recommendations and principles for people with diabetes mellitus. *Diabetes Care* 22:S42–S45.

American Diabetes Association. 1999c. Translation of the diabetes nutrition recommendations for health care institutions. *Diabetes Care* 22:S46–48.

Bitzen PO, Melander A, Schersten B, Svensson M. 1988. Efficacy of dietary regulation in primary health care patients with hyperglycemia detected by screening. *Diabet Med* 5:640–647.

Brown SA. 1988. Effects of educational interventions and outcomes in diabetic adults: A meta-analysis revisited. *Nurs Res* 37:223–230.

Brown SA. 1990. Studies of educational interventions in diabetes care: A meta-analysis of findings. *Patient Edu Counseling* 16:189–215.

DCCT (Diabetes Control and Complications Trial) Research Group. 1993. The effect of intensive treatment of diabetes on the development and progression of long-term complications in insulin-dependent diabetes mellitus. *N Engl J Med* 329:977–986.

Delahanty LM, Halford BM. 1993. The role of diet behaviors in achieving improved glycemic control in intensively treated patients in the Diabetes Control and Complications Trial. *Diabetes Care* 16:1453–1458.

Delahanty L, Simkins SW, Camelon K. 1993. Expanded role of the dietitian in the Diabetes Control and Complications Trial: Implications for clinical practice. *J Am Diet Assoc* 93:758–762.

Fonseca V, Wall J. 1995. Diet and diabetes in the elderly. *Clin Geriatr Med* 11:613–624.

Franz MJ, Monk A, Barry B, McClain K, Weaver T, Cooper N, Upham P, Bergenstal R, Mazze RS. 1995. Effectiveness of medical nutrition therapy provided by dietitians in the management of non-insulin-dependent diabetes mellitus: A randomized, controlled clinical trial. *J Am Diet Assoc* 95:1009–1017.

Funnell MM, Arnold MS, Fogler J, Merrit JH, Anderson LA. 1997. Participation in a diabetes education and care program: Experience from the Diabetes Care for Older Adults Project. *Diabetes Educ* 23:163–167.

García R, Suárez R. 1996. Diabetes education in the elderly: A 5-year follow-up of an interactive approach. *Patient Educ Couns* 29:87–97.

Gilden, JL, Hendryx M, Casia C, Singh S. 1989. The effectiveness of diabetes education programs for older patients and their spouses. *J Am Geriatr Soc* 37:1023–1030.

Glasgow RE, Toobert DJ, Hampson SE, Brown JE, Lewinsohn PM, Donnelly J. 1992. Improving self-care among older patients with type II diabetes: The Sixty Something Study. *Patient Educ Couns* 19:61–74.

Halter J, Anderson L, Herman W, Fogler J, Merritt J, Funntell M, Arnold M, Brown M, Davis W. 1993. Intensive treatment safely improves glycemic control of elderly patients with diabetes mellitus. *Diabetes* 42:146A.

HCFA (Health Care Financing Administration). 1999. Medicare program: Expanded coverage for outpatient diabetes self-management training services. *Fed Reg* 64:6827–6852.

Kulkarni K, Castle G, Gregory R, Holmes A, Leontos C, Powers M, Snetselaar L, Splett P, Wylie-Rosett J. 1998. Nutrition practice guidelines for type 1 diabetes mellitus positively affect dietitian practices and patient outcomes. *J Am Diet Assoc* 98:62–72.

LaPorte RE, Matsushima M, Chang Y-F. 1995. Prevalence and incidence of insulin-dependent diabetes. In: *Diabetes in America,* 2nd ed. Publication No. 95-1468. Bethesda, Md.: National Institutes of Health, National Institute of Diabetes and Digestive and Kidney Diseases.

Ohkubo Y, Kishikawa H, Araki E, Miyata T, Isami S, Motoyoshi S, Kojima Y, Furuyoshi N, Shichiri M. 1995. Intensive insulin therapy prevents the progression of diabetic microvascular complications in Japanese patients with non-insulin-dependent diabetes mellitus: A randomized prospective 6-year study. *Diabetes Res Clin Pract* 28:103–117.

Padgett D, Mumford E, Haynes M, Carter R. 1988. Meta-analyses of the affects of educational and psychosocial interventions on management of diabetes mellitus. *J Clin Epidemiol* 41:1007–1030.

Reichard P, Nilsson B-Y, Rosenqvist U. 1993. The effect of long-term intensified insulin treatment on the development of microvascular complications of diabetes mellitus. *N Engl J Med* 329:304–309.

UKPDS (UK Prospective Diabetes Study) Group. 1995. U.K. prospective diabetes study 16. Overview of 6 years' therapy of type II diabetes: A progressive disease. *Diabetes* 44:1249–1258.

UKPDS (UK Prospective Diabetes Study) Group. 1998. Intensive blood-glucose control with sulphonylureas or insulin compared with conventional treatment and risk of complications in patients with type 2 diabetes (UKPDS 33). *Lancet* 352:837–853.

World Health Organization. 1994. *Management of Diabetes Mellitus: Standards of Care and Clinical Practice Guidelines.* Geneva: World Health Organization.

7

Renal Disease

In the past, the development of severe renal disease signaled certain death within a short period of time. With the launch of hemodialysis for the management of end-stage renal disease (ESRD) in 1960 and subsequent developments such as peritoneal dialysis, home hemodialysis, and renal transplantation, the survival period for persons with severe renal disease has markedly increased. While the prognosis for persons with ESRD has improved, the number of patients continues to grow. As of December 31, 1995, the point prevalence of ESRD was 257,266 individuals (USRDS, 1997). As of December 31, 1997, the point prevalence grew to 304,083 (USRDS, 1999). Table 7.1 provides the demographic distribution of new cases of ESRD in 1997.

The above estimates indicate that the future economic burden will be great. In 1999, the total cost of care for patients with ESRD was approximately $15.64 billion (USRDS, 1999). This cost includes federal, state, and private sources of payment but does not include the cost of disability or Social Security monthly benefits. The estimated cost per person per year is $43,000 (USRDS, 1999).

Patients with ESRD experience significant morbidity and mortality and consume considerable health care resources. In 1995, dialysis patients over the age of 65 spent an average of 11.4 days per year in the hospital (USRDS, 1997). Medicare patients in general spent a mean of 7.1 days in the hospital per year (HCFA, 1999). Despite recent improvements in survival rates, the expected lifetime of a dialysis patient still ranges between 16 and 37 percent of the age-, gender-, and race-matched U.S. population

TABLE 7.1 Renal Disease Population as of December 31, 1997

	End-Stage Renal Disease Patients		Dialysis Patients	
	Number	Percent	Number	Percent
Total	304,083	100	221,596	100
Age Group				
0–19	5,480	2	1,768	1
20–44	76,018	25	39,398	18
45–64	117,865	39	81,904	37
65–74	63,197	21	57,316	26
≥75	41,523	14	41,210	18
Race				
Native American	4,614	2	3,663	2
Asian/Pacific Islander	10,795	4	7,885	4
African American	97,503	32	82,624	37
Caucasian	186,341	61	123,269	56
Other	4,830	2	4,155	2
Gender				
Male	165,176	54	115,902	52
Female	138,907	46	105,694	48
Cause of ESRD				
Diabetes	100,892	33	84,076	38
Hypertension	72,961	24	61,673	28
Glomerulonephritis	52,229	17	29,433	13
Other	78,001	26	46,414	21

SOURCE: USRDS (1999).

(USRDS, 1997). The high morbidity and mortality among dialysis patients has stimulated research into potentially correctable factors that are associated with increased risk of death. The search for antecedent factors requires consideration of earlier stages of chronic renal disease.

Renal disease is marked by a decrease in the ability of the kidney to excrete metabolic waste and a subsequent build up of urea and other nitrogenous waste in the blood. For the purpose of this report, three stages of chronic renal disease are considered: chronic renal insufficiency, ESRD, and post-renal transplantation. Chronic renal insufficiency (CRI) is defined as the stage of renal disease associated with a reduction in renal function not severe enough to require dialysis or transplantation (glomerular filtration rate [GFR] 13–50 ml/min/1.73 m^2). ESRD is defined as chronic renal disease that necessitates treatment by dialysis or renal transplantation. Lastly, patients who have received a renal transplant are considered. Although many transplant recipients also have CRI, since the level of renal function usually remains subnormal after transplantation, for the purpose of this report, these patients are considered separately from those who have CRI, without a history of renal transplantation.

As described below, three key findings suggest that nutrition therapy may substantially lessen or delay the burden of chronic renal disease. First, dietary protein restriction in CRI may slow the onset of ESRD. Second, malnutrition during CRI is a major risk factor for death after the onset of ESRD. Third, patients at all stages of chronic renal disease are at high risk of cardiovascular disease, which may be prevented, in part, by treatment of traditional cardiovascular disease risk factors, such as hypertension, hyperlipidemia and diabetes.

CHRONIC RENAL INSUFFICIENCY

CRI can be detected and treated prior to the onset of ESRD. An elevation in serum creatinine concentration of approximately 1.5 mg/dL or greater indicates this stage of CRI. Diagnostic coding for individuals with CRI is not uniform and for this reason, the cost of providing care for these patients has not been analyzed.

Debate surrounds the question of the effectiveness of dietary protein restriction as a treatment for patients with moderate or early renal disease and as a method to delay the onset of ESRD. While convincing evidence in rats with reduced renal mass shows that deterioration is slowed with restriction of dietary protein (Ibels et al., 1978; Kleinknecht et al., 1979; Laouari et al., 1982), human studies have been less certain. During the past decade, a number of clinical trials on protein restriction in patients with CRI have been carried out.

Studies Including Patients with Diabetes

While more extensive experience is available in patients with non-diabetic renal disease, a few trials have been performed in patients with type 1 diabetes. Zeller and colleagues (1991) conducted a randomized trial in patients with type 1 diabetes ($n = 35$) who had greater than 1.0 g/day urine protein excretion. Results demonstrated a slower decline in GFR in patients randomized to a low protein diet. Walker and colleagues (1989) also demonstrated a similar slowing in GFR decline in a sequential (non-randomized) trial of patients with type 1 diabetes ($n = 19$). Pedrini et al. (1996) performed a meta-analysis including these two studies, plus three others, which demonstrated a uniform finding of reduced progression of renal disease in patients assigned to dietary protein restriction.

Despite the results, the authors recommended caution because of the small number of patients included in the clinical trials and because of variation in study design and endpoints.

Modification of Diet in Renal Disease Study

Implemented in 1989, the Modification of Diet in Renal Disease (MDRD) Study was the largest clinical trial designed to determine the effects of a reduced protein and phosphorus diet on the progression of renal disease. While the multicenter, randomized trial included some persons over 65, the average age was 52 years (range 18–70 years). The MDRD Study was the first randomized clinical trial designed to determine the effects of a reduced protein and phosphorus diet on the progression of renal disease. It included two studies related to nutrition and the progression of renal disease:

- Study A assessed low protein diets (0.58 g/kg body weight per day) combined with low phosphorus intakes (5 to 10 mg/kg body weight per day) in comparison to usual protein diets (1.3 g/kg body weight per day) combined with low phosphorus intakes (16 to 20 mg/kg body weight per day).
- Study B assessed very low protein diets (0.28 g/kg body weight per day) combined with a low phosphorus intake (4 to 9 mg/kg body weight per day) in comparison to low protein diets (0.58 g/kg body weight per day) alone. The very low protein diet was supplemented with ketoacids, raising the total equivalent protein intake to 0.58 g/kg body weight per day.

In Study A, 585 patients with moderate renal disease, defined as a baseline GFR ranging from 25 to 55 mL/min per 1.73 m^2 were randomly allocated to a low protein diet or a usual protein diet. Study B included 255 patients with advanced renal disease and a GFR of 13 to 24 ml/min per 1.73 m^2 randomly assigned to a low protein diet or a very low protein diet. The primary outcome measure was the rate of change in GFR (Klahr et al., 1994).

This trial allowed careful monitoring of dietary potassium, sodium, and calcium intakes as well as corresponding biological indicators. For maximum patient adherence, participants were asked to record protein intake alone (MDRD Study Group, 1994). If phosphorus intakes were found by the dietitian to be out of range, he/she suggested changes in types of foods to reduce elevated levels. When other nutrient levels required adjustment, the nutritionist used laboratory values and food record intakes to help patients change their types of foods in order to bring nutrient values back to normal ranges (Milas et al., 1995).

Initial results of the study showed that low protein dietary intervention was not conclusive in delaying the progression of renal disease (Klahr et al., 1994). For patients in Study A, the rate of decline in GFR over 36 months was not significantly different between the diet groups. It is proposed that this might be attributed to a nonlinear decline in GFR and a follow-up period that ended too quickly for dietary effects to be observed. For many patients, the MDRD diet was initially very difficult to follow. Many patients needed several months to acclimate to major changes in dietary habits. Data in Figure 7.1 show that patients in the low protein group demonstrated a faster rate of GFR decline in the first 4 months than those in the usual protein group. On the other hand, after 4 months the mean decline in GFR was slower in the low protein group compared to the usual protein group.

One of the limitations of the MDRD Study was the exclusion of subjects with diabetes. Presently, 38 percent of all ESRD patients have diabetes. A second limitation of the Study was its short duration, with an average intervention time of only 2.2 years.

Many have interpreted the failure of the MDRD Study to demonstrate a beneficial effect of protein restriction over a 2- to 3-year period as proving that low protein diets do not slow renal disease. Levey and coworkers (1999) state that this is an incorrect view and a result of misinterpretation of the inconclusive result as evidence in favor of the null hypothesis.

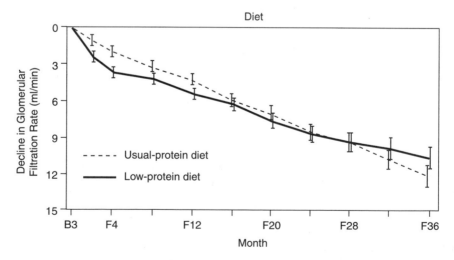

FIGURE 7.1 Estimated mean (±SE) decline in the glomerular filtration rate from base line (B) to selected follow-up time (F).

Following the initial analysis of MDRD Study data, secondary analyses have clarified the effect of protein restriction on the rate of decline in renal function, urine protein excretion, and onset of ESRD (Levey et al., 1999). Early analyses of patients in study B had showed a trend ($p = 0.07$) toward a slower progression of renal disease in the very low protein diet group versus the low protein group. Levey and colleagues (1996) conducted a secondary analysis of those Study B patients with advanced renal disease and demonstrated a correlation between achieving low protein intake and rate of decline in GFR. In this study, patients who complied very well with the diet were compared to those who had lower adherence. As described earlier, dietary intervention in MDRD included individualized counseling using feedback from dietary self-monitoring and laboratory data, modeling with low protein products, and dietitian support (Gillis et al., 1995).

More recently, a meta-analysis of five studies (Pedrini et al., 1996), which included the MDRD Study A, reported a beneficial effect of a low protein diet on the incidence of renal failure or death (relative risk [RR] = 0.67, 95 percent confidence interval [CI] = 0.50–0.89, $p \leq 0.01$). All studies had a follow-up of more than 1 year, and information about the number of patients who died or developed renal failure was available. The prescribed protein intake in the low protein diet arms of these studies ranged from 0.4 to 0.6 g/kg per day. These results are consistent with those from an earlier meta-analysis (odds ratio [OR] = 0.54, 95 percent CI = 0.37–0.79, $p < 0.002$) (Fouque et al., 1992).

In a third meta-analysis, Kasiske and colleagues (1998) focused specifically on the rate of decline in renal function. In results pooled from 13 randomized, controlled trials along with 11 other nonrandomized, controlled trials, the effect of dietary protein restriction on rate of decline in renal function (GFR decreases in treatment subjects minus decrease in control subjects) was significantly less ($p < 0.05$) in randomized versus nonrandomized trials (regression coefficient 5.2 mL/min per year, 95 percent CI = –7.8 to –2.5 mL/min per year), relatively greater among patients with diabetes than those without (5.4 mL/min per year; 95 percent CI = 0.3–10.5 mL/min per year, $p < 0.05$); and although not statistically significant, demonstrated a trend toward greater effect with each additional year of follow-up (2.1 mL/min per year, 95 percent CI = –0.05 to 4.2 mL/min per year, $p > 0.05$) (Kasiske et al., 1998).

Meta-analysis of randomized trials of protein restriction has both advantages and disadvantages. One advantage is the larger number of patients compared to results from a single clinical trial. Use of outcome measures such as ESRD or death can be used as a primary outcome measure, thus avoiding the problems of using surrogate outcomes based on the rate of decline in measures of renal function (Levey et al., 1999). Lastly, using a time-to-event analysis may have more statistical meaning than comparisons of the rate of decline in renal function (Greene et al., 1995).

Potential disadvantages also exist in meta-analyses that use the onset of ESRD or death as the primary outcome. The disadvantage is that the analysis gives weight to patients with advanced renal disease or rapidly declining renal function. This occurs because these patients will develop ESRD more quickly during the relatively short follow-up times of these studies. A second disadvantage is that patients who are randomized to the low protein intervention group may be diagnosed with ESRD later than persons assigned to the usual protein intervention group. This results because the low protein intervention masks the symptoms of uremia or because of investigator bias in these unmasked studies. Finally, two well-recognized disadvantages of meta-analysis result from the possibility of non-uniformity of studies and publication bias (Levey et al., 1999).

Based on secondary analyses of the MDRD study results in conjunction with data from other randomized trials, it has been recommended that a protein intake of 0.6 g/kg/day for patients with chronic renal disease should be recommended (Levey et al., 1999). Because older individuals make up a large fraction of those with renal insufficiency and because there is motivation to follow this rather restricted diet because of the negative quality of life associated with dialysis treatment, older adults with renal insufficiency should be included in dietary treatment recommendations.

Nutritional Management of Chronic Renal Insufficiency Consensus Recommendations

In 1994, a conference in Bethesda, Maryland, supported by the National Institutes of Health, was held for the purpose of developing management recommendations for chronic renal disease. Panels of nephrology experts from around the world reviewed literature and developed practical recommendations for the prevention of progression of various stages of chronic renal disease. Recommendations for the nutritional management of CRI were as follows (Striker, 1995):

Nutritional Management, GFR 25–55 mL/min/1.73 m^2

The evidence that the prescription of a low-protein diet slows the progression of renal failure in this group of patients is still inconclusive. Data from an additional year's follow-up of the MDRD cohort shows even stronger trends in the direction of the benefit of a low-protein intake. However, until definitive information is available from longer-term studies, further group analysis of the MDRD or additional data from other studies, a standard protein intake should be prescribed (>0.8 g/kg per day). If there is evidence of the progression of renal insufficiency or the development of uremic symptoms, an intake of 0.8 g/kg per day is appropriate.

Nutritional Management, GFR 13–25 ml/min/1.73 m^2

Those who adhere to a diet containing 0.6 g/kg per day of protein have a reduced rate of loss of renal function, and the time to reach ESRD is prolonged. In addition, dietary protein restriction delays the onset of the uremic syndrome.

Nutritional Status during Chronic Renal Insufficiency

As will be discussed later, protein–energy undernutrition is a well-described important risk factor for morbidity and mortality in patients maintained on dialysis. Many studies have demonstrated a high prevalence of protein–energy undernutrition in patients beginning dialysis, suggesting that this disorder begins during the stage of CRI.

The causes of protein–energy undernutrition in patients with CRI are similar to those in ESRD (reviewed later). Of particular importance is decreased protein and energy intake. A recent cross-sectional analysis of the large number of patients enrolled in the MDRD Study baseline cohort clearly demonstrated reduced protein and energy intake in patients with GFRs as high as 50 ml/min per 1.73 m^2, which became progressively impaired with further reduction in GFR (Kopple et al., in press). Progressive reduction in parameters of nutritional status including body weight, serum albumin and transferrin concentrations, skinfold thickness, arm muscle area, and urinary creatinine excretion accompanied these changes. These findings are particularly important because patients with type 1 diabetes and severe cardiovascular disease were excluded from this study. Thus, decreased nutrient intake and nutritional status did not appear to be the result of other coexisting conditions.

These data suggest that protein and energy intake, as well as nutritional status, begin to decline early during the stage of CRI, and worsen progressively as patients approach ESRD. It is reasonably hypothesized, but not yet proven, that preventing the development of malnutrition during this phase of CRI may reduce the consequences of malnutrition during ESRD. Thus, attention to diet in CRI is essential, not only to slow the progression of renal disease, but also to maintain nutritional status. Restriction of dietary protein, while maintaining adequate intakes of quality protein and total energy requires appropriate dietary prescription, counseling, and follow-up by a trained dietitian.

Renal Insufficiency as a Risk Factor for Cardiovascular Disease

Cardiovascular disease is the leading cause of death in patients with ESRD. In the general population, cardiovascular disease morbidity and mortality have declined substantially over the past three decades through risk-factor identification and reduction and more effective treatment of coronary artery disease. In 1997, the National Kidney Foundation convened a task force, consisting of experts in cardiovascular disease epidemiology, clinical trials, clinical cardiology, and nephrology, to consider whether strategies for the prevention and treatment of cardiovascular disease in the general population were applicable to patients with chronic renal disease. The task force considered four target populations of patients with chronic renal disease: patients with CRI, patients with ESRD treated by hemodialysis, patients with ESRD treated by peritoneal dialysis, and renal transplant recipients. Recommendations of the task force (Levey et al., 1998) especially relevant to consideration of nutrition therapy for Medicare beneficiaries with chronic renal disease follow:

Epidemiology of Cardiovascular Disease in Chronic Renal Disease

Patients with chronic renal disease should be considered in the highest risk group for subsequent cardiovascular disease events. They have a high prevalence of coronary artery disease and left ventricular hypertrophy, which are precursors of cardiovascular disease mortality and morbidity. They also have a high prevalence of congestive heart failure, which is an independent predictor of death in chronic renal disease. Treatment recommendations based on cardiovascular disease risk stratification should consider the "highest risk status" of patients with chronic renal disease.

Risk Factors

The excess risk for cardiovascular disease in chronic renal disease is caused, in part, by a higher prevalence of conditions that are recognized as risk factors for cardiovascular disease in the general population, such as older age, hypertension, hyperlipidemia, diabetes, and physical inactivity. The excess risk may also be caused, in part, by hemodynamic and metabolic factors characteristic of chronic renal disease, including proteinuria, increased extracellular fluid volume, electrolyte imbalance, anemia, and higher levels of thrombogenic factors and homocysteine than in the general population. Strategies for risk factor identification and reduction should target both the traditional coronary risk factors and specific factors related to chronic renal disease.

Recent studies have highlighted the excess risk of cardiovascular disease in patients with CRI, as well as in ESRD. A prospective study of

246 patients with CRI in France determined that the coronary artery disease event rates were three times higher than in the general population (Jungers et al., 1997). A cross-sectional study of 175 patients showed that the prevalence of left ventricular hypertrophy was inversely correlated with the level of renal function. The prevalence of left ventricular hypertrophy was 27 percent, 31 percent, and 45 percent, respectively, among patients with creatinine clearance of greater than 50, 25 to 50, and less than 25 ml/min (Levin et al., 1996). These studies suggest that CRI is a risk factor for both coronary artery disease and left ventricular hypertrophy.

CRI is also a risk factor for cardiovascular disease mortality. Secondary analysis of the Hypertension Detection and Follow-Up Program (a randomized clinical trial of two levels of blood pressure control in essential hypertension) found that an elevated serum creatinine concentration was an independent risk factor for total and cardiovascular disease mortality (Shulman et al., 1989). In that study, cardiovascular mortality was almost three times higher than mortality due to renal disease. Similar findings were reported in secondary analyses of the Program on the Surgical Control of the Hyperlipidemias (a randomized controlled trial of partial ileal bypass surgery versus medical therapy for hypercholesterolemic survivors of myocardial infarction) (Matts et al., 1993), and the Cardiovascular Health Study (a community-based observational study of factors associated with cardiovascular disease) (Fried et al., 1998). Preliminary data from the Framingham Study (a community-based observational study of factors associated with cardiovascular disease) also document an increased risk of fatal and nonfatal cardiovascular disease events in participants with elevated serum creatinine concentration, although the relationship was strongly related to age and coexisting cardiovascular disease risk factors (Culleton et al., 1999). Interpretation of these secondary analyses is limited by the diverse study populations, and the possibility of unique effects of the underlying disease on serum creatinine concentrations. Nonetheless, there appears to be consensus that an elevated serum creatinine concentration is a risk factor for cardiovascular disease.

Nutrition therapy is widely recommended as part of the medical regimen for the secondary prevention of cardiovascular disease in patients with hypertension, hyperlipidemia, and diabetes. The above data provide a strong basis for targeting patients with CRI for similar secondary preventive measures.

Chronic Renal Insufficiency:
Summary and Recommendations

Overall the findings from the above randomized, controlled clinical trial in adults suggest that there may be a beneficial effect over the long term from nutrition therapy in delaying the progression of renal disease. Two meta-analyses also support the benefits of nutrition therapy for these patients. Dietary interventions for patients with moderate renal disease, however, have not been widely adopted.

The committee recommends that dietary interventions be used in patients who are at risk for progression of renal failure in diabetic as well as in non-diabetic renal disease. Trained renal nutrition specialists are needed as part of the renal team and should be involved in the education and the monitoring of nutritional status for these patients. In addition, nutrition therapy is necessary to maintain adequate energy intake to prevent the onset of malnutrition, which is a risk factor for death after the onset of ESRD. Finally, nutrition therapy is necessary to address risk factors for cardiovascular disease which are highly prevalent in patients with CRI and ESRD.

Summary of Evidence—Nutrition Therapy for Chronic Renal Insufficiency (Pre-End Stage Disease)

Consensus statements:	Recommended by 1994 consensus conference (Striker, 1995)
Observational studies:	Supportive evidence in animal studies (3 studies: Ibels et al., 1978; Kleinknecht et al., 1979; Laouari et al., 1982)
Randomized trials:	Supportive evidence (2 large studies: Klahr et al. 1994; Zeller et al., 1991; and numerous small studies)
Meta-analysis of trials:	Supportive evidence (3 studies: Fouque et al., 1992; Kasiske et al., 1998; Pedrini et al., 1996)
Systematic reviews:	Supportive recent evidence (Levey et al., 1999)

END-STAGE RENAL DISEASE

ESRD requires complex nutritional management, which may include the modification of dietary intake of protein, sodium, potassium, phosphorus, magnesium, calcium, vitamin D, several other vitamins, trace minerals, and fluid (Renal Dietitians Dietetic Practice Group of the American Dietetic Association, 1993). Because many ESRD patients have underlying diabetes, hypertension, or cardiovascular disease, modification of calorie, carbohydrate, and fat intake is often required as well. Thus, the dietary interventions for ESRD patients are complex and are challenging for most to learn and follow. The consequences of dietary noncompliance include increased frequency and duration of dialysis, increased morbidity, and possibly mortality.

The nutritional needs of patients may change as ESRD progresses and thus modifications of the diet prescribed are frequently required. For example, predialysis patients may need to restrict protein. On the other hand, patients who are stable on dialysis will require almost twice the amount of protein as predialysis patients. Depending on the adequacy of dialysis, underlying medical conditions, and patient compliance issues, protein intake may need to be adjusted periodically over the course of dialysis. Adjustments may also be necessary for other nutrients (e.g., sodium and potassium). Because of the complexity of the diet, each change in the dietary prescription requires reeducation of the patient and family. Patients dependent on dialysis may also need adjustments in nutrition therapy for other nutrition-related problems such as anemia, aluminum toxicity, and interactions between nutrients and medications. A number of complex interactions between medications and nutrients require close monitoring of medication administration and nutrition therapy (Sanders et al., 1994).

Undernutrition is common among patients with renal disease, especially those who are dependent on dialysis (Schoenfeld et al., 1983; Young et al., 1991). Several possible etiologies of undernutrition in renal failure have been explored, including the low protein diet restrictions (MDRD Study Group, 1994), altered taste in uremia resulting in anorexia (Atkin-Thor et al., 1978), and reduced energy intake (Monteon et al., 1986). The elevated risk of undernutrition may be related to losses of protein (Ikizler et al., 1994; Wolfson et al., 1982), carbohydrate (Gutierrez et al., 1994), and vitamins (Wolfson, 1988) during the dialysis procedure.

It has been suggested that dialysis is itself a catabolic process contributing to undernutrition (Borah et al., 1978). This hypothesis is supported by the work of Kopple and colleagues (1969, 1986) who found increased protein and possibly energy needs in dialysis patients compared to the normal population. Others have suggested that metabolic acidosis in renal failure may be associated with protein catabolism and that correction of the acidosis may reduce protein breakdown (Reaich et al., 1993).

Undernutrition has been identified as a predictor of mortality for patients dependent on dialysis. The prevalence of undernutrition in ESRD patients is appreciable. In a prospective study of 15,245 ESRD patients, 5,177 patients with a serum albumin concentration of less than 3.5 mg/dL on initiation of dialysis died within 91 days. A death rate of 29 percent has been reported for patients with a serum albumin concentration of less than 3.0 mg/dL (Soucie and McClellan, 1996). Although this is the largest study of this type, several smaller studies have reported similar findings (Canada-USA Peritoneal Dialysis Study Group, 1996; Iseki et al., 1993).

(Chapter 4 documents the limited utility of albumin as a nutritional status indicator. Since albumin is a strong proxy indicator of disease, inflammation, and injury, it is not surprising that dialysis patients with lower serum albumin concentrations face greater mortality risk.)

Dietitians have played a role in the nutritional management of ESRD patients since the inception of dialysis programs. As the knowledge regarding the effectiveness of nutrition intervention during dialysis has evolved, nutrition therapy has become increasingly complex. The advent of urea kinetic modeling has further contributed to the complexity of nutritional assessment and monitoring. Dietitians have also taken on roles as physician extenders in monitoring iron status, response to medication, and dosing of calcium, trace element supplements, and erythropoietin.

The expanding role of the dietitian has not always been accompanied by increased time to perform these tasks. A review of data submitted to the Health Care Financing Administration (HCFA) showed a decline in dietitian hours per renal patient from 0.315 to 0.245 (a decrease of 22 percent) from 1982 to 1987 (Held et al., 1990).

There are limited data concerning nutrition therapy providers for ESRD patients. Since the need for the involvement of dietitians in the provision of nutrition therapy to patients with ESRD was recognized before current reimbursement for services was implemented, there has been little incentive to study the provision of nutrition therapy. In one uncontrolled report, however, patients seemed to respond positively to individualized nutritional intervention by a dietitian (Hoover and Connelly, 1985). There are also small studies suggesting that counseling for appropriate protein intake may result in improved nutritional status (Borah et al., 1978; Kopple, 1994). Further studies are needed to identify the most appropriate diet for patients with ESRD, and to determine the frequency, type, and duration of nutrition therapy. Until further data are available, it is recommended that nutrition services be continued at their present level and that surveillance efforts continue to ensure that there are adequate numbers of trained renal nutrition specialists available to meet the needs of ESRD patients.

Enteral[1] and Parenteral[2] Nutrition in Dialysis Patients

Supplemental essential amino acids are available for dialysis patients, however limited data are available to support their use. One study found improved plasma amino acid levels in a small series of patients who

---

[1]Delivery of nutrients through a feeding tube into the gastrointestinal tract.
[2]Delivery of nutrients intravenously rather than through the gastrointestinal tract.

received essential amino acid supplementation, but the study did not control for the protein intake of subjects (Phillips et al., 1978). A later study found no advantage to supplementing a 1 g/kg protein diet with essential amino acids (Hecking et al., 1978). More recently, liquid meal replacement formulas with lowered electrolyte levels have been marketed. Like essential amino acid supplements, these products are too expensive for many ESRD patients to purchase. No randomized trials of their use in augmenting the nutrition intake of undernourished patients with renal disease were available to review. Such trials should be conducted before use of these products is recommended.

Although undernourished ESRD patients should be candidates for enteral nutrition, this therapeutic modality has largely been ignored. Since no trials of enteral feeding in patients with ESRD were found, it is recommended that randomized, controlled trials of this therapy be conducted. The use of parenteral nutrition for acute renal failure patients in the acute hospital setting is discussed in chapter 10.

Intradialytic parenteral nutrition (IDPN) has been subject to preliminary study for use with ESRD patients receiving hemodialysis. A concentrated solution containing modest amounts of amino acids, dextrose, fat, electrolytes, vitamins, and minerals is typically administered several times weekly by infusion during hemodialysis treatments. The rationale for its development and use was to supplement the nutrient intake of patients at risk of undernutrition due to inadequate nutrient intake. Prospective case series suggest that there is opportunity for improved nutritional status in patients receiving IDPN, but none of these series include more than 21 patients, none were adequately controlled, and all were of short duration. One nonrandomized, retrospective review of 81 patients found improved survival (RR = 1.34, $p < 0.01$) in 50 patients receiving IDPN (Capelli et al., 1994). A large, retrospective analysis of 1,679 chronic hemodialysis patients (Chertow et al., 1994) found a decreased risk of death (OR for death = 3.14 in the IDPN group versus 4.93 in the untreated group, $p < 0.01$) in undernourished hemodialysis patients receiving IDPN. Prospective, appropriately randomized trials of IDPN in carefully selected patients should be conducted before Medicare reimbursement for IDPN is considered.

Economic and Regulatory Considerations

Presently, nutrition services for dialysis patients are provided by qualified dietitians who are employed by, or in a contractual relationship with, the ESRD facility. HCFA currently specifies that in consultation with the attending physician, the dietitian is responsible for assessing the nutritional needs of each ESRD patient, recommending therapeutic diets, counseling patients and their families on prescribed diets, and monitoring adherence and response to diets. Dietitians are not currently reimbursed for services; rather, they are included through the monthly capitation payment. Medicare considers the provision of nutritional services to ESRD patients a "minimal services requirement," which is a condition for coverage as part of comprehensive interdisciplinary care.

End-Stage Renal Disease: Summary and Recommendations

It is recommended that nutrition therapy for dialysis patients be continued at the present level and that surveillance continue to document that ESRD patients receive adequate nutrition therapy provided by a trained renal nutrition specialist.

NUTRITION THERAPY AFTER TRANSPLANTATION

There are many situations following kidney transplantation in which patients may benefit from nutrition therapy. The need for complex nutrient modifications is not always ameliorated with renal transplantation. Although individuals who have had a successful kidney transplant need encouragement to eat a normal diet, recommendations for nutrient intake will vary according to the posttransplant duration. The acute posttransplant phase lasts for 1 to 2 months. The chronic posttransplant phase follows. No difference in nutritional management is described; however, if graft failure occurs, further diet modifications are likely to be needed. In addition, several nutrition-related complications may occur in patients following transplant. These include obesity, hyperlipidemia, hypertension, hyperkalemia, and steroid-induced diabetes mellitus as well as bone disease and possibly hypervitaminosis (Rosenberg, 1986). Protein requirements also may change with adjustments in steroid dosing (Cogan et al., 1981; Seagraves et al., 1986). Corticosteroid medications (usually prednisone) cause decreases in lean body mass (due to increased gluconeogenesis) and increases in body fat deposition, glucose intolerance, hyperlipidemia, osteoporosis, hyperphagia, and steroid-induced diabetes.

Most posttransplant patients are at risk for excessive weight gain. In a study of 263 patients following transplant, Merion and colleagues (1991) found that each experienced weight gain. Results showed that in the 6 to 12 month period following transplant, the net 1-year weight gain was 14.2 ± 2.2 kg for obese patients (defined as > 120 percent of ideal body weight) and 8.9 ± 0.6 kg for nonobese patients.

Hyperlipidemia following kidney transplantation has been described

(Kritchevsky, 1987). In a survey of 500 patients treated with cyclosporine, 38 percent had hypercholesterolemia (> 250 mg/dL) and 15 percent had hypertriglyceridemia (> 300 mg/dL) (Rosenberg, 1986). The hyperlipidemia is thought to be steroid induced, but the withdrawal of steroids was not shown to change the total cholesterol-high-density lipoprotein (HDL) cholesterol ratio in a 2-month study (Hricik et al., 1992). A small trial by Shen and colleagues (1983) showed that diet modification may be helpful in decreasing cholesterol and triglyceride levels. Total cholesterol, but not HDL cholesterol or low-density lipoprotein cholesterol, was changed in another small study. Clearly, larger studies are needed to confirm the value of nutrition therapy, as are studies comparing dietary management with drug therapy.

As many as 19 percent of 173 posttransplant patients developed diabetes (Boudreaux et al., 1987). This observation was confirmed by Sumrani and colleagues (1991). It has been noted that the incidence of diabetes was greater in obese patients (Holley et al., 1990).

In patients who have been on dialysis for a long period of time before receiving a kidney transplant, dietary restrictions have become habitual and patients must re-establish normal eating patterns during the posttransplantation period. Given the short length of hospital stay following kidney transplantation (3 days), it is generally not feasible to adequately address nutrition counseling during the hospitalization. In addition, the need for nutrition interventions following transplantation often necessitates access to a nutrition professional for in-depth nutrition counseling.

Nutrition Therapy after Transplantation: Summary and Recommendations

The potential for nutrition-related complications following renal transplant, as well as the potential change in nutritional needs, makes this patient population a candidate that would likely benefit from nutritional therapy. Given the complexity of combined dietary modifications, nutrition therapy should be provided by a trained renal nutrition specialist. Insufficient data are available at this time to determine the appropriate type and frequency of nutritional intervention to maximize the nutritional status in these patients.

FUTURE AREAS OF RESEARCH

Randomized, controlled clinical trials designed to test interventions to maintain optimal nutrition status in predialysis, dialysis, and posttransplant patients are needed. Also necessary are prospective, randomized trials of IDPN in carefully selected undernourished patients before coverage for IDPN can be considered further. Specific research subjects to be addressed include the following:

- although the calorie and protein needs of dialysis patients have been studied, there are gaps in knowledge about the optimum amounts of these and other nutrients in the diet of patients with renal disease;
- the development of undernutrition as ESRD progresses in patients highlights the priority for further investigation of the underlying causes; the optimum type and frequency of nutrition intervention for these patients should be investigated;
- the appropriate roles of oral nutritional supplements and enteral nutrition have not been defined and should be the focus of well-conceived clinical trials; and
- large-scale, randomized trials of parenteral nutrition as a component of treatment for renal disease with clearly defined outcomes should be conducted.

REFERENCES

Atkin-Thor E, Goddard BW, O'Nion J, Stephen RL, Kolff WJ. 1978. Hypogeusia and zinc depletion in chronic dialysis patients. *Am J Clin Nutr* 31:1948–1951.

Borah MF, Schoenfeld PY, Gotch FA, Sargent JA, Wolfson M, Humphreys MH. 1978. Nitrogen balance during intermittent dialysis therapy of uremia. *Kidney Int* 14:491–500.

Boudreaux JP, McHugh L, Canafax DM, Asher N, Sutherland DE, Payne W, Simmons RL, Najarian JS, Fryd DS. 1987. Cyclosporine, combination immunosuppression, and post-transplant diabetes mellitus. *Transplant Proc* 19:1811–1813.

Canada-USA Peritoneal Dialysis Study Group. 1996. Adequacy of dialysis and nutrition in continuous peritoneal dialysis: Association with clinical outcomes. *J Am Soc Nephrol* 7:198–207.

Capelli JP, Kushner H, Camiscioli TC, Chen S-M, Torres MA. 1994. Effect of intradialytic parenteral nutrition on mortality rates in end-stage renal disease care. *Am J Kidney Dis* 23:808–816.

Chertow GM, Ling J, Lew NL, Lazarus JM, Lowrie EG. 1994. The association of intradialytic parenteral nutrition administration with survival in hemodialysis patients. *Am J Kidney Dis* 24:912–920.

Cogan MG, Sargent JA, Yarbrough SG, Vincenti F, Amend WJ Jr. 1981. Prevention of prednisone-induced negative nitrogen balance. Effect of dietary modification on urea generation rate in patients on hemodialysis receiving high-dose glucocorticoids. *Ann Intern Med* 95:158–161.

Culleton BF, Larson MG, Evans JC, Wilson PW, Barrett BJ, Parfrey PS, Levy D. 1999. Prevalence and correlates of elevated serum creatinine levels: The Framingham Heart Study. *Arch Intern Med* 159:1785–1790.

Fouque D, Laville M, Boissel JP, Chifflet R, Labeeuw M, Zech PY. 1992. Controlled low protein diets in chronic renal insufficiency: Meta-analysis. *Brit Med J* 304:216–220.

Fried LP, Kronmal RA, Newman AB, Bild DE, Mittelmark MB, Polak JF, Robbins JA, Gardin JM. 1998. Risk factors for 5-year mortality in older adults: The Cardiovascular Health Study. *J Am Med Assoc* 279:585–592.

Gillis BP, Caggiula AW, Chiavacci AT, Coyne T, Doroshenko L, Milas C, Nowalk MP, Scherch LK. 1995. Nutrition intervention program of the Modification of Diet in Renal Disease Study: A self-management approach. *J Am Diet Assoc* 95:1288–1294.

Greene T, Beck GJ, Kutner MH, Paranandi L, Wang S, MDRD Study Group, 1995. AASK Study Group: Comparison of time-to-event and slope-based analyses in nephrology clinical trials. *Controlled Clin Trials* 16:65S.

Gutierrez A, Bergström J, Alvestrand A. 1994. Hemodialysis-associated protein catabolism with and without glucose in the dialysis fluid. *Kidney Int* 46:814–822.

HCFA (Health Care Financing Administration). 1999. HCFA statitics: Utilization, Table 38. Available at: http://www.hcfa.gov/stats/hstats96/blustat3.htm. Accessed July 1999.

Hecking E, Köhler H, Zobel R, Lemmel EM, Mader H, Opferkuch W, Prellwitz W, Keim HJ, Muller D. 1978. Treatment with essential amino acids in patients on chronic hemodialysis: A double blind cross over study. *Am J Clin Nutr* 31:1821–1826.

Held PJ, Brunner F, Odaka M, García JR, Port FK, Gaylin DS. 1990. Five-year survival for end-stage renal disease patients in the United States, Europe, and Japan, 1982 to 1987. *Am J Kidney Dis* 15:451–457.

Holley JL, Shapiro R, Lopatin WB, Tzakis AG, Hakala TR, Starzl TE. 1990. Obesity as a risk factor following cadaveric renal transplantation. *Transplantation* 49:387–389.

Hoover H, Connelly SV. 1985. The effect of diet intervention on 31 chronic hemodialysis patients. *J Nephrol Nurs* 2:244–249.

Hricik DE, Bartucci MR, Mayes JT, Schulak JA. 1992. The effects of steroid withdrawal on the lipoprotein profiles of cyclosporine-treated kidney and kidney-pancreas transplant recipients. *Transplantation* 54:868–871.

Ibels LS, Alfrey AC, Haut L, Huffer WE. 1978. Preservation of function in experimental renal disease by dietary restriction of phosphate. *N Engl J Med* 298:122–126.

Ikizler TA, Flakoll PJ, Parker RA, Hakim RM. 1994. Amino acid and albumin losses during hemodialysis. *Kidney Int* 46:830–837.

Iseki K, Kawazoe N, Fukiyama K. 1993. Serum albumin is a strong predictor of death in chronic dialysis patients. *Kidney Int* 44:115–119.

Jungers P, Massy ZA, Khoa TN, Fumeron C, Labrunie M, Lacour B, Descamps-Latscha B, Man NK. 1997. Incidence and risk factors of atherosclerotic cardiovascular accidents in predialysis chronic renal failure patients: A prospective study. *Nephrol Dial Transplant* 12:2597–2602.

Kasiske BL, Lakatua JD, Ma JZ, Louis TA. 1998. A meta-analysis of the effects of dietary protein restriction on the rate of decline in renal function. *Am J Kidney Dis* 31:954–961.

Klahr S, Levey AS, Beck GJ, Caggiula AW, Hunsicker L, Kusek JW, Striker G. 1994. The effects of dietary protein restriction and blood-pressure control on the progression of chronic renal disease. *N Engl J Med* 330:877–884.

Kleinknecht C, Salusky I, Broyer M, Gubler M-C. 1979. Effect of various protein diets on growth, renal function, and survival of uremic rats. *Kidney Int* 15:534–541.

Kopple JD. 1994. Effect of nutrition on morbidity and mortality in maintenance dialysis patients. *Am J Kidney Dis* 24:1002–1009.

Kopple JD, Shinaberger JH, Coburn JW, Sorensen MK, Rubini ME. 1969. Optimal dietary protein treatment during chronic hemodialysis. *Trans Am Soc Artif Intern Organs* 15:302–308.

Kopple JD, Monteon FJ, Shaib JK. 1986. Effect of energy intake on nitrogen metabolism in nondialyzed patients with chronic renal failure. *Kidney Int* 29:734–742.

Kopple et al. In press. *J Am Soc Nephrol*.

Kritchevsky D. 1987. Atherosclerosis: Diet and risk factors. *Transplantation Proc* 19:53–56.

Laouari D, Kleinknecht C, Gubler M-C, Ravet V, Broyer M. 1982. Importance of proteins in the deterioration of the remnant kidneys, independently of other nutrients. *Int J Pediatr Nephrol* 3:263–269.

Levey AS, Adler S, Caggiula AW, England BK, Greene T, Hunsicker LG, Kusek JW, Rogers NL, Teschan PE. 1996. Effects of dietary protein restriction on the progression of advanced renal disease in the Modification of Diet in Renal Disease Study. *Am J Kidney Dis* 27:652–663.

Levey AS, Beto JA, Coronado BE, Eknoyan G, Foley RN, Kasiske BL, Klag MJ, Mailloux LU, Manske CL, Meyer KB, Parfrey PS, Pfeffer MA, Wenger NK, Wilson PW, Wright JT Jr. 1998. Controlling the epidemic of cardiovascular disease in chronic renal disease: What do we know? What do we need to learn? Where do we go from here? *Am J Kidney Dis* 32:853–906.

Levey AS, Greene T, Beck GJ, Caggiula AW, Kusek JW, Hunsicker LG, Klahr S. 1999. Dietary protein restriction and the progression of chronic renal disease: What have all the results of the MDRD study shown? *J Am Soc Nephrol* 10:2426–2439.

Levin A, Singer J, Thompson CR, Ross H, Lewis M. 1996. Prevalent LVH in the predialysis population. Identifying opportunities for intervention. *Am J Kidney Dis* 27:347–354.

Matts JP, Karnegis JN, Campos CT, Fitch LL, Johnson JW, Buchwald H. 1993. Serum creatinine as an independent predictor of coronary heart disease mortality in normotensive survivors of myocardial infarction. POSCH Group. *J Fam Pract* 36:497–503.

MDRD (Modification of Diet in Renal Disease) Study Group. 1994. Reduction of dietary protein and phosphorus in the Modification of Diet in Renal Disease Feasibility Study. *J Am Diet Assoc* 94:986–990.

Merion RM, Twork AM, Rosenberg L, Ham JM, Burtch GD, Turcotte JG, Rocher LL, Campbell DA Jr. 1991. Obesity and renal transplantation. *Surg Gynecol Obstet* 172:367–376.

Milas NC, Nowalk MP, Akpele L, Castaldo L, Coyne T, Doroshenko L, Kigawa L, Korzec-Ramirez D, Scherch LK, Snetselaar L. 1995. Factors associated with adherence to the dietary protein intervention in the Modification of Diet in Renal Disease Study. *J Am Diet Assoc* 95:1295–1300.

Monteon FJ, Laidlaw SA, Shaib JK, Kopple JD. 1986. Energy expenditure in patients with chronic renal failure. *Kidney Int* 30:741–747.

Pedrini MT, Levey AS, Lau J, Chalmers TC, Wang PH. 1996. The effect of dietary protein restriction on the progression of diabetic and nondiabetic renal diseases: A meta-analysis. *Ann Intern Med* 124:627–632.

Phillips ME, Havard J, Howard JP. 1978. Oral essential amino acid supplementation in patients on maintenance hemodialysis. *Clin Nephrol* 9:241–248.

Reaich D, Channon SM, Scrimgeour CM, Daley SE, Wilkinson R, Goodship THJ. 1993. Correction of acidosis in humans with CRF decreases protein degradation and amino acid oxidation. *Am J Physiol* 265:E230–E235.

Renal Dietitians Dietetic Practice Group of the American Dietetic Association. 1993. *National Renal Diet: Professional Guide*. Chicago, Ill.: The American Dietetic Association.

Rosenberg ME. 1986. Nutrition and transplantation. *Kidney* 18:19–22.

Sanders HN, Rabb HA, Bittle P, Ramirez G. 1994. Nutritional implications of recombinant human erythropoietin therapy in renal disease. *J Am Diet Assoc* 94:1023–1029.

Schoenfeld PY, Henry RR, Laird NM, Roxe DM. 1983. Assessment of nutritional status of the National Cooperative Dialysis Study population. *Kidney Int* 23:S80–S88.

Seagraves A, Moore EE, Moore FA, Weil R 3rd. 1986. Net protein catabolic rate after kidney transplantation: Impact of corticosteroid immunosuppression. *J Parenter Enteral Nutr* 10:453–455.

Shen SY, Lukens CW, Alongi SV, Sfeir RE, Dagher FJ, Sadler JH. 1983. Patient profile and effect of dietary therapy on post-transplant hyperlipidemia. *Kidney Int* 24:S147–S152.

Shulman NB, Ford CE, Hall WD, Blaufox MD, Simon D, Langford HG, Schneider KA. 1989. Prognostic value of serum creatinine and effect of treatment of hypertension on renal function. Results from the hypertension detection and follow-up program. The Hypertension Detection and Follow-up Program Cooperative Group. *Hypertension* 13:I80–I93.

Soucie JM, McClellan WM. 1996. Early death in dialysis patients: Risk factors and impact on incidence and mortality rates. *J Am Soc Nephrol* 7:2169–2175.

Striker GE. 1995. Report on a workshop to develop management recommendations for the prevention of progression in chronic renal disease Bethesda (MD) April 1994. *Nephrol Dial Transplant* 10:290–292.

Sumrani NB, Delaney V, Ding ZK, Davis R, Daskalakis P, Friedman EA, Butt KM, Hong JH. 1991. Diabetes mellitus after renal transplantation in the cyclosporine era—an analysis of risk factors. *Transplantation* 51:343–347.

USRDS (U.S. Renal Data System). 1997. *1997 Annual Data Report*. Bethesda, Md.: National Institute of Diabetes and Digestive and Kidney Diseases.

USRDS (U.S. Renal Data System). 1999. *1999 Annual Data Report*. Bethesda, Md.: National Institute of Diabetes and Digestive and Kidney Diseases.

Walker JD, Bending JJ, Dodds RA, Mattock MB, Murrells TJ, Keen H, Viberti GC. 1989. Restriction of dietary protein and progression of renal failure in diabetic nephropathy. Lancet 2:1411–1415.

Wolfson M. 1988. Use of water soluble vitamins in patients with chronic renal failure. *Semin Dial* 1:28–32.

Wolfson M, Jones MR, Kopple JD. 1982. Amino acid losses during hemodialysis with infusion of amino acids and glucose. *Kidney Int* 21:500–506.

Young GA, Kopple JD, Lindholm B, Vonesh EF, De Vecchi A, Scalamogna A, Castelnova C, Oreopoulos DG, Anderson GH, Bergstrom J, DiChiro J, Gentile D, Nissenson A, Sakhrani L, Brownjohn AM, Nolph KD, Prowant BF, Algrim CE, Martis L, Serkes KD. 1991. Nutritional assessment of continuous ambulatory peritoneal dialysis patients: An international study. *Am J Kidney Dis* 17:462–471.

Zeller K, Whittaker E, Sullivan L, Raskin P, Jacobson HR. 1991. Effect of restricting dietary protein on the progression of renal failure in patients with insulin-dependent diabetes mellitus. *N Engl J Med* 324:78–84.

8

Osteoporosis

Osteoporosis is a common disorder that affects approximately 10 million people in the United States. Although the prevalence varies considerably according to gender and race, being less common in men, African Americans, and Hispanic Americans, 25 to 30 percent of Caucasian women over age 65 suffer from osteoporosis. Recent data suggests that this diagnosis may also be common among older men who suffer from either absolute or relative androgen insufficiency (Ebeling, 1998).

The World Health Organization (1994) has defined osteoporosis and its precursor, osteopenia, as follows: osteopenia is defined as having a bone density one or more standard deviations below the gender-specific mean for a normal 25 year old; osteoporosis is defined as greater than 2.5 standard deviations below the same mean; severe osteoporosis is defined as greater than 2.5 standard deviations below the mean with clinical fractures. It should be noted that these definitions are not based on a pathologic classification of the disease but merely attempt to quantitate the degree of the problem according to relative bone mineral density (BMD), as measured by dual-energy x-ray absorptiometry scanning.

Although BMD is not a perfect intermediate outcome measure, several studies have demonstrated a good relationship between BMD and the risk of future fracture development (Cummings et al., 1993; Melton et al., 1993). Therefore, a decrease in BMD is the most frequent outcome measure in recent studies of osteoporosis, while clinically relevant end points such as fracture incidence are less commonly determined.

Osteoporosis is associated with considerable morbidity and mortality. The National Osteoporosis Foundation estimates that there are approximately 1.5 million osteoporosis-related fractures each year: 300,000 at the hip, 700,000 at the spine, 250,000 at the wrist, and 300,000 at other sites (National Osteoporosis Foundation, 1999). The impact of hip fractures on the mortality of the Medicare-age population is significant. A hip fracture is associated with a 20 to 25 percent 1-year mortality rate in women (higher in men), a 25 percent rate of admission to a long-term care setting, and a less than 50 percent likelihood of regaining baseline functional status (National Osteoporosis Foundation, 1999). In 1995, the cost of hip fractures in individuals over 45 years of age were estimated to be $8.7 billion in the United States (Ray et al., 1997). It has also been predicted that these costs could double in the next 30 years (Cummings et al., 1990). While fractures at sites other than the hip are less likely to be associated with mortality, their association with functional impairment, pain, fear, isolation, and depression may not be easily measured but should not be underestimated.

Multiple risk factors for osteoporosis have been defined, and include: (1) estrogen/testosterone deficiency, (2) Caucasian or Asian race, (3) small or thin body habitus, (4) inactivity, (5) alcohol and tobacco use, (6) chronic renal/liver disease, hyperthyroidism, and diabetes, (7) chronic use of pharmacological agents such as glucocorticoids, barbiturates, and phenytoin, (8) inadequate calcium intake, and (9) vitamin D deficiency. This chapter focuses on these last two risk factors, reviewing the role of diet and nutritional supplementation in preventing, delaying, and treating osteoporosis.

ROLE OF DIET IN ONSET AND TREATMENT OF OSTEOPOROSIS

Assessing Dietary Intake of Calcium

Most studies assessing the dietary intakes of free-living (community-dwelling) elderly populations (greater than 65 years of age) in the United States indicate that few individuals are consuming the level of calcium intake recommended as adequate for those over 50 years of age, 1,200 mg/day (IOM, 1997). Indeed, estimates of calcium intake in older women in the United States in 1994 (ARS, 1997) showed an adjusted median intake of 571 mg/day for women 51 to 70 years of age, and a median intake of 517 mg/day for those 71 years and older (IOM, 1997). Only 1 percent of those over age 50 were reported to consume this recommended intake. These estimated intakes are in all likelihood underestimates because the Continuing Survey of Food Intakes by Individuals did not include calcium intakes from supplements or from foods recently available in the market that may have been fortified with calcium.

While it is recognized that such national surveys may underreport intakes by as much as 20 percent (Mertz et al., 1991), a recent evaluation of the Third National Health and Nutrition Examination Survey data suggested that only 2 percent of people over age 50 took any calcium supplement (Bendich et al., 1999), while the National Health Interview Survey (Moss et al., 1989) suggested that close to 21 percent of people over age 65 had taken a calcium supplement within the last 2 weeks. In any case, it is clear that at present, average intakes of calcium by those over age 50 in the United States are far below the recommended 1,200 mg/day (IOM, 1997). This has been borne out in most of the randomized controlled trials discussed below where baseline calcium intake was almost uniformly below 800 mg/day. It should be noted, however, that in some studies, subjects were specifically selected for average reported daily intakes of less than 1,000 mg of calcium.

Calcium Supplementation

Many studies have assessed the extent to which increased calcium intake can mitigate the bone loss seen in the elderly and therefore decrease the risk and sequelae of osteoporosis. Most of the studies conducted have measured BMD, a widely available and useful technique to screen for osteoporosis and osteopenia. Most of the studies have enhanced calcium intake by providing calcium supplements because of the presence of confounding variables related to changes in intake of food with different amounts of calcium.

Because of substantial improvements in the technology for measuring BMD in the last decade, this review focuses only on the most recent randomized controlled trials. However, it should be noted that a review of calcium supplementation studies prior to 1991 (Dawson-Hughes, 1991) in general supports the more recent findings.

Aloia and colleages (1994) compared 70 healthy women in the United States treated for 3 years with either a placebo, a supplement of 1,700 mg of calcium alone or a combination of 1,700 mg of calcium supplement with hormone replacement therapy (HRT). All subjects were given 10 mg (400 IU) of vitamin D as a supplement. At baseline, calcium intake was reported to average about 500 mg/day, with 90 percent of the subjects consuming less than 800 mg/day. At the end of the study the calcium-only group lost less total body and femoral neck bone mass compared to the placebo group; however, there was no difference seen at the spine or proximal radius sites. The calcium and HRT group had the best outcome during the 3-year study, having less change in total body calcium and femoral neck BMD than the placebo group.

A 4-year study from New Zealand (Reid et al., 1995) examined 78 healthy white women who were at least 3 years postmenopausal. This was a 2-year continuation of a previously reported 2-year investigation in which subjects were provided either a 1,000 mg/day of calcium supplement or a placebo. At baseline, and throughout the 4 years, usual dietary intake of calcium was approximately 750 mg/day for each group. This study found that the positive effect of calcium supplementation on total BMD that had been noted during years 1 and 2 of the study continued in years 3 and 4. Bone loss at specific sites (lumbar spine, proximal femur, trochanter) tended to be reduced most in the supplemented group during the first year of the study, but an overall difference at 4 years was still detected. Significantly fewer incident fractures were noted in the calcium-supplemented group.

Recker and colleagues (1996) evaluated the effect of a daily supplement of 1,200 mg of calcium on spine fractures in older women with and without previous spinal fractures. At baseline, dietary calcium intake was estimated to be less than 500 mg/day. After the 4-year follow-up period, calcium supplementation significantly reduced the incidence of new fractures in the group with prior spine fractures and greatly reduced bone loss compared to the placebo control group. No significant difference in incident fractures was found in the group without prior fractures at baseline compared to control subjects.

A long-term follow-up study in Australia evaluated the effect of a daily 1,000 mg calcium supplement compared to a placebo for 4 years in women who were at least 10 years postmenopause at baseline (Devine et al., 1997). The baseline dietary intake in this study was estimated to be close to 1,000 mg/day. Thus, the actual comparison was between 1,000 and 2,000 mg/day. Investigators found a significant reduction in bone loss at every site in the supplemented group compared to placebo. Of interest, when a subgroup of subjects were compared (who were noncompliant with the calcium supplement during the last 2 years and thus averaged only 1,000 mg/day of total calcium intake per day in years 3–4), they lost more bone than the more compliant subjects.

A recent study looked at the effect of 1,000 mg/day of calcium supplementation for 2 years on seasonal bone loss in nonosteoporotic women over age 65 living in the state of Maine, with an estimated baseline calcium intake of less than 800 mg/day (Storm et al., 1998). The investigators compared a placebo control group to two different calcium supplementation regimens: (1) milk (four 8 ounce glasses/day) and (2) calcium carbonate ($CaCO_3$) tablets (500 mg of calcium twice daily). The milk group was unable to maintain the expected supplementation level and had an estimated total calcium intake of 1,000 mg/day; this was an intermediate total daily intake between the placebo (700 mg/day) and $CaCO_3$ (1,700 mg/day) groups. The reduction in bone loss seen was related to the total daily calcium intake, but only the $CaCO_3$ group was different from the placebo group at the spine, femoral neck, and greater trochanter. The $CaCO_3$ supplemented group was noted to have an increase in bone density after 2 years. It is interesting to note that after the first year, the milk supplemented group experienced an even larger percent increase in greater trochanter BMD than the $CaCO_3$ group despite a lower total calcium intake (1,600 versus 1,000 mg/day).

Most of the bone loss in the greater trochanter and femoral neck occurred during the winter months and was halted with $CaCO_3$ or milk (in the case of the greater trochanter) treatment. In addition, winter was associated with a 20 percent decline in vitamin D levels. The importance of calcium supplementation at a level greater than 1,000 mg/day is underscored in this study since the high-calcium supplement group lost less bone in most sites than the milk drinkers who were also receiving vitamin D supplementation in their milk.

Vitamin D Supplementation

Other studies have recently looked at the effect of vitamin D intake as part of an overall approach to maintaining bone mass. It has been demonstrated that primary vitamin D deficiency, diagnosed as serum 25-hydroxyvitamin D [25-(OH)D] concentrations below 10 ng/mL (25 mmol/L), is common in older individuals, especially during the winter months, and in those living at more northern latitudes or with little direct sun exposure (Gloth and Tobin, 1995; Kinyamu et al., 1997). Elderly groups confined indoors have been shown to have low serum 25-(OH)D concentrations in 45 percent of individuals, with vitamin D intakes estimated to range from 3 to 7 mg (121–282 IU) per day (Gloth and Tobin, 1995). A recent report of older patients in a U.S. hospital found that 66 percent had low serum 25-(OH)D levels (Thomas et al., 1998). Furthermore, 46 percent of those taking a multiple vitamin, frequently supplying 10 mg (400 IU) of vitamin D, were still found to have low serum levels. Although this hospitalized population might have had diseases or had been taking drugs that could have negatively affected their vitamin D status, inadequate intake, winter season, and homebound status were all independent predictors of inadequate vitamin D level. This high percentage of probable vitamin D deficiency is supported by an earlier study that found low vitamin D levels in almost 80 percent of older Dutch women (Lips et al., 1988).

There is strong evidence that these low serum 25-(OH)D levels are more than just an innocuous biochemical abnormality. Indeed, serum vitamin D concentration is inversely associated with parathyroid hormone levels and markers of accelerated bone turnover (Chapuy et al.,

1996), and has been inversely linked to the occurrence of hip fractures (LeBoff et al., 1999). Most importantly, clinical trials now suggest that oral supplementation of vitamin D can reduce bone loss. In a 2-year trial in healthy postmenopausal women living in a northern latitude of the United States, whose estimated baseline dietary intake of vitamin D was only 2.5 mg (100 IU) per day, supplementation with an additional 2.5 mg (100 IU) or 17.5 mg (700 IU) was compared (Dawson-Hughes et al., 1995). Both groups received a calcium supplement of 500 mg/day in addition to their usual dietary calcium intake of about 450 mg/day. The higher dose of vitamin D (17.5 mg) reduced femoral neck bone loss by more than 50 percent, with much of the benefit occurring during the winter and spring months. Spine and whole body BMD did not differ between the groups.

A 36-month follow-up study of over 3,000 elderly French women (mean age 84 years) living in nursing homes compared fracture incidence in a group receiving both calcium (1,200 mg/day) and vitamin D (20 mg [800 IU] per day) supplementation to a double placebo control group (Chapuy et al., 1994). The calcium and vitamin D supplemented group had 29 percent fewer hip fractures and 24 percent fewer nonvertebral fractures (odds ratio of 0.7 for both).

A study of similar design (500 mg additional calcium and 17.5 mg [700 IU] vitamin D per day versus double-placebo) has recently been reported in a younger, healthier U.S. population (Dawson-Hughes et al., 1997). The supplemented groups, with average ages of 70 (males) and 71 (females), had less bone loss at all sites after year 1, but the groups (supplemented versus double-placebo) differed significantly only in total BMD after years 2 and 3. The cumulative incidence of a first fracture was 6 percent in the treatment group and 13 percent in the placebo group by the end of the study (relative risk = 0.5). In the men, supplementation significantly reduced bone loss from the spine, hip, and total body. In the women, the reduction was significant from the total body only. As expected, most of the fractures occurred in the women. The effect of supplementation on fracture rates in men has not been demonstrated.

As is evident in reviewing these studies, not all studies agree; a large study of Dutch women (receiving no calcium supplementation) found no effect of added vitamin D supplementation (Lips et al., 1996).

COST AND QUALITY-OF-LIFE CONSIDERATIONS

Recent studies have attempted to evaluate the potential economic and quality-of-life effects of treating osteoporosis. Given the high rate of expenditure for osteoporosis-related problems and the substantial data demonstrating that treatment can significantly reduce both bone loss and fracture rate, it is not surprising that these studies support economic benefits due to therapeutic management of osteoporosis. In one study that specifically evaluated the effect of calcium supplementation, the predicted cost for avoiding one hip fracture was $33,000 when treating all men and women over 65 years of age (male and female), $14,000 for treating all women over 75 years of age, and $8,000 for treating all women over 85 (Bendich et al., 1999). This study probably overestimates the true cost of dietary intervention for preventing osteoporosis, since the cost of nonhip fractures is not included.

It should be noted that this estimate is greatly influenced by the percentage of the population already taking calcium supplementation (estimated between 2 and 21 percent, see above). It should also be noted that there are other, possible non-osteoporosis-related benefits of increased calcium intake. Although not yet determined to be a primary indication for calcium supplementation, some recent studies suggest positive influences of higher calcium intakes on blood pressure (Griffith et al., 1999) and colon tumors (Baron et al., 1999).

Studies have also attempted to evaluate the cost of treating osteoporosis per quality-adjusted life year (QALY). This type of evaluation is important because of the tremendous overall impact that osteoporosis can have on quality of life. These models, while complicated, generally assume a given level of fracture reduction and also assume a utility figure describing the trade-off value between years with a condition and years of perfect health. Nevertheless, the estimate in one study of $30,000 per QALY for treating osteoporosis is similar to that estimated for treating hypertension (Tosteson, 1997). An earlier study also suggested that the cost per QALY for treating osteoporosis is similar to that for treating hypertension (Jonsson et al., 1995; see chapter 14 for economic analyses related to osteoporosis for Medicare).

FUTURE AREAS OF RESEARCH

There are considerable data supporting the effectiveness of treatments for osteoporosis in reducing bone loss and subsequent fracture rate. While there is not total agreement, many recent studies strongly support a role for calcium and vitamin D as part of this treatment strategy. These studies include multiple randomized, controlled trials; reviews and meta-analyses; and consensus opinions from professional organizations. However, gaps remain in the understanding of this important issue that deserve future attention:

- There are relatively few published intervention studies in men and non-Caucasian women.
- There is a need for better dose–response data to determine the

lowest levels of intake or supplementation that are necessary and to evaluate the interactions between estrogen, calcium, and vitamin D with respect to determining minimum levels necessary.

- The importance of seasonal vitamin D and/or calcium intake should be examined further.
- There is a need for more studies demonstrating clinically relevant outcome measures such as fracture incidence. In addition, newer intermediate outcome measures such as microstructure of bone (by computed tomography) may help to reduce the variance noted in the relationship between changes in bone mass and fracture.
- Better evaluation is needed of the long-term potential side effects of calcium and vitamin D supplementation.
- Population-based estimates of the QALY utility value have to be developed to define more accurately the true cost per QALY models.
- Studies are needed to assess behavior related to the use of calcium and vitamin D-fortified foods and supplements by individuals to chronically enhance calcium and vitamin D intake and the long-term efficacy of such interventions. This is especially important because of the potential added value of consuming foods that contain other nutrients and components thought to be beneficial to health as opposed to pure supplement forms. The development of culturally appropriate calcium and vitamin D-fortified foods may also be indicated to increase intake.

SUMMARY AND RECOMMENDATIONS

Enhanced intake of calcium and vitamin D for both the prevention and treatment of osteoporosis in the at-risk Medicare population is strongly supported by a considerable body of data including multiple randomized controlled trials. It must be noted that adequate calcium and vitamin D are also critical for the accretion of maximal bone mass, which occurs much earlier in life. The exact amounts of calcium and vitamin D intake that are necessary and safe have been reviewed at length (IOM, 1997) and are not specifically addressed in this report.

While consumption of calcium and vitamin D through food is the preferred route, it is recognized that the variability in food habits and preferences makes this a less reliable source of calcium and vitamin D to those at increased risk of osteoporosis. Although a variety of calcium-fortified foods continue to be introduced into the U.S. food supply (e.g., juices, cereals), there is currently a lack of data suggesting that those at risk for osteoporosis are able to maintain an adequate calcium and vitamin D intake without the use of supplements.

The more important and germane issue is whether counseling by a nutrition professional versus basic nutrition education by a variety of health professionals (e.g., physicians and nurses) improves the probability of meeting adequate calcium and vitamin D intake. Current data is lacking, rather than suggestive for any specific health care provider to counsel patients regarding the use of calcium or vitamin D supplements. While a relatively simple history of the intake of calcium rich foods and supplements is indicated to ensure against the intake of excess levels of calcium (>2,500 mg/day) (IOM, 1997), such a history could be obtained by physicians, nurses, or other staff and would not likely require a comprehensive nutritional assessment by a dietitian. However, for individuals who would prefer to meet and sustain adequate intakes of calcium and vitamin D without supplements, nutrition counseling by a nutrition professional with training equivalent to that of a dietitian may be warranted, particularly for individuals with other nutrient restrictions or unique meal planning circumstances.

Summary of Evidence:
Nutrition Intervention[1] for Osteoporosis

Consensus statements: Recommended as part of the standard of care by the World Health Organization (1994) and the National Osteoporosis Foundation (1999)

Observational studies: Strongly supportive (e.g., Chapuy et al., 1994, 1996; LeBoff et al., 1999)

Randomized trials: Strongly supportive (Aloia et al., 1994; Dawson-Hughes et al., 1995, 1997; Devine et al., 1997; Recker et al., 1996; Reid et al., 1995; Storm et al., 1998)

Systematic review: Several (e.g., Dawson-Hughes, 1991)

---

[1]This summary of evidence pertains to nutrition intervention through increased calcium and vitamin D intake, but not specifically for nutrition therapy as a means to increase intake of calcium or vitamin D intake through either supplements or food.

REFERENCES

Aloia JF, Vaswani A, Yeh JK, Ross PL, Flaster E, Dilmanian FA. 1994. Calcium supplementation with and without hormone replacement therapy to prevent postmenopausal bone loss. *Ann Intern Med* 120:97–103.

ARS (Agricultural Research Service), U.S. Department of Agriculture. 1997. *Results from USDA's 1994–1996 Continuing Survey of Food Intakes by Individuals and 1994–1996 Diet and Knowledge Health Survey.* Beltsville, Md.: U.S. Department of Agriculture.

Baron JA, Beach M, Mandel JS, van Stolk RU, Haile RW, Sandler RS, Rothstein R, Summers RW, Snover DC, Beck GJ, Bond JH, Greenberg ER. 1999. Calcium supplements for the prevention of colorectal adenomas. Calcium Polyp Prevention Study Group. *N Engl J Med* 340:101–107.

Bendich A, Leader S, Muhuri P. 1999. Supplemental calcium for the prevention of hip fracture: Potential health-economic benefits. *Clin Ther* 21:1058–1072.

Chapuy MC, Arlot ME, Delmas PD, Meunier PJ. 1994. Effect of calcium and cholecalciferol treatment for three years on hip fractures in elderly women. *Br Med J* 308:1081–1082.

Chapuy MC, Schott AM, Garnero P, Hans D, Delmas PD, Meunier PJ, Epidos Study Group. 1996. Healthy elderly French women living at home have secondary hyperparathyroidism and high bone turnover in winter. *J Clin Endocrinol Metab* 81:1129–1133.

Cummings SR, Rubin SM, Black D. 1990. The future of hip fractures in the United States. Numbers, costs, and potential effects of postmenopausal estrogen. *Clin Orthop* 252:163–166.

Cummings SR, Black DM, Nevitt MC, Browner W, Cauley J, Ensrud K, Genant HK, Palermo L, Scott J, Vogt TM. 1993. Bone density at various sites for prediction of hip fractures. The Study of Osteoporotic Fractures Research Group. *Lancet* 341:72–75.

Dawson-Hughes B. 1991. Calcium supplementation and bone loss: A review of controlled clinical trials. *Am J Clin Nutr* 54:274S–280S.

Dawson-Hughes B, Harris SS, Krall EA, Dallal GE, Falconer G, Green CL. 1995. Rates of bone loss in postmenopausal women randomly assigned to one of two dosages of vitamin D. *Am J Clin Nutr* 61:1140–1145.

Dawson-Hughes B, Harris SS, Krall EA, Dallal GE. 1997. Effect of calcium and vitamin D supplementation on bone density in men and women 65 years of age or older. *N Engl J Med* 337:670–676.

Devine A, Dick IM, Heal SJ, Criddle RA, Prince RL. 1997. A 4-year follow-up study of the effects of calcium supplementation on bone density in elderly postmenopausal women. *Osteoporosis Int* 7:23–28.

Ebeling PR. 1998. Osteoporosis in men. New insights into aetiology, pathogenesis, prevention and management. *Drugs Aging* 13:421–434.

Gloth FM III, Tobin JD. 1995. Vitamin D deficiency in older people. *J Am Geriatr Soc* 43:822–828.

Griffith LE, Guyatt GH, Cook RJ, Bucher HC, Cook DJ. 1999. The influence of dietary and nondietary calcium supplementation on blood pressure: An updated metaanalysis of randomized controlled trials. *Am J Hypertens* 12:84–92.

IOM (Institute of Medicine). 1997. *Dietary Reference Intakes for Calcium, Phosphorus, Magnesium, Vitamin D, and Fluoride.* Washington, D.C.: National Academy Press.

Jonsson B, Christiansen C, Johnell O, Hedbrandt J. 1995. Cost-effectiveness of fracture prevention in established osteoporosis. *Osteoporos Int* 5:136–142.

Kinyamu HK, Gallagher JC, Balhorn KE, Petranick KM, Rafferty KA. 1997. Serum vitamin D metabolites and calcium absorption in normal young and elderly free-living women and in women living in nursing homes. *Am J Clin Nutr* 65:790–797.

LeBoff MS, Kohlmeier L, Hurwitz S, Franklin J, Wright J, Glowacki J. 1999. Occult vitamin D deficiency in postmenopausal U.S. women with acute hip fracture. *J Am Med Assoc* 281:1505–1511.

Lips P, Wiersinga A, van Ginkel FC, Jongen MJ, Netelenbos JC, Hackeng WH, Delmas PD, van der Vijgh WJ. 1988. The effect of vitamin D supplementation on vitamin D status and parathyroid function in elderly subjects. *J Clin Endocrinol Metab* 67:644–650.

Lips P, Graafmans WC, Ooms ME, Bezemer PD, Bouter LM. 1996. Vitamin D supplementation and fracture incidence in elderly persons. A randomized, placebo-controlled clinical trial. *Ann Intern Med* 124:400–406.

Melton LJ 3rd, Atkinson EJ, O'Fallon WM, Wahner HW, Riggs BL. 1993. Long-term fracture prediction by bone mineral assessed at different skeletal sites. *J Bone Miner Res* 8:1227–1233.

Mertz W, Tsui JC, Judd JT, Reiser S, Hallfrisch J, Morris ER, Steele PD, Lashley E. 1991. What are people really eating? The relation between energy intake derived from estimated diet records and intake determined to maintain body weight. *Am J Clin Nutr* 54:291–295.

Moss AJ, Levy AS, Kim I, Park YK. 1989. *Use of Vitamin and Mineral Supplementation in the United States: Current Users, Types of Products and Nutrients*. Advance Data, Vital and Health Statistics, No. 174. Hyattsville, Md.: National Center for Health Statistics.

National Osteoporosis Foundation. 1999. Osteoporosis fast facts. Available at: http://www.nof.org/osteoporosis/stats.htm. Accessed November 4, 1999.

Ray NF, Chan JK, Thamer M, Melton LJ 3rd. 1997. Medical expenditures for the treatment of osteoporotic fractures in the United States in 1995: Report from the National Osteoporosis Foundation. *J Bone Miner Res* 12:24–35.

Recker RR, Hinders S, Davies KM, Heaney RP, Stegman MR, Lappe JM, Kimmel DB. 1996. Correcting calcium nutritional deficiency prevents spine fractures in elderly women. *J Bone Miner Res* 11:1961–1966.

Reid IR, Ames RW, Evans MC, Gamble GD, Sharpe SJ. 1995. Long-term effects of calcium supplementation on bone loss and fractures in postmenopausal women: A randomized controlled trial. *Am J Med* 98:331–335.

Storm D, Eslin R, Porter ES, Musgrave K, Vereault D, Patton C, Kessenich C, Mahon S, Chen T, Holick MF, Rosen CJ. 1998. Calcium supplementation prevents seasonal bone loss and changes in biochemical markers of bone turnover in elderly New England women: A randomized placebo-controlled trial. *J Clin Endocrinol Metab* 83:3817–3825.

Thomas MK, Lloyd-Jones DM, Thadhani RI, Shaw AC, Deraska DJ, Kitch BT, Vamvakas EC, Dick IM, Prince RL, Finkelstein JS. 1998. Hypovitaminosis D in medical inpatients. *N Engl J Med* 338:777–783.

Tosteson AN. 1997. Quality of life in the economic evaluation of osteoporotic prevention. *Spine* 22:58S–62S.

WHO (World Health Organization). 1994. *Assessment of Fracture Risk and Its Application to Screening for Postmenopausal Osteoporosis*. Technical Report Series 843. Geneva: WHO.

Section III

Nutrition Services Along the Continuum of Care

9

Nutrition Services in the Acute Care Setting

In 1967, inpatient hospital costs comprised close to 63 percent of all Medicare payments, while the combined payments to skilled nursing facilities (SNFs), home health agencies (HHAs), and outpatient services were less than 9 percent. During the past two decades, Medicare payment reforms and cost containment initiatives have changed the proportion of payments to inpatient hospitals. By 1996, inpatient hospital costs had dropped to 48 percent of Medicare payments and SNF, HHA, and outpatient services had increased to almost 26 percent of total Medicare payments. However, Medicare spending was concentrated on a relatively small percentage of enrollees. In 1996, approximately 12 percent of Medicare enrollees accounted for more than 75 percent of Medicare payments. The three groups of high-cost users were those with end-stage renal disease, beneficiaries who died (services became more intense as they approached death), and beneficiaries who required an inpatient hospital stay. The leading diagnoses for hospitalized beneficiaries, in terms of Medicare dollars spent, were malignant neoplasms, heart disease, fractures, pneumonia, and cerebrovascular disease (Health Care Financing Administration, 1998). Nutrition is involved in the primary, secondary, and/or tertiary prevention of each of these diseases or conditions.

MEDICARE REIMBURSEMENT IN ACUTE CARE, SHORT-STAY HOSPITALS

A prospective payment system is used by Medicare to reimburse for inpatient hospital costs. This system is based on diagnosis-related groups.

Coverage includes room, meals, nursing services, operating and recovery rooms, intensive care, inpatient prescription drugs, laboratory tests, and x-rays. Professional nutrition services, formulas, and parenteral solutions are also included in this payment.

ROLE OF THE NUTRITION PROFESSIONAL

Licensing standards require that hospitals employ a registered dietitian full-time, part-time, or on a consulting basis. Nutritional needs of patients must be met in accordance with recognized dietary practices and in agreement with orders of the practitioner responsible for the care of the patient (Code of Federal Regulations, 1998).

The Joint Commission on Accreditation of Health Care Organizations (JCAHO) requires that all patients are screened for nutrition problems and, when a problem exists, there is appropriate nutrition intervention. This is an interdisciplinary process. Examples of the roles that various health care providers play can be found in Box 9.1. JCAHO standards also require that a patient's readiness to learn be evaluated and that discharge planning and good transitional care begins when the patient is admitted to the hospital. The JCAHO designates the geriatric population as a high-risk group and has emphasized nutrition in its inspections during the last few years (JCAHO, 1996).

Identification of Nutrition Problems at Admission

Because of the JCAHO standards, most acute care hospitals have procedures to identify or screen patients for nutrition problems within 24 hours of admission. This may be done by the nurse, dietetic technician, or dietitian. The most common criteria used in this evaluation are diagnosis, weight, weight change, need for diet modification or education, problems with chewing or swallowing, diarrhea, constipation, and food dislikes or intolerance. The screening tool may also include specific laboratory values, such as serum albumin and cholesterol concentrations, and hematologic values such as hemoglobin and total lymphocyte count.

Nutrition Assessment

If a problem is identified in the screening, the patient is to be evaluated further by the dietitian. In-depth nutrition assessments may include such things as evaluation of anthropometric, biochemical, and clinical data; evaluation of energy and nutrient intake at home or in the hospital; evaluation of access to food at home; calculation or measurement of energy and nutrient needs; and assessment of learning needs. All of this is done within the context of the patient's disease or condition and any other treatment received. Interventions may include diets that are modified in macro- or micronutrients, diets that are modified in consistency, nutrient or energy supplementation using liquid dietary supplements, vitamin and mineral supplements, enteral or parenteral nutrition support, or nutrition counseling.

Continuum of Care

The nature of nutrition counseling has changed with decreased lengths of stay in acute care facilities. For the most part, patient education in hospitals involves teaching "survival skills" and linking the patient with a dietitian in the ambulatory setting where conditions are more conducive to helping people make long-term behavior changes. However, the lack of reimbursement for nutrition services in the ambulatory setting often limits the resources available to people once they have been discharged from the hospital. Patient education and the ability of people to manage their own care has been reported to be negatively impacted by short stays and inadequate ambulatory nutrition services (Weinberger et al., 1988).

Hospital dietitians also work with discharge planners, attempting to provide a smooth transition between the hospital and nutrition services in skilled nursing facilities or home care. However, few dietitians work in home care and the hospital dietitian is often called upon to advise home care agencies or home infusion companies about patients long after they have been discharged from the hospital.

Hospital dietitians may also refer patients with continuing nutrition or food assistance needs to community agencies, such as food banks, congregate feeding programs, and home-delivered meals.

Older People Needing Intervention for Undernutrition

Hospitalized people have more complicated and costly illnesses today than they did 20 years ago (Duffy and Farley, 1995). Although the overall length of stay has decreased, those patients with the most complex nutrition problems often have longer stays than the average patient and use more nutrition services during their hospital stay. The 24-hour requirement by JCAHO for screening is unrealistic and labor intensive. The methods adopted by many institutions to meet this requirement lack validity in the identification of undernourished patients, often depending on information that is unreliable (see chapter 4) or unavailable.

Some patients are discharged before screening and intervention can take place. Others do not receive the care needed because human re-

BOX 9.1 Roles of Health Care Professionals Providing Nutrition Care in Short-Stay, Acute Care Hospitals

Health Care Professional	Role in Nutrition Care
Physician	Overall responsibility for patient care, including identification of nutrition problems on physical examination (e.g., weight or lean body mass loss, abnormal lab values), ordering, monitoring and evaluating nutrition care. The physician needs to recognize how other kinds of therapy affect nutritional status.
Registered Nurse	Overall responsibility for coordinating patient care. Administering nutrition support regimens. Ongoing monitoring and reporting of effects of nutrition care on patient (e.g., food intake, weight, blood glucose monitoring, food intolerances, other complications), reinforces patient education. Supervises feeding and observation of food intake.
Registered Dietitian	Assessment of nutritional status. Planning, implementing, and evaluating nutrition care for high-risk patients. Integrates nutrition care with other forms of care (e.g., drug food interactions). Oversees work of support personnel (e.g., dietetic technician).
Dietetic Technician	Screens patients for nutrition problems. Provides nutrition care for patients at moderate risk. Plans modi-

sources are tied up with a mandatory screening process that is cumbersome and ineffective. The screening process may need to be simplified and focused on those patients with the most complex nutrition problems. The deadline for completion may also need to be extended so that screening of short-stay patients with the least complex nutrition problems does not overwhelm the limited resources available. Human resources could also be better used to help those patients with the most complex problems, including those needing help with food choices, feeding, or monitoring food intake.

There is also evidence in the literature that intervention for many older people in acute care hospitals is inadequate. Burns and Jensen (1995) reviewed the medical records of 268 "young" (aged 65 to 80 years) and "old" (over 80 years) elderly patients from seven admitting services in a tertiary care teaching hospital. Data in the medical record were used to evaluate the patients' nutritional and functional status, hospital mortality, readmission, and disposition outcome. Data that were needed to

	fied diets. Helps patients choose appropriate foods. Liaison with food service. Monitors and calculates nutrient intake.
Pharmacist	Identifies potential drug-nutrient/food interactions, particularly as they relate to drug bioavailability. Works with dietitian, nurse, physician to order and monitor parenteral nutrition support.
Respiratory Therapist	Observes effects of respiratory problems on food intake or effects of poor nutritional status on respiratory function. May measure and help interpret energy expenditure.
Social Worker	Coordinates transition from hospital to home or other level of care (e.g., provides assistance to patients about community agencies that can help with food access, home nutrition support).
Clergy	Identifies food preferences related to religion.
Rehabilitation— Occupational Therapy Speech Therapy Physical Therapy	Identifies and evaluates limitations in functional status that may affect food intake (e.g., dysphagia, immobility).

SOURCE: University of California at San Francisco Medical Center (1998).

evaluate nutritional status were found in most of the medical records (i.e., serum albumin [31 percent of records]; total lymphocyte count [95 percent of records]; percent ideal body weight [90 percent of records]). Even though investigators found that severe malnutrition was common in this elderly population, there was little evidence that the patient's physicians had identified or documented this. The presence of a positive malnutrition index was associated with older age, impaired functional status, and greater mortality. Patients with malnutrition also required more subsequent health care based on hospital readmissions or referrals to skilled nursing or home care.

Mowé and Bøhmer (1991) studied 121 hospitalized, older patients in Norway. Using anthropometric data (height, weight, triceps skinfold, and midarm circumference measurements), they determined that more than 50 percent of the patients had protein–energy undernutrition. No patients had been given a diagnosis of malnutrition, only a few were characterized as malnourished, and only two of the most undernourished patients received nutrition support while they were in the hospital.

A sample of 250 older patients, admitted to a Department of Veterans Affairs hospital was studied prospectively beginning at hospital admission (Sullivan et al., 1989). A medical and nutritional profile was developed based on information extracted from each patient's chart. This included admitting diagnosis, secondary diagnoses, laboratory values at admission or when first obtained in the hospital, and the physician's and dietitian's work-up. Patients were classified as low risk (44 percent of patients), moderate risk (24 percent), and very high risk (15 percent) of having protein–energy undernutrition, based on serum albumin, total lymphocyte count, and weight for height or body mass index. The rest of the patients (17 percent) had so little data that nutritional status could not be determined. During the entire study period only 36 percent of the study patients and 44 percent of the at-risk patients received a formal evaluation by a dietitian. Dietary intake data for the patients at risk were questionable and nurses reported having inadequate time to monitor nutrient intakes. Patients at risk for protein–energy undernutrition were significantly older and had longer hospital stays.

The most commonly cited reason that nutrition problems are not addressed in the hospital is lack of education or understanding of the importance of nutrition by physicians (Burns and Jensen, 1995; Mowé and Bøhmer, 1991; Sullivan et al., 1989).

EFFECTS OF UNDERNUTRITION ON FUNCTIONAL STATUS IN THE ELDERLY

In 1994, more than one-third of the admissions to nonfederal acute care, short-stay hospitals were for people at least 65 years old. Functional status in the elderly may be lost during acute care hospitalization (Sager et al., 1996). In a large study, the Hospital Outcomes Project for the Elderly, activities of daily living such as bathing and dressing, deteriorated significantly between baseline admission to an acute care hospital and discharge. Forty-one percent of the older individuals were reported to have a continued decline in functional status 3 months after hospitalization; they were unable to recover from hospital-acquired disabilities and had developed additional ones since discharge (Riedinger and Robbins, 1998). The functional decline was attributed to the illness, medical and surgical treatment, and adverse events associated with hospitalization, such as drug events and bed rest or reduced mobility (Sager et al., 1996). Older patients often enter the hospital in an undernourished state which is then exacerbated by changes in diet or inadequate intake as the patient undergoes various diagnostic and therapeutic procedures (Palmer et al., 1998; Riedinger and Robbins, 1998).

FUTURE AREAS FOR RESEARCH

Although the optimal method for identification of undernutrition in hospitalized older people has not been determined, the methods currently employed lack validity and are cumbersome and resource intensive. Additional research needs to be conducted in this area.

SUMMARY

Acute care hospitalizations are associated with a decline in functionality of older people. Poor nutritional status at admission and inadequate nutrient intake during hospitalization may contribute to this decline. Evidence in the literature indicates that identification and intervention for nutrition problems in older patients may be inadequate. Education in the hospital setting is often limited to teaching patients "survival skills" and referring them to the ambulatory setting for additional counseling. However, lack of reimbursement in ambulatory settings limits the resources available to people once they have been discharged from the hospital. Hospital dietitians often provide guidance to home health agencies and home infusion companies who may not have adequate staffing of qualified nutrition professionals.

RECOMMENDATIONS

• Current standards for screening and assessing nutritional status in hospitalized Medicare beneficiaries need to be reassessed and revised. JCAHO requirements for hospital-based nutrition screening, assessment, intervention, and surveillance warrant comprehensive review. In particular, the methods adopted by many institutions to meet 24-hour screening requirements lack validity in the identification of undernourished patients, often depend upon information that is unreliable or unavailable, and are cumbersome and resource intensive.

• Changes in reimbursement have to be made in the ambulatory and home-health settings to provide additional nutrition resources for individuals once they have been discharged from the hospital (see chapters 11 and 12).

REFERENCES

Burns JT, Jensen GL. 1995. Malnutrition among geriatric patients admitted to medical and surgical services in a tertiary care hospital: Frequency, recognition, and associated disposition and reimbursement outcomes. *Nutrition* 11:245–249.

Code of Federal Regulations. 1998. Health Care Financing Administration. Conditions of participation for hospitals. 42CFR482.28. Washington, D.C.: U.S. Government Printing Office.

Duffy SQ, Farley DE. 1995. Patterns of decline among inpatient procedures. *Publ Health Rep* 110:674–681.

Health Care Financing Administration. 1998. *Health Care Financing Review, 1998 Statistical Supplement*. Baltimore, Md.: U.S. Department of Health and Human Services.

JCAHO (Joint Commission on Accreditation of Healthcare Organizations). 1996. *Comprehensive Accreditation Manual for Hospitals. The Official Handbook*. Oakbrook Terrace, Ill.: JCAHO.

Mowé M, Bøhmer T. 1991. The prevalence of undiagnosed protein-calorie undernutrition in a population of hospitalized elderly patients. *J Am Geriatr Soc* 39:1089–1092.

Palmer RM, Counsell S, Landefeld CS. 1998. Clinical intervention trials: The ACE unit. *Clin Geriatr Med* 14:831–849.

Riedinger JL, Robbins LJ. 1998. Prevention of iatrogenic illness: Adverse drug reactions and nosocomial infections in hospitalized older adults. *Clin Geriatr Med* 14:681–698.

Sager MA, Franke T, Inouye SK, Landefeld CS, Morgan TM, Rudberg MA, Siebens H, Winograd CH. 1996. Functional outcomes of acute medical illness and hospitalization in older persons. *Arch Intern Med* 156:645–652.

Sullivan DH, Moriarty MS, Chernoff R, Lipschitz DA. 1989. Patterns of care: An analysis of the quality of nutritional care routinely provided to elderly hospitalized veterans. *J Parenter Enteral Nutr* 13:249–254.

University of California at San Francisco Medical Center. 1998. *Policies and Procedures for Nutrition Services*. San Francisco, Calif.: University of California at San Francisco Medical Center.

Weinberger M, Ault KA, Vinicor F. 1988. Prospective reimbursement and diabetes mellitus. Impact upon glycemic control and utilization of health services. *Med Care* 26:77–83.

10

Nutrition Support

Nutrition support, defined as the provision of enteral or parenteral nutrition, has made great strides over the past three decades. Enteral nutrition includes oral ingestion of foods or supplements as well as the non-volitional administration of nutrients by tube into the gastrointestinal tract. Parenteral nutrition is the intravenous administration of nutrients into the bloodstream, by either peripheral or central venous access routes. Nutrition administered by the peripheral route is termed peripheral parenteral nutrition, and by the central route total parenteral nutrition (TPN). Improvements in enteral and parenteral techniques, equipment, nutrient formulations, and gastrointestinal and venous access devices have enabled the provision of nutrients to many patients who might otherwise have received inadequate or inappropriate nutrition. Reflecting shifting health care demographics in America, Medicare beneficiaries comprise a substantial proportion of all adult patients who receive parenteral or enteral nutrition in hospitals.

Although it is generally accepted that adequate nutrition plays an important role in maintaining optimal health, many hospitalized patients have compromised nutrient intakes for extended periods (Sullivan et al., 1999). Studies document a prevalence of protein–energy undernutrition among hospitalized older persons that exceeds one-third of all admissions (Constans et al., 1992; Mowé and Bøhmer, 1991; Sullivan et al., 1989). Many elderly are undernourished prior to hospitalization (Mowé et al., 1994). The nutritional status of older patients at hospital discharge is also predictive of the need for early nonelective readmission to the hospital (Friedmann et al., 1997; Sullivan, 1992).

The indications for providing nutrients by the enteral or parenteral route have not been well defined, and the efficacy of nutrition support is unproven in many circumstances. Nutrition support is most frequently used as short-term therapy for hospitalized patients with protein–energy undernutrition. The consequences of protein–energy undernutrition include depletion of body cell mass and decline of vital tissue and organ functions (see chapter 4). Compromise in host defense and wound-healing functions can result in suboptimal response to medical and surgical therapies. Complications may include hospital-acquired infections and wound breakdown. Adverse outcomes that may result include increased morbidity and mortality with associated increased length of hospital stay and increased use of health care resources (Friedmann et al., 1997; Incalzi et al., 1998; Jensen et al., 1997; Marinella and Markert, 1998; Sullivan et al., 1999).

The rationale for the provision of nutrition support includes (1) to mitigate the effects of semi-starvation, and (2) to favorably alter the natural history or response to treatment for a disease. Nutrition support is clearly indicated when food intake or nutrient assimilation will be compromised for an extended period, since starvation and death will otherwise result. Such patients may include those with inadequate gastrointestinal function (e.g., short-bowel syndrome or chronic intestinal obstruction), as well as those with severe oropharyngeal dysfunction or permanent neurological impairment.

Enteral and parenteral nutrition support of shorter duration can also prevent and treat protein–energy undernutrition among other selected Medicare beneficiaries in the hospital setting. Complications can be reduced among patients who are either undernourished or at high risk of becoming undernourished. Such patients may include those who have suffered major abdominal trauma or who undergo major elective abdominal surgery (Heyland, 1998; Kudsk et al., 1992; Moore et al., 1992; Müller et al., 1982; Senkal et al., 1997; VA TPN Cooperative Study Group, 1991). Reported benefits have included decreased rates of septic and wound complications, with resulting reductions in number of hospital days and cost.

There are also risks associated with enteral and parenteral nutrition support that must be taken into consideration. Serious complications include aspiration of enteral feedings and infectious and thrombotic events related to parenteral venous access (Cataldi-Betcher et al., 1983; Ryan et al., 1974). Appreciable under- or overfeeding can result in adverse metabolic consequences (Dark et al., 1985; Keys et al., 1950). Feeding intolerance, derangement of fluid balance, and laboratory abnormalities may be observed with refeeding of the undernourished patient (Solomon and Kirby, 1990; Weinsier and Krumdieck, 1981). Such complications can also be associated with increased lengths of hospital stay and health care expenditures.

LITERATURE REVIEW

The Committee on Nutrition Services for Medicare Beneficiaries sought to critically review the available nutrition support literature according to the guidelines of the Agency for Healthcare Research and Quality (formerly the Agency for Health Care Policy and Research). The committee was greatly assisted in this process by the availability of several recent review articles of this literature that served as a strong foundation (ASPEN, 1993; Heyland et al., 1998; Klein et al., 1997; Pillar and Perry, 1990; Souba, 1997). In addition to systematic examination of the literature used to support these reviews, relevant new material was examined from the past 5 years, corresponding to more than 1,500 parenteral and 2,000 enteral citations from Medline in both the English and the non-English scientific literature. The general approach taken by the committee was to clarify the type of evidence available and to specifically highlight evidence in relation to persons 65 years of age or older. When there was no specific evidence available in relation to older persons, the committee attempted to ascertain what might reasonably be generalized from studies of middle-aged adults. Both the types of evidence and any relevant assumptions are clearly highlighted for each section. The limitations of current data and future research needs and recommendations are summarized for each indication for nutrition support.

INDICATIONS FOR THE USE OF NUTRITION SUPPORT

GASTROINTESTINAL DISEASES

Short-Bowel Syndrome

Extensive resection of the small intestine can result in inadequate intestinal length and/or function to maintain normal fluid, electrolyte, and nutritional homeostasis. Short-bowel syndrome is characterized by severe malabsorption and resulting dehydration, electrolyte losses, metabolic abnormalities, and undernutrition (Purdum and Kirby, 1991). Since clinical experience has demonstrated the clear efficacy of nutrition support in this setting, prospective randomized trials that include nonintervention arms have not been and are unlikely to be conducted. No studies have focused specifically on older persons with short-bowel syndrome, but many of the patients who have benefited from nutrition support intervention for this condition are Medicare eligible. Indeed 21 percent of all registrants in the North American Home Parenteral and Enteral Nutrition Patient Registry with a diagnosis of motility disorder were Medicare beneficiaries (Howard and Malone, 1997).

Patients with substantial intestinal resection will often require TPN temporarily until adequate adaptation of the remaining intestine occurs to facilitate transition to enteral feedings by tube or mouth. The use of TPN in these patients hastens rehabilitation and transition to the home care setting. Some patients with profound malabsorption require indefinite parenteral support for survival. The degree of impairment of nutrient assimilation is determined by the remaining bowel anatomy and function.

The least favorable anatomical alteration is to have combined resections of both the small and the large intestines and resulting decreased function (Gouttebel et al., 1986; Nightingale et al., 1990). Nonetheless, even in the setting of long-term TPN dependence, it is sometimes possible with aggressive enteral nutritional supplementation and rehydration therapies, in combination with pharmacologic interventions, to modulate gut secretions and transit in order to obviate the need for parenteral support (Cosnes et al., 1985; Lennard-Jones, 1990). The applications of specific hormonal and nutrient growth factors to increase intestinal mass and absorptive function are being tested in active research and may offer important therapeutic opportunities (Byrne et al., 1995).

Enterocutaneous Fistulas

Case series demonstrate a high prevalence of undernutrition among fistula patients and suggest that the most undernourished patients have the worst clinical outcomes (Chapman et al., 1964; Dudrick et al., 1999; Rose et al., 1986; Soeters et al., 1979). Prior to the use of nutrition support, many of these patients suffered severe dehydration, electrolyte derangements, and undernutrition. The role of nutrition intervention is primarily supportive care to prevent further deterioration.

Retrospective analysis of clinical experience with patients having small-bowel fistulas found that those patients who received nutrition support had lower mortality rates, higher rates of spontaneous fistula closure, and superior surgical closure outcomes (Himal et al., 1974). Prospective randomized trials have not been conducted that rigorously evaluate the role of nutrition support in the treatment of enterocutaneous fistulas, and older patients have not been specifically investigated. Such studies are unlikely to be undertaken because it appears likely that medical therapy that includes TPN in conjunction with bowel rest and pharmacologic intervention (i.e., octreotide and histamine receptor antagonists) favors spontaneous fistula closure and improved clinical outcomes (di Costanzo et al., 1987; Dudrick et al., 1999; Meguid and Campos, 1996). Spontaneous closure will occur within 5 weeks in 40 to 60 percent of patients treated with this approach, and if surgical intervention to close the fistula proves necessary then nutritional status will be maintained. Although elemental diets have been successfully used for enteral feeding in patients with fistulas, there are no randomized prospective studies that contrast this approach with TPN (Dudrick et al., 1999; Meguid and Campos, 1996).

Inflammatory Bowel Disease

Protein–energy undernutrition and specific nutrient deficiencies are common among patients with inflammatory bowel disease. Even patients with long-standing Crohn's disease in remission demonstrate a variety of nutritional deficiencies (Geerling et al., 1998). Sequelae of inflammatory bowel disease and related treatment interventions can result in decreased nutrient intake, malabsorption, enteropathy, and drug–nutrient interactions. Although nutrition therapy is often part of the overall management plan, its role in primary therapy remains controversial. However, in those patients who suffer inadequate intestinal length or function as a result of surgery or complications associated with inflammatory bowel disease (short-bowel syndrome or enterocutaneous fistula), nutrition support clearly will be efficacious.

A number of randomized prospective trials have examined the roles of bowel rest and TPN in inducing remission in patients with active Crohn's disease (Greenberg et al., 1988; Lochs et al., 1984; Wright and Adler, 1990). None of these studies focused specifically on older persons. Bowel rest alone, independent of nutritional support, did not appear necessary to achieve clinical remission, and long-term outcome was not affected. There was also no apparent role for TPN as primary therapy in the specific treatment of Crohn's disease or ulcerative colitis (Dickinson et al., 1980; McIntyre et al., 1986). Patients randomized to bowel rest and TPN had no better outcomes than those assigned to enteral feedings (González-Huix et al., 1993).

Enteral diets using elemental formula[1] have been suggested to be as effective as glucocorticoid therapy in inducing remission of Crohn's disease, but the majority of randomized prospective trials suffer from small size, heterogeneous participants, variable diet composition and intake,

---

[1]A liquid formula designed for easy digestion and absorption and leaves minimal residue in the bowel.

and disproportionate withdrawals among the enteral treatment arm (Bernstein and Shanahan, 1996). Again no studies focus specifically on older persons. Meta-analysis of prospective randomized trials suggests that enteral nutrition may not be as effective as corticosteroids (Fernández-Bañares et al., 1995; Griffiths et al., 1995; Trallori et al., 1996). Since there are no studies that randomize to enteral feedings versus placebo, it is not possible to discern the therapeutic benefit of enteral feeding alone.

Pancreatitis

No studies of nutrition support in pancreatitis have focused specifically on older persons. The potential benefits of nutrition support for patients with acute pancreatitis may be best determined by the severity of the disease. The majority of patients with acute pancreatitis have mild or moderate disease. Prospective randomized trials indicate that the provision of enteral or parenteral nutrition does not alter the natural history of pancreatitis in this setting (Sax et al., 1987). Indeed, the administration of TPN to patients with pancreatitis resulted in greater insulin requirements and higher prevalence of catheter-related sepsis than that observed in a control group who received only intravenous fluids (Sax et al., 1987). McClave and coworkers (1997) found that enteral feedings were well tolerated in such patients and that clinical outcomes were comparable to TPN. Beneficial effects of aggressive nutrition support on morbidity or mortality have not been realized and hospital costs are elevated in those who receive TPN.

Although most patients with mild or moderate pancreatitis require only routine supportive measures, it is not clear how long such patients will tolerate semistarvation. If the course is protracted, severe, or complicated, nutrition support may be indicated (Baron and Morgan, 1999; Wyncoll, 1999). Recent prospective trials have randomized patients with severe pancreatitis to enteral feeding versus TPN (Kalfarentzos et al., 1997; Windsor et al., 1998). The enteral feedings were well tolerated and had no adverse clinical effects. There were fewer total and infectious complications, and the acute-phase response and disease severity scores were favorably attenuated with enteral nutrition.

Liver Disease

Although many patients with chronic liver disease suffer protein–energy undernutrition (Lautz et al., 1992; Mendenhall et al., 1984), the efficacy of nutrition support for these patients is not yet established. Older persons with liver disease have not been specifically evaluated in this regard. Whereas some laboratory measures of liver function appear to be improved with the provision of enteral or parenteral nutrition to patients with chronic alcoholic liver diseases, other outcomes are less clear (Mizock, 1999). Some prospective randomized trials have observed improved survival among patients with chronic alcoholic liver diseases who receive enteral or parenteral nutrition (Cerra et al., 1985), while others have not (Nasrallah and Galambos, 1980; Naveau et al., 1986; Naylor et al., 1989).

Meta-analysis of prospective randomized trials that evaluated TPN formulations enriched with branched-chain amino acids suggests that recovery from acute hepatic encephalopathy may be hastened (Naylor et al., 1989). The follow-up for these studies was, however, of short duration, and many of the control subjects received TPN that contained no amino acids. In a prospective randomized trial that included control patients who received TPN with a standard amino acid formulation, a beneficial effect of branched-chain amino acids was not observed (Michel et al., 1985).

Enteral nutrition is well-tolerated by many patients with liver diseases (Cabré et al., 1990; Hirsch et al., 1993; Kearns et al., 1992) and clinical trials suggest that simple casein-based enteral feeding may be efficacious in promoting recovery from acute hepatic encephalopathy (Christie et al., 1985; Horst et al., 1984; Kearns et al., 1992).

Gastrointestinal Disease Summary

Short-Bowel Syndrome. Provision of enteral and parenteral nutrition support has established efficacy in the prevention of life-threatening undernutrition for patients with inadequate intestinal length and/or function.

Enterocutaneous Fistulas. Parenteral nutrition in combination with bowel rest and pharmacologic intervention to diminish gastrointestinal secretions appears likely to improve the opportunity for spontaneous fistula closure and more favorable clinical outcomes. Studies are insufficient to address the role of enteral nutrition in fistula management.

Inflammatory Bowel Disease. Enteral and parenteral nutrition support is likely to be indicated for inflammatory bowel disease patients who suffer undernutrition related to compromised intestinal length and/or function. Although enteral nutrition may have a therapeutic role in the treatment of Crohn's disease, it appears that corticosteroids are more effective. In addition, the use of TPN is not supported as primary therapy.

Pancreatitis. The routine use of enteral and parenteral nutrition is not indicated in patients with mild or moderate pancreatitis. If the course is protracted or severe, nutrition support may be considered. Studies are inadequate to clarify the optimal timing, feeding route, or formulation for this indication. Enteral feedings may be well tolerated in selected patients.

Liver Disease. Enteral and parenteral nutrition may improve some laboratory measures of liver function in patients with chronic alcoholic liver diseases. Studies are conflicting with regard to whether there are associated improvements in survival. It is also unclear whether branched-chain amino acid-enriched formulations offer advantage in accelerated recovery from acute hepatic encephalopathy.

Gastrointestinal Disease Recommendations

- There is a need for well-designed clinical trials of nutrition support interventions for gastrointestinal disease. Studies should include older persons. Indications for nutrition support require further clarification for inflammatory bowel disease, pancreatitis, and liver diseases. The use of specific nutrients, growth factors, and modified nutrient formulations warrants further investigation.
- The use of enteral and parenteral nutrition is recommended as life-sustaining and supportive therapy for patients with short-bowel syndrome and enterocutaneous fistula.

HUMAN IMMUNODEFICIENCY VIRUS AND ACQUIRED IMMUNE DEFICIENCY SYNDROME

Even though the incidence of acquired immune deficiency syndrome (AIDS) is higher among younger age groups, persons aged 50 years or older accounted for 11 percent of all AIDS cases in the United States in 1996 (CDC, 1998). The Centers for Disease Control and Prevention (CDC) estimated that newly reported AIDS cases among persons ages 50 years and older increased by 12.6 percent (from 55,819 to 62,874) from mid-1996 to mid-1997 (CDC, 1997). This increase is alarming since the number of new AIDS cases reported annually is declining among younger persons. Because many older persons do not perceive themselves to be at risk for human immunodeficiency virus (HIV)/AIDS, they may delay testing and be diagnosed at a later stage of disease, placing them at increased risk of malnutrition associated with AIDS. AIDS-related malnutrition is associated with loss of lean body mass, which in turn can lead to reduced functional capacity and diminished quality of life (Grinspoon et al., 1999;

Wilson and Cleary, 1997). In two studies (Turner et al., 1994; Wilson and Cleary, 1997), loss of lean body mass, resulting in fatigue and weakness, was closely associated with functional status, an important aspect of quality of life. Although wasting is less common, significant loss of lean body mass occurs even in patients who are receiving highly active antiretroviral therapy (Grinspoon et al., 1997). Moreover, highly active antiretroviral therapy may contribute to deleterious fat redistribution, as well as the premature development of cardiovascular disease and diabetes mellitus in some patients (Carr et al., 1998; Dubé et al., 1997; Henry et al., 1998). Other studies have documented a correlation between weight loss and more rapid disease progression, increased risk for hospitalization and opportunistic infections, and reduced tolerance of and response to treatments (Rivera et al., 1998; Wheeler et al., 1998; Wilson and Cleary, 1997).

A growing body of evidence suggests that nutrition counseling and/or nutrition support may improve nutritional status in persons with HIV/AIDS. In a 6-week randomized, controlled trial, Rabeneck and colleagues (1998) found that nutrition counseling, with or without oral supplementation, achieved a substantial increase in energy intake in nearly half of their malnourished HIV-infected patients. Compared to the counseling-only group, the supplement group had greater increases in fat-free mass and grip strength. A study by Stack and colleagues (1996) found that HIV-infected patients without secondary infections were able to maintain or gain weight with a high-energy, high-protein supplement used in conjunction with nutrition counseling. Studies of omega-3 fatty acid supplementation have shown that fish oil may be efficacious in lowering hypertriglyceridemia and increasing lean body mass (Bell et al., 1996; Hellerstein et al., 1996). Studies of oral and enteral supplements designed especially for HIV/AIDS indicate that these products are associated with greater weight gain when compared to standard supplements (Pichard et al., 1998; Süttmann et al., 1996). The majority of weight gain in these studies was fat, however, as opposed to lean body mass. In a randomized study comparing total parenteral nutrition to dietary counseling in severely malnourished men (loss of more than 10 percent usual body weight and concomitant diarrhea), weight increased by a mean of 8 kg in the parenteral nutrition group and decreased by a mean of 3 kg in the dietary counseling group (Melchior et al., 1996). The administration of TPN increased body cell mass in men with AIDS wasting and malabsorption and gastrointestinal disease, but those with secondary infections continued to lose body cell mass despite TPN administration. A recent study by Kotler et al. (1998) compared TPN to a semielemental diet given to AIDS patients with malabsorption syndrome. Patients receiving TPN consumed more calories and gained more weight than patients receiving the oral formula; however, weight gain was a function of total calorie intake. As in other studies, the composition of weight gained was predominantly fat. In this study, the semielemental diet was less costly than TPN and associated with improvement in quality of life, specifically functional status.

In summary, there are limited but consistent data that nutrition counseling and support in HIV/AIDS are associated with greater calorie intake and weight gain. Because the weight gain was due to fat deposition as opposed to lean body mass accrual in some of the studies, exercise and pharmacologic agents may be indicated as adjuncts to nutrition interventions to produce an increase in lean body mass. Further research is needed to identify optimum combinations of nutrition interventions, pharmacologic approaches, and exercise that will maximize nutritional status and clinical outcomes in HIV/AIDS in a cost-effective manner, particularly in persons aged 50 years and older. Methodological problems of the studies discussed in this section include the short-term nature of the nutrition interventions, the lack of inclusion of clinical outcome measures (e.g., functional status, quality of life) that may respond to nutrition therapy, and the homogeneity of the study populations which consist of mostly younger, homosexual white males.

HIV/AIDS Summary

Weight loss in patients with AIDS is correlated with more rapid disease progression, increased risk of hospitalization and opportunistic infections, and reduced tolerance of and response to treatments. Loss of lean body mass is correlated with diminished functional status, a component of quality of life. There are limited, but consistent, data that nutrition counseling and oral, enteral, and parenteral nutrition promote calorie intake and weight gain in AIDS patients who have experienced significant weight loss or have malabsorption, but who do not have secondary infections. There are limited data which indicate that total parenteral nutrition may be more costly and associated with lower quality of life than either oral or enteral nutrition.

HIV/AIDS Recommendations

• Nutrition therapy to improve caloric intake and weight gain in persons with AIDS is recommended using a multidisciplinary team of nutrition support professionals. Parenteral nutrition is costly and may therefore be indicated only in select cases.

• Further research should focus on the development of the most effective combinations of nutrition and adjunctive (e.g., exercise) therapies which increase lean body mass, especially in persons with AIDS who are aged 50 years and older.

CANCER AND BONE MARROW TRANSPLANTATION

Chemotherapy and Radiation Therapy

The CDC (1999) estimated that there were 1,374,000 cancer-related hospital discharges in 1996, with an average length of stay of 7 days. More than two-thirds of cancer patients lose weight during their disease course (Rowan Chlebowski, Harbor-UCLA Medical Center, personal communication, 1999). Since 60 percent of all cancers occur in older adults who may already have preexisting special nutritional needs, this is a significant problem. Studies of nutrition support during cancer chemotherapy, radiation therapy, and bone marrow transplantation report mixed results. Three meta-analyses that examined the use of TPN in cancer patients undergoing chemotherapy or radiation therapy reported no benefit of TPN in terms of tumor response, treatment tolerance, or survival. Moreover, TPN administration in these patient populations was associated with higher rates of pneumonia and sepsis (ACP, 1989; Klein et al., 1986; McGeer et al., 1990). Systematic reviews have also indicated that enteral and parenteral nutrition may not be efficacious for cancer patients undergoing these particular treatments (Klein and Koretz, 1994; Klein et al., 1997). However, the reviews point out that serious shortcomings in study design and methods make it difficult to draw definitive conclusions from the data.

Since these reviews (Klein and Koretz, 1994; Klein et al., 1997), a few studies have evaluated the use of nutrition support in cancer patients treated with chemotherapy. In one clinical trial, malnourished gastrointestinal cancer patients who received both parenteral nutrition and chemotherapy preoperatively had fewer complications and more tumor sensitivity to chemotherapy than patients without nutrition support (Jin et al., 1999). In another trial involving metastatic cancer patients treated with high doses of interleukin-2, a brief course of TPN during treatment corrected calorie and protein undernutrition, improved control of serum electrolytes, and was well tolerated (Samlowski et al., 1998). A prospective study of nutrition support in patients receiving antineoplastic therapy indicated that parenteral nutrition successfully maintained the body weight of patients who were unable to receive enteral nutrition (Lees, 1997). A retrospective study of chemotherapy and TPN for advanced ovarian cancer patients with bowel obstruction found that median survival was 17 days longer ($p < 0.05$) for patients who received chemotherapy with TPN than for patients who received chemotherapy alone (Abu-Rustum et al., 1997). In a retrospective study of nutrition support during chemoradiation therapy in esophageal cancer, parenteral nutrition facilitated the administration of complete chemoradiation doses (Sikora et al., 1998).

Bone Marrow Transplantation

With increasing frequency, bone marrow transplantation (BMT) is used in treating patients with hematologic malignancies who are over the age of 65 years. Due to the severe gastrointestinal side effects of total body irradiation and chemotherapy, BMT patients are frequently unable to eat for 2 or more weeks following transplantation. TPN traditionally has been used to meet the nutritional needs of the BMT patient population (Aker et al., 1982). In a systematic review of studies involving bone marrow transplant patients, the use of standard TPN was generally not found to be associated with improved clinical outcomes (Klein et al., 1997). One exception occurred in a prospective study of 137 patients (age greater than 1 year) who were randomized to either a TPN or a no-TPN group (Weisdorf et al., 1987). They found that patients receiving short-term TPN had increased long-term survival (more than 6 months), decreased rate of tumor relapse, and increased energy intake when compared to the no-TPN control group. More recently, the effects of a lipid-based versus a glucose-based TPN solution on 66 randomly assigned bone marrow transplant patients were evaluated (Muscaritoli et al., 1998). The results suggest that the use of a lipid-based TPN solution was associated with a lower incidence of acute graft-versus-host disease and hyperglycemia. However, the lack of a control group makes the study findings difficult to interpret.

Szeluga and colleagues (1987) randomized patients to TPN versus an enteral-oral feeding program and found that the nutritional needs of 23 of 30 patients could be met with the enteral feeding program. The safety of enteral feeding in bone marrow transplant patients was also documented in a small group of patients undergoing autologous BMT (Mulder et al., 1989).

A few studies have focused on the benefit of oral or parenteral feedings supplemented with the amino acid glutamine. Forty-five patients (aged 20 to 49) were randomly assigned to a double-blind, controlled trial of glutamine-supplemented versus standard TPN (Ziegler et al., 1992). They found that patients whose TPN was supplemented with glutamine had significantly greater nitrogen balance, fewer infections, less bacterial colonization, and shortened hospital stay compared to patients who received standard TPN. A significantly reduced hospital stay, as well as significantly less fluid retention, was reported in 29 patients (average age 35 years) who were randomly assigned to a similar TPN protocol with or without glutamine (Schloerb and Amare, 1993). MacBurney and colleagues (1994) calculated hospital charges for patients in the 1992 Ziegler et al. study and found significantly lower charges ($51,484 versus $61,591, $p = 0.02$) in the group of patients receiving the glutamine-supplemented formula. However, Schloreb and Skikne (1999) randomly assigned 48 patients (aged 26 to 56) to oral and parenteral glutamine or isocaloric and isonitrogenous oral and parenteral therapy without glutamine. They concluded that glutamine is of limited benefit to bone marrow transplant patients.

Cancer and Bone Marrow Transplantation Summary

There is insufficient evidence to suggest that nutrition support has been shown to be efficacious in cancer patients undergoing chemotherapy or radiation therapy. The limitations of the available data, however, do not rule out the possible utility of nutrition support in older cancer patients undergoing chemotherapy or radiation therapy. In bone marrow transplantation, enteral nutrition is safe and can be used to meet energy needs. In addition to various methodological flaws, none of the studies explicitly studied older persons. Many of the cancer trials are conducted with younger subjects even though older persons comprise the majority of cancer patients.

Cancer and Bone Marrow Transplantation Recommendations

• Until additional data, including data specific to the elderly, become available, nutrition support should be used selectively in malnourished cancer patients undergoing radiation therapy and/or chemotherapy.

• Enteral nutrition may be considered for bone marrow transplantation patients who are unable to eat due to the side effects of chemoradiation. TPN is recommended for those who have protracted gastrointestinal dysfunction.

• More prospective, randomized clinical trials of older cancer patients are necessary to determine whether a relationship exists between nutrition support and clinical outcomes. Additional studies are needed before recommendations can be made concerning the efficacy of specific amino acid formulations in bone marrow transplant patients.

ACUTE RENAL FAILURE

Hospitalized patients with acute renal failure will often have serious underlying comorbid disease and may be critically ill and in a catabolic state (Ikizler and Himmelfarb, 1997). Protein–energy undernutrition is highly prevalent among acute renal failure patients and is associated with increased likelihood of death, complications, and use of health care resources (Fiaccadori et al., 1999). Since anorexia, nausea, vomiting, and metabolic derangement are common, these patients may suffer compromised nutritional intakes for extended periods. When clinically indicated, the initiation of acute hemodialysis or ultrafiltration facilitates the provision of adequate amino acids or protein but also promotes nutrient losses (Ikizler et al., 1994; Mehta, 1994; Wolfson et al., 1982).

There have been no prospective randomized trials of enteral nutrition in the setting of acute renal failure. A number of studies with modest subject numbers and variable control groups have examined the use of TPN. None of these investigations have explicitly studied older persons. Only one well-designed randomized trial with 53 subjects has detected a significant improvement in recovery from acute renal failure among patients treated with parenteral glucose and essential amino acids in comparison to glucose alone (Abel et al., 1973). Two smaller studies of similar design did not observe an accelerated recovery of renal function with essential amino acid treatment (Feinstein et al., 1981; Leonard et al., 1975). Improved survival rates have also been described for patients who received essential amino acids in TPN in comparison to glucose alone, but these did not achieve statistical significance (Abel et al., 1973; Feinstein et al., 1981). Other randomized studies of TPN with small numbers of subjects have tested formulations enriched in essential amino acids in comparison to formulations containing both essential and nonessential amino acids (Feinstein et al., 1981, 1983; Mirtallo et al., 1982). While recovery and survival rates favored the essential amino acid formulations, statistically significant differences were not observed.

Acute Renal Failure Summary

Although parenteral formulations enriched in essential amino acids may improve patient outcomes in acute renal failure, data are insufficient to make conclusions regarding clinical efficacy. The limited data from younger adults are insufficient to make any generalizations about specific nutrition support therapy to be used in the older person with acute renal failure.

Acute Renal Failure Recommendations

• Well-conceived clinical trials of nutrition support interventions are needed in patients with acute renal failure.
• Studies should include older persons.
• The role of specific nutrient supplementation must be clarified in studies with adequate control groups and methodology.

For a discussion of the efficacy of nutrition therapy for chronic renal failure, see chapter 7.

CRITICAL ILLNESS

Nutrition support is often used in patients with critical illness, although benefit has been difficult to demonstrate given the great diversity of patient conditions and variable severity of illness. Studies have suffered from the inability to acquire adequate samples of homogeneous patients, inadequately controlled designs, concurrent treatments, and ill-defined outcome measures. Older persons have been excluded from many of the clinical trials that have examined the role of nutrition support in critical illness. Heyland and colleagues (1998) recently presented a meta-analysis of 26 randomized trials comparing the use of TPN with standard care (usual oral diet and intravenous dextrose) in 2,211 pooled patients with critical illness or surgery. It was concluded that TPN does not influence overall mortality rate or major complication rates in critically ill patients. Post-hoc subgroup analyses suggested that TPN might reduce the complication rate in malnourished patients. Unfortunately, this benefit was limited to studies published prior to 1989, studies that did not use intravenous lipids, and studies of surgical patients. These findings are likely confounded by the unsound methodology used in the older studies and the general limitations of studies of critical illness described above.

There has been a growing emphasis on enteral feeding when feasible for patients with critical illness because the provision of nutrients via the gastrointestinal lumen appears to help maintain mucosal structure and function of the intestine (Buchman et al., 1995; Hadfield et al., 1995; Hernandez et al., 1999). The "gut injury" hypothesis suggests that a breakdown in mucosal barrier function associated with the lack of luminal nutrients when giving TPN may facilitate the translocation of intestinal flora and their associated endotoxin, thereby fueling inflammatory pathways (Deitch, 1990). Enteral feeding of critically ill patients has numerous proponents but remains controversial (Lipman, 1998; Minard and Kudsk, 1998; Moore and Moore, 1996). Unfortunately there are so few studies that directly contrast carefully matched enteral and parenteral nutrition that a meta-analysis comparing these interventions across the spectrum of critical illness is not feasible.

Patients with major trauma, including major blunt or penetrating trauma, head injury, or burn, are at high risk of protein–energy undernutrition. These patients are often hypermetabolic with ongoing injury response. They may be unable to eat for extended periods and may have compromise to intestinal function. They may also have complex wounds that require repeated surgical interventions. Clinical trials of nutrition support in trauma patients have not included appreciable numbers of older persons. Nonintervention controls are also lacking. A number of trials have found enteral nutrition to be superior to parenteral nutrition in reducing septic complications in abdominal trauma patients (Kudsk et al., 1992; Moore and Jones, 1986; Moore et al., 1989, 1992). It is not evident whether there is a specific benefit to enteral nutrition or alternatively whether TPN is associated with increased risk of infections. Thus, the benefits of nutrition support in trauma have not been clearly established.

Nutrition support should offer benefit for patients with severe head injury since they will otherwise be subject to protracted semistarvation. While early studies (Rapp et al., 1983) suggested that parenteral nutrition had more favorable outcomes when head-injured patients received greater parenteral than enteral nutrition, more recent clinical trials have observed equivalent outcomes with enteral or parenteral nutrition when nutrient intakes are comparable (Borzotta et al., 1994; Grahm et al., 1989; Norton et al., 1988).

A number of small prospective randomized trials have examined assorted nutrition support interventions in patients with burns (Alexander et al., 1980; Brown et al., 1990; Chiarelli et al., 1990; Herndon et al., 1987; Liljedahl et al., 1982), but in the absence of rigorous clinical trials, the guidelines for intervention are largely empiric. Enteral feedings have been shown to be well tolerated by burn patients and modified nutrient formulations have been shown to diminish the rate of infection (Garrel et al., 1995; Gottschlich et al., 1990).

New strategies are being tested to modulate immune functions in critical illness using modified enteral formulations that have been enriched in nutrients which may have immune-enhancing or preserving functions. Nutrients tested include arginine, nucleotides, glutamine, and omega-3 fatty acids. Prospective randomized trials have suggested potential benefits such as reductions in infectious complications and hospital length of stay when such modified enteral formulas are compared to standard enteral feedings (Bower et al., 1995; Brown et al., 1994; Daly et al., 1992; Moore et al., 1994). These studies, however, have been questioned as to their conclusions because of the inclusion of multiple nutrients that may impact immune functions, the mismatching of control feedings for nitrogen and/or energy, and the extensive use of post-hoc subgroup analysis. More recent trials have attempted to address these concerns, and have found benefit to groups receiving the modified formulas (Atkinson et al., 1998; Daly et al., 1995; Houdijk et al., 1998; Kudsk et al., 1996; Senkal et al., 1997). An evidence-based review by Zaloga (1998) found that 12 of 13 prospective randomized clinical trials attributed beneficial outcomes to immune-enhancing enteral formulas and that evidence for their use among critically ill patients would meet level I recommendation criteria. A meta-analysis by Heys and colleagues (1999) examined 11 prospective randomized trials of enteral nutritional supplementation with formulations containing key nutrients felt to favor immune function. The control subjects received standard enteral formulas. There were a total of 1,009 evaluable subjects who were critically ill patients with trauma or burn or were patients who had surgery for gastrointestinal cancer. Findings suggested that enteral feeding with formulas with a combination of possible immune-enhancing nutrients added resulted in a significant reduction in the risk of infectious complications and reduced the length of overall hospital stay in patients with critical illness and patients with gastrointestinal cancer. There was, however, no effect on mortality. Although older persons are subject to relative decline in immunocompetence with aging and might accrue benefit from such modified feeding formulations, these feedings have not yet been rigorously evaluated for efficacy among older, critically ill patients.

Critical Illness Summary

The benefits of enteral versus parenteral nutrition support have not been clearly established for patients with critical illness. The preponderance of recent research suggests that trauma patients fed enteral nutrition have fewer complications than those given TPN. Nutrient formulations modified with specific nutrients which may preserve or promote immune or other vital functions have shown promise in preliminary trials with critically ill patients, but studies among older persons are inadequate to draw definitive conclusions for the Medicare population at this time.

Critical Illness Recommendations

• There is a need for prospective randomized trials of enteral versus parenteral nutrition in well-characterized subgroups of critically ill patients. Older persons should be included and, when safe and appropriate, nonintervention controls should be considered.

• The efficacy of supplementation with specific nutrients in regard to immune or other vital functions in the critically ill warrants further investigation with well-designed prospective randomized trials that focus on single nutrients and include appropriate controls.

PERIOPERATIVE NUTRITION SUPPORT

The effect of perioperative nutritional support—that is, nutrition support given before and/or after surgery—has been evaluated in a number of prospective randomized clinical trials, in meta-analyses, and by expert groups. These evaluations indicate that perioperative nutrition support is efficacious in selected surgical populations such as gastrointestinal cancer surgery patients and elderly hip fracture patients. In addition, there is current evidence and expert opinion supporting the use of nutritional support in severely malnourished patients undergoing major elective surgery and in surgical patients unable to eat for more than 1 to 2 weeks pre- and/or postoperatively.

Gastrointestinal Surgery

Enteral Nutrition

A meta-analysis of six randomized, controlled clinical trials of gastrointestinal cancer surgery patients treated postoperatively with enteral supplements enriched with selected nutrients (Heys et al., 1999) revealed a significant reduction in the risk of developing infectious complications and in length of stay in the treatment patients compared to patients receiving standard enteral nutrition. The enriched enteral nutrition formulas had no effect on incidence of pneumonia or death.

One large study included in the meta-analysis was a multicenter trial conducted in Germany (Senkal et al., 1997). Within 12 hours of upper gastrointestinal cancer surgery, patients were randomized to receive an enteral formula enriched with arginine, dietary nucleotides, and omega-3 fatty acids (n = 77, mean age 65 years) or a standard formula with identical calorie and protein content (n = 77, mean age 66 years). Early feeding was well tolerated by both patient groups. Patients who received the enriched formula experienced significantly fewer late (more than 5 days after surgery) infectious and wound-healing complications compared with the standard enteral group. The costs for treating the complications were substantially less in the enriched-formula group compared to the standard-formula group.

Another large study included in the meta-analysis reported similar findings (Braga et al., 1998). Gastrointestinal surgery patients (n = 166, mean age 62 years) were randomized into one of three groups: a standard-formula group, an enriched-formula group, or a TPN group. In all three groups, nutrition support was initiated 12 hours after surgery. Early enteral feeding was well tolerated by both groups given enteral formulas. In a subgroup of malnourished and transfused patients, the enriched-formula group had significantly less severe infectious complications and a shorter hospital stay compared to the TPN group.

In a related study, the effects of three different nutrition support techniques on 260 patients following major abdominal surgery were evaluated (Gianotti et al., 1997). Patients were randomly assigned to receive a standard enteral formula; an enteral formula enriched with arginine, omega-3 fatty acids, and RNA; or TPN. All of the nutritional support regimens contained equal amounts of calories and protein and were started 6 hours after surgery. Compared with patients who received either standard enteral nutrition or TPN, patients who received the enriched enteral formula had significantly better immune measures, fewer complications, and a shorter length of hospital stay.

Recent trials have also examined the efficacy of standard enteral formulas versus placebo formulas or regular oral diets. A two-phase clinical trial evaluated the effects of oral dietary supplements versus a regular diet in 100 marginally nutritionally depleted gastrointestinal surgery patients (Keele et al., 1997). Patients were randomly assigned to either a control group (mean age 60 years) or an oral supplement group (mean age 64 years). In phase 1, the inpatient phase, the treatment group had significantly better nutritional intake, fewer complications, less fatigue, and less weight loss when compared to the control group. In the outpatient phase, phase 2, patients in the treatment group continued to have better nutritional intakes, but measures of nutritional status and well-being were not significantly different from the control group. An earlier study (Beier-Holgersen and Boesby, 1996) had similar results. After major abdominal surgery, patients (n = 30) were randomly assigned to receive either enteral feeding or a placebo (flavored water) through a naso-duodenal feeding tube. Patients in the enteral feeding group had a significantly lower rate ($p < 0.001$) of infectious complications than patients in the placebo group. Considering the substantial costs associated with treating infectious complications and of administering TPN, coupled with the costs of longer hospital stays, the use of early enteral nutrition has implications for reducing overall hospital costs.

Total Parenteral Nutrition

Estimates from a pooled analysis of 13 prospective randomized clinical trials have indicated that TPN given to "malnourished" gastrointestinal cancer patients, as defined by weight loss, plasma proteins, or prognostic indices, for 7 to 10 days before surgery reduced the overall risk of postoperative complications by approximately 10 percent. In contrast, a pooled analysis of nine prospective randomized clinical trials in a similar population indicated that postoperative TPN increased the overall risk of postoperative complications by approximately 10 percent (Klein et al., 1997).

A key study in the pooled analysis, the Veterans Affairs Total Parenteral Nutrition Cooperative Study Group (VA TPN Cooperative Study Group, 1991) evaluated the use of TPN in 395 patients (mean age 63 years) undergoing thoracoabdominal surgery. Patients were randomly assigned either to receive TPN for 7 to 15 days before surgery and 3 days after surgery or to a regular diet. Patients who were randomized to TPN and who were identified as severely malnourished (weight loss >10 percent, albumin <2.8g/dL, nutrition risk index <83.5) had fewer noninfectious complications compared to similar malnourished patients randomly assigned to a regular diet. Patients who were mildly malnourished and received TPN had more infectious complications than patients who received a regular diet.

A second study in the pooled analysis had a comparable design and findings. Gastrointestinal cancer surgery patients (n = 125) who received preoperative parenteral nutrition had fewer postoperative complications, better serum protein and immune parameters, and a lower mortality rate than patients who received a regular diet (Müller et al., 1982). Similarly, Fan and colleagues (1994) reported significantly less postoperative pneumonia and diuretic use in a group of surgical patients with hepatic cancer who received perioperative parenteral nutrition versus patients who received a regular diet.

Five to 7 days of postoperative parenteral nutrition was compared to feeding with 5 percent glucose infusion in a large number of patients (n = 678) undergoing major elective abdominal surgery (Doglietto et al., 1996). They concluded that the two groups of patients did not significantly differ in terms of complications or mortality rates. In another study of postoperative parenteral nutrition, patients (n = 300) who received parenteral nutrition for 14 days after surgery had higher complication and mortality rates compared to patients who received glucose infusions (Sandström et al., 1993).

Several investigations have tested the effects of enriched TPN solutions in patients following major abdominal surgery. TPN enriched with omega-3 fatty acids improved selected immune status parameters in 40 gastrointestinal surgery patients (Wachtler et al., 1997). While these findings were not associated with significant changes in the rate of postoperative complications, they provide evidence that enriched TPN solutions can modulate immune function. Twenty-eight elective abdominal surgery patients (mean age 68 years) were randomly assigned to either standard TPN or TPN supplemented with glutamine dipeptide (Morlion et al., 1998). The use of supplemented TPN resulted in improved nitrogen balance, improved immune parameters, and shortened hospital stay.

Taken together, these results suggest that (1) TPN should be reserved for severely malnourished patients, (2) short-term therapy with glucose infusions does not complicate recovery from surgery, (3) early enteral nutrition is preferable to TPN in the postoperative period, and (4) enriched parenteral solutions may have beneficial effects.

Hip Surgery

Studies that have evaluated the use of oral and enteral nutritional supplementation after surgical repair of hip fracture in frail elderly patients consistently report beneficial effects. In two studies, supplemental nutrition following surgery reduced postoperative complications and shortened rehabilitation time and hospital stay (Bastow et al., 1983; Delmi et al., 1990). Elderly women (n = 744) who had undergone hip fracture surgery were divided into three groups based on nutritional status: well nourished, thin, and very thin (Bastow et al., 1983). Patients who were thin or very thin were randomly assigned to receive overnight tube feedings in addition to a regular diet. Enteral supplementation was associated with improvements in nutritional and serum protein status in both groups. In addition, patients in the very thin group had shorter rehabilitation times and hospital stays compared to those who did not get the nightly tube feedings.

Similar results with oral supplemental feeding in elderly patients (mean age 82 years) with femoral neck fracture were reported (Delmi et al., 1990). Patients who were randomly assigned to receive a daily oral nutrition supplement had significantly lower rates of complications and shorter hospital stays compared to nonsupplemented patients. These findings are also similar to a clinical trial in elderly subjects (mean age 81 years) (Schürch et al., 1998). In a 6-month randomized, double-blind trial, 82 patients with recent hip fractures were randomly assigned to receive protein supplementation (20 g per day) or an isocaloric placebo. Patients who were given supplemental protein had significantly shorter hospital stays and attenuated proximal femur bone loss. In another study, 18 elderly male hip fracture patients who received supplemental nightly enteral nutrition (mean age 76.5 years) during hospitalization had lower mortality rates within 6 months of surgery compared to control patients (mean age 74.5 years) (Sullivan et al., 1998). No differences between supplemented patients and control patients were found in relation to postoperative complications and in-hospital mortality.

Perioperative Nutrition Support Summary

Consistent data show that enriched enteral nutrition administered in the postoperative period reduces the incidence of infectious complications and length of hospital stay in gastrointestinal cancer surgery patients. There are extensive data to suggest that preoperative TPN administered for 7 to 10 days decreases postoperative complications in these patients.

There are limited, but consistent data to suggest that postoperative oral and enteral supplementation decreases complications and length of stay and speeds rehabilitation in elderly hip fracture patients.

Perioperative Nutrition Support Recommendations

• Enriched enteral nutrition may be considered for older patients following gastrointestinal cancer surgery.

• Postoperative enteral nutrition is recommended for undernourished hip fracture patients.

• Further studies are needed to evaluate the safety and benefits of enteral and parenteral nutrition, including the use of early enteral nutrition and modified enteral formulas, in well-characterized groups of older surgical patients.

LIMITATIONS OF NUTRITION SUPPORT EVIDENCE

Table 10.1 summarizes available studies on the role of nutrition support. As can be seen, there have been few clinical trials of nutrition support with elderly subjects. Some observations may be reasonably generalized from studies of middle-aged adults, but limitations in design, inadequate sample size, the inclusion of heterogeneous subjects of variable nutritional risk, and inappropriate clinical outcome measures often preclude this possibility. Information is therefore insufficient to draw specific conclusions regarding some of the possible indications for use of enteral and parenteral nutrition for Medicare beneficiaries. The absence of broad-based evidence that nutrition support favorably impacts diverse outcomes for older persons does not, however, condemn its use.

Although most patients do not appear to require enteral or parenteral nutrition support interventions, clear benefits have been established for selected subgroups of patients. Those individuals with inadequate intestinal length or function or those with severe oropharyngeal dysfunction or permanent neurological impairment are striking examples. In order to avoid complications of semistarvation, it also appears prudent to consider nutrition support in selected patients who will otherwise be unable to eat or to assimilate adequate nutrition for more than 7 to 10 days. Patients who are undernourished at baseline and/or highly stressed may not, however, tolerate this duration of starvation. Such patients may include those with major trauma or severely undernourished patients who undergo major elective surgical procedures. The frail older person with hip fracture is an example of an appropriate candidate for nutrition support intervention.

The need for skilled nutrition professionals to oversee the safe and appropriate administration of enteral and parenteral nutrition in the hospital has been repeatedly emphasized in the nutrition literature. The requirement for skilled nutrition personnel is supported by three observations: (1) the need for appropriate patient selection to accrue benefit and justify risk, (2) the potential for serious complications that require close surveillance, and (3) the appreciable costs that can be associated with these interventions and their related complications.

DELIVERY OF NUTRITION SUPPORT

Parenteral and enteral nutrition support are complex medical nutrition therapies that may result in significant morbidity or mortality if administered inappropriately. Parenteral and enteral nutrition support have traditionally been administered by a multidisciplinary team consisting of a physician, registered nurse, registered dietitian, and registered pharmacist. Several models exist for the organization of a nutrition support service. In one model, a free-standing department operates with a physician-, dietitian-, pharmacist-, or nurse-director, and an appropriate number of employees. In another more common model, clinicians retain appointments in their primary departments and consult as needed with other team members. Institutions with fewer resources or fewer patients receiving enteral or parenteral nutrition may function with a nutrition support committee. The model in place in any institution depends upon available resources, local practice patterns, and institutional tradition. Many clinicians express strong opinions about the preferred model, but there is little documentation that one model is superior to another.

In some institutions, nutrition support teams have been established to reduce inappropriate resource utilization, increase revenue, and/or improve patient care. Initially, teams were supported by revenue generated from the provision of parenteral nutrition. As revenue from parenteral nutrition has declined, nutrition support teams have been under pressure to or have already downsized. Some institutions have eliminated nutrition support teams based on the rationale that the work they perform can be done by less specialized staff. However, most of the work performed by the nutrition support team members (assessment of nutritional status, implementation of enteral and parenteral nutrition therapy, monitoring response to therapy, patient education, and quality assurance monitoring) is a necessary part of quality patient care. Thus, the true cost of a nutrition support team is probably limited to the expenses needed for coordination of team activities. Most regulatory agencies and many hospitals accept the multidisciplinary nutrition support team as the standard of care for provision of enteral and parenteral nutrition.

TABLE 10.1 Hospital Settings: Evaluation of Nutrition Support Interventions

Intervention	Observational Studies[a]		Consensus Document		Systematic Review	
	GP[b]	Elderly	GP	Elderly	GP	Elderly
Gastrointestinal						
Short bowel						
Enteral	✓	–	✓	–	✓	–
Parenteral	✓	–	✓	–	✓	–
Fistulas						
Enteral	✓	–	✓	–	✓	–
Parenteral	✓	–	✓	–	✓	–
Inflammatory bowel disease						
Enteral	✓	–	✓	–	✓	–
Parenteral	✓	–	✓	–	✓	–
Pancreatitis						
Enteral	✓	–	✓	–	✓	–
Parenteral	✓	–	✓	–	✓	–
Liver disease						
Enteral	✓	–	✓	–	✓	–
Parenteral	✓	–	✓	–	✓	–
HIV/AIDS						
Enteral	✓	–	–	–	–	–
Parenteral	✓	–	–	–	–	–
Cancer Therapy						
Chemotherapy						
Enteral	✓	–	✓	–	✓	–
Parenteral	✓	–	✓	–	✓	–
Radiation Therapy						
Enteral	✓	–	✓	–	✓	–
Parenteral	✓	–	✓	–	✓	–
Renal Failure						
Acute						
Enteral	–	–	–	–	–	–
Parenteral	✓	–	–	–	–	–
Chronic						
Enteral	✓	–	–	–	–	–
Parenteral	✓	–	–	–	–	–
Critical Illness						
Enteral	✓	–	✓	–	–	–
Parenteral	✓	–	✓	–	✓	–
Perioperative						
Abdominal						
Enteral	–	✓	–	–	✓	–
Parenteral	✓	✓	–	–	✓	–
Hip fracture						
Enteral	–	✓	–	–	–	–
Parenteral	–	–	–	–	–	–

[a] This category includes case series, case-control studies, cohort studies and nonrandomized trials of nutrition-based therapies including nonhuman studies.

[b] GP = general population.

Some Clinical Trial Evidence		Extensive Clinical Trial Evidence		Overall Strength of Evidence Supporting Nutrition Therapy for Elderly Persons
GP	Elderly	GP	Elderly	
–	–	–	–	Efficacious
–	–	–	–	Efficacious
–	–	–	–	Insufficient data
–	–	–	–	Efficacious
✓	–	–	–	Insufficient data
✓	–	–	–	Not primary therapy
✓	–	–	–	Insufficient data
✓	–	–	–	Insufficient data
✓	–	–	–	Insufficient data
✓	–	–	–	Insufficient data
✓	–	–	–	Insufficient data
✓	–	–	–	Insufficient data
✓	–	–	–	Not supported
✓	–	–	–	Not supported
✓	–	–	–	Not supported
✓	–	–	–	Not supported
–	–	–	–	Insufficient data
✓	–	–	–	Insufficient data
–	–	–	–	Insufficient data
–	–	–	–	Not supported
✓	–	–	–	Insufficient data
✓	–	–	–	Insufficient data
✓	–	–	–	Selected efficacy
✓	–	–	–	Selected efficacy
–	✓	–	–	Efficacious
–	–	–	–	Insufficient data

In instances where nutrition support teams have been eliminated, the work formerly performed by dietitians, pharmacists, and nurses must then be performed by physicians, which may actually increase costs. The literature suggests that without the aid of a nutrition support team, patients receiving nutrition support are subjected to increased complications and increased costs in the form of unnecessary therapy. A discussion of these studies follows.

Early studies justified nutrition support teams based on their role in reducing catheter sepsis during parenteral nutrition (Dalton et al., 1984; Faubion et al., 1986; Hickey et al., 1979; Jacobs et al., 1984; Nehme, 1980; Sanders and Sheldon, 1976; Traeger et al., 1986). Several of these studies attributed positive results to trained nursing staff who used standard protocols for dressing changes and catheter care. However, none of these trials were randomized, only two were prospective, and results are difficult to aggregate due to inconsistent definitions of catheter sepsis.

Several studies have looked at the role of the nutrition support team in reducing electrolyte abnormalities in patients receiving TPN. In an early study of 382 patients, Nehme (1980) found fewer electrolyte abnormalities in patients whose parenteral nutrition was managed by a team.

However, in a retrospective review of 31 patients prior to team formation and a prospective review of 9 patients following team formation, no significant difference was found in the number of electrolyte abnormalities (Hickey et al., 1979). Jacobs and coworkers (1984) reported similar findings in a retrospective review of 78 patients. In both of these studies, the team functioned by team members making recommendations to the referring physician who managed his/her own patients, which could have inhibited team effectiveness.

These two studies (Hickey et al., 1979; Jacobs et al., 1984) described the method of practice during the initiation phase of a nutrition support team and may not represent the practice of an established team. In a later study of 206 patients (mean age 53 years, range 18–88 years) significantly less hypokalemia (12 percent versus 3 percent, $p < 0.05$) and hyperglycemia (47 percent versus 22 percent, $p < 0.01$) were found when cohorts of team-managed patients from 1992 and 1979 were compared (ChrisAnderson et al., 1996). The authors attributed this improvement in practice over time to established protocols as well as educational efforts. A significant reduction in metabolic complications of TPN (34 percent versus 66 percent, $p < 0.005$) was reported in a study ($n = 209$) when team-managed patients were compared with non-team-managed patients (Trujillo et al., 1999).

Team management of enteral nutrition has also resulted in significantly fewer metabolic abnormalities (Brown et al., 1987; Hassell et al., 1994; Powers et al., 1986). In a prospective study of 101 patients (mean age

64 years, ± 16 years) 513 metabolic abnormalities in non-team-managed patients were documented compared to 131 in team-managed patients ($p < 0.05$) (Powers et al., 1986) Formula modifications to correct abnormalities were made significantly more often (30 percent versus 9.8 percent, $p < 0.05$) by the nutrition support team. In a similar study of 102 patients, 49 percent of enterally fed patients managed by a nutrition support team had metabolic abnormalities compared to 72 percent of the non-team-managed patients ($p < 0.01$) (Brown et al., 1987). Thus, it appears that nutrition support team management has resulted in fewer metabolic abnormalities, particularly for patients receiving enteral feeding.

Nutrition support teams are also more effective with respect to nutrition outcomes. Team-managed patients received more nutritional assessments (Traeger et al., 1986), and significantly more patients achieved nutrition goals (Powers et al., 1986; Traeger et al., 1986). Hassell and colleagues (1994) found that team-managed enteral patients had significantly fewer metabolic, pulmonary, and gastrointestinal complications despite significantly higher acuity. In general, patients followed by nutrition support teams were monitored more frequently for laboratory abnormalities. More frequent monitoring was probably the reason that one team identified a higher incidence of hypomagnesemia as the team gained experience (ChrisAnderson et al., 1996).

Many nutrition support teams have a role in cost reduction by identifying and implementing the most cost-effective therapy. For example, a retrospective study of 31 patients compared costs of nutrition therapy for patients when nutrition support team recommendations were followed versus when they were not (O'Brien et al., 1986). In 14 cases, the referring physician did not comply with the recommendations of the nutrition support team. In 12 of these cases, a less expensive form of therapy (enteral nutrition) was recommended. Cost comparisons were based on 1984 patient charges which included overhead. Differences in the cost of therapy received and the cost of the therapy recommended by the nutrition support team were calculated and a potential cost saving of $72,270 was identified.

A prospective review of 50 patients (average age 63 ± 4 years) who received parenteral nutrition identified inappropriate or avoidable days of parenteral nutrition (Maurer et al., 1996). Independent review by two clinicians followed by a quality assurance subcommittee was used to determine inappropriate and avoidable TPN. Of 469 days of parenteral nutrition, 22 percent were inappropriate and half of the days were avoidable. Most avoidable days of TPN (184) were due to failure to access the gastrointestinal tract. Based on estimated costs to the hospital to provide TPN, the authors projected a savings of approximately $220,000 annually if a multidisciplinary oversight group had eliminated the use of avoidable or inappropriate TPN. Costs of monitoring and alternate therapy were not included in the study, and overhead was not calculated for anything other than the TPN preparation.

In a similar study, 209 patients who were started on TPN over a 4-month period were prospectively followed (Trujillo et at., 1999). Of the 209 starts, 62 percent were indicated, 23 percent were preventable, and 15 percent were not indicated. Standards established by the American Society for Parenteral and Enteral Nutrition were used to determine whether TPN was "indicated" or "not indicated." TPN was considered to be preventable when the gastrointestinal tract was functioning. For patients followed by the nutrition support team, 82 percent of the starts were indicated. For patients not followed by the nutrition support team, 56 percent of the starts were not indicated ($p < 0.005$). Avoidable charges were calculated based on a charge of $301 per day for parenteral nutrition. Avoidable charges per parenteral nutrition day averaged $20.57 for nutrition support team-managed patients versus $94.57 per day for non-nutrition support team patients. Reduced charges of approximately $430,000 annually could be projected based on the above data. These charges do not take into consideration the cost of overhead, costs of substitute therapy, or team management of patients. However, these data point to the role of a multidisciplinary nutrition support team in reducing charges to the patient.

Perhaps the most impressive economic data are those of Hassell et al. (1994) who studied 136 elderly patients (mean age 72 years) receiving enteral nutrition support for more than 24 hours. Cost calculations included salaries for clinicians and support personnel to provide care using a team or non-team model. Benefit was calculated based on dollar savings resulting from reduced length of hospital stay applied to the deficit shown between hospital costs and expected reimbursement. Of the surviving patients, 41 received care provided by the nutrition support team and 53 received care from non-team staff members. Mean patient acuity score assigned by the Pittsburgh Research Institute Patient Management Category System was 3.02 for the nutrition support team group and 1.83 for the non-team group ($p < 0.001$) with the average score of a hospitalized patient being 1.00. Patients managed by the nutrition support team had a hospital stay 2.43 days shorter than non-team patients, which was not statistically significant. However, the net savings (reduction in length-of-stay personnel costs associated with care) was $1,174 per patient which translated into a benefit of $4.20 for every $1 invested in salaries of nutrition support team personnel.

Role of the Dietitian

The role of the dietitian in parenteral and enteral nutrition has been widely expanded beyond the early descriptions of Wade (1977). Initially, dietitians focused only on the assessment of nutritional status, selection of enteral feedings, and transition to oral intake. Dietitians today measure body composition, perform indirect calorimetry, monitor the metabolic response to enteral and parenteral nutrition therapy, and in some cases order parenteral and enteral nutrition. In a 1996 survey by Olree and Skipper (1997), dietitians were found to have increased their role in parenteral nutrition and in monitoring drug–nutrient interactions when compared to a similar study conducted by Jones et al. (1986) a decade earlier.

Significantly improved enteral feeding tolerance ($p < 0.05$) was demonstrated in patients for whom dietitian recommendations for enteral feeding were implemented (Braunschweig et al., 1988). The same study showed that the goal rate of enteral formula delivery was achieved sooner (4 versus 7 days) when recommendations by the dietitian were implemented. Another study found that 56 percent of dietitian recommendations for parenteral nutrition were implemented (Skipper et al., 1994), which is comparable to the data of O'Brien and colleagues (1986) previously cited for recommendations made by a multidisciplinary team.

Specialty credentials based on role delineation studies are available for dietitians involved with parenteral and enteral nutrition. While the number of credentialed dietitians is increasing, surveys indicate that nutrition support positions for dietitians have declined often disproportionately to other workers (Compher and Colaizzo, 1992; Compher et al., 1989). The effect of these declines has not been measured. However, the requirements for nutrition assessment are increasing, and with decreasing hospitalizations, the percentage of malnourished patients would logically remain the same or increase. Therefore, regulatory agencies should be encouraged to ensure that sufficient qualified staff are available to monitor patients receiving enteral and parenteral nutrition.

Delivery of Nutrition Support Recommendations

• A multidisciplinary team approach to the provision of nutrition support is recommended for Medicare beneficiaries in the hospital setting. A variety of team models may fulfill this need and the approach chosen by an individual acute care hospital may be best determined by institutional resources and policy.

• The dietitian should be a key member of the multidisciplinary team. Optimally it would also include a physician, pharmacist, and nurse, irrespective of the model chosen.

• Medicare reimbursement to hospitals for nutrition support-related activities should be continued and periodically re-evaluated for adequacy.

REFERENCES

Abel RM, Beck CH Jr, Abbott WM, Ryan JA Jr, Barnett GO, Fischer JE. 1973. Improved survival from acute renal failure after treatment with intravenous essential L-amino acids and glucose. Results of a prospective, double-blind study. *N Engl J Med* 288:695–699.

Abu-Rustum NR, Barakat RR, Venkatraman E, Spriggs D. 1997. Chemotherapy and total parenteral nutrition for advanced ovarian cancer with bowel obstruction. *Gynecol Oncol* 64:493–495.

ACP (American College of Physicians). 1989. Parenteral nutrition in patients receiving cancer chemotherapy. *Ann Intern Med* 110:734–736.

Aker SN, Cheney CL, Sanders JE, Lenssen PL, Hickman RO, Thomas ED. 1982. Nutritional support in marrow graft recipients with single versus double lumen right atrial catheters. *Exp Hematol* 10:732–737.

Alexander JW, MacMillan BG, Stinnett JD, Ogle C, Bozian RC, Fischer JE, Oakes JB, Morris MJ. 1980. Beneficial effects of aggressive protein feeding in severely burned children. *Ann Surg* 192:505–517.

ASPEN (American Society for Parenteral and Enteral Nutrition). 1993. Guidelines for the use of parenteral and enteral nutrition in adult and pediatric patients. *J Parenter Enteral Nutr* 17:1SA–52SA.

Atkinson S, Sieffert E, Bihari D. 1998. A prospective, randomized, double-blind, controlled clinical trial of enteral immunonutrition in the critically ill. *Crit Care Med* 26:1164–1172.

Baron TH, Morgan DE. 1999. Acute necrotizing pancreatitis. *N Engl J Med* 340:1412–1417.

Bastow MD, Rawlings J, Allison SP. 1983. Benefits of supplementary tube feeding after fractured neck of femur: A randomised controlled trial. *Br Med J* 287:1589–1592.

Beier-Holgersen R, Boesby S. 1996. Influence of postoperative enteral nutrition on postsurgical infections. *Gut* 39:833–835.

Bell SJ, Chavali S, Bistrian BR, Connolly CA, Utsunomiya T, Forse RA. 1996. Dietary fish oil and cytokine and eicosanoid production during human immunodeficiency virus infection. *J Parenter Enteral Nutr* 20:43–49.

Bernstein CN, Shanahan F. 1996. Critical appraisal of enteral nutrition as primary therapy in adults with Crohn's disease. *Am J Gastroenterol* 91:2075–2079.

Borzotta AP, Pennings J, Papasadero B, Paxton J, Mardesic S, Borzotta R, Parrott A, Bledsoe F. 1994. Enteral versus parenteral nutrition after severe closed head injury. *J Trauma* 37:459–468.

Bower RH, Cerra FB, Bershadsky B, Licari JJ, Hoyt DB, Jensen GL, Van Buren CT, Rothkopf MM, Daly JM, Adelsberg BR. 1995. Early enteral administration of a formula (Impact®) supplemented with arginine, nucleotides, and fish oil in intensive care unit patients: Results of a multicenter, prospective, randomized, clinical trial. *Crit Care Med* 23:436–449.

Braga M, Gianotti L, Vignali A, Cestari A, Bisagni P, Di Carlo V. 1998. Artificial nutrition after major abdominal surgery: Impact of route of administration and composition of the diet. *Crit Care Med* 26:24–30.

Braunschweig CL, Raizman DJ, Kovacevich DS, Kerestes-Smith JK. 1988. Impact of the clinical nutritionist on tube feeding administration. *J Am Diet Assoc* 88:684–686.

Brown RO, Carlson SD, Cowan GS Jr, Powers DA, Luther RW. 1987. Enteral nutritional support management in a university teaching hospital: Team vs. nonteam. *J Parenter Enteral Nutr* 11:52–56.

Brown RO, Buonpane EA, Vehe KL, Hickerson WL, Luther RW. 1990. Comparison of modified amino acids and standard amino acids in parenteral nutrition support of thermally injured patients. *Crit Care Med* 18:1096–1101.

Brown RO, Hunt H, Mowatt-Larssen CA, Wojtysiak SL, Henningfield MF, Kudsk KA. 1994. Comparison of specialized and standard enteral formulas in trauma patients. *Pharmacotherapy* 14:314–320.

Buchman AL, Moukarzel AA, Bhuta S, Belle M, Ament ME, Eckhert CD, Hollander D, Gornbein J, Kopple JD, Vijayaroghavan SR. 1995. Parenteral nutrition is associated with intestinal morphologic and functional changes in humans. *J Parenter Enteral Nutr* 19:453–460.

Byrne TA, Persinger RL, Young LS, Ziegler TR, Wilmore DW. 1995. A new treatment for patients with short-bowel syndrome. Growth hormone, glutamine, and a modified diet. *Ann Surg* 222:243–254.

Cabré E, González-Huix F, Abad-Lacruz A, Esteve M, Acero D, Fernández-Bañares. 1990. Effect of total enteral nutrition on the short-term outcome of severely malnourished cirrhotics. A randomized controlled trial. *Gastroenterology* 98:715–720.

Carr A, Samaras K, Chisholm DJ, Cooper DA. 1998. Pathogenesis of HIV-1-protease inhibitor-associated peripheral lipodystrophy, hyperlipidaemia, and insulin resistance. *Lancet* 352:1881–1883.

Cataldi-Betcher EL, Seltzer MH, Slocum BA, Jones KW. 1983. Complications occurring during enteral nutrition support: A prospective study. *J Parenter Enteral Nutr* 7:546–552.

CDC (Centers for Disease Control and Prevention). 1997. AIDS cases by sex, age at diagnosis, and race/ethnicity, reported through June 1997, United States. *HIV/AIDS Surveill Rep* 9:13.

CDC (Centers for Disease Control and Prevention). 1998. AIDS among persons aged greater than or equal 50 years—United States, 1991–1996. *Morb Mortal Wkly Rep* 47:21–27.

CDC (Centers for Disease Control and Prevention). 1999. Fastats: Cancer. Available at: http://www.cdc.gov/nchswww/fastats/cancer.htm. Accessed July 21, 1999.

Cerra FB, Cheung NK, Fischer JE, Kaplowitz N, Schiff ER, Dienstag JL, Bower RH, Marry CD, Leevy CM, Kiernan T. 1985. Disease-specific amino acid infusion (F080) in hepatic encephalopathy: A prospective, randomized, double-blind, controlled trial. *J Parenter Enteral Nutr* 9:288–295.

Chapman R, Foran R, Dunphy JE. 1964. Management of intestinal fistula. *Am J Surg* 108:157–164.

Chiarelli A, Enzi G, Casadei A, Baggio B, Valerio A, Mazzoleni F. 1990. Very early nutrition supplementation in burned patients. *Am J Clin Nutr* 51:1035–1039.

ChrisAnderson D, Heimburger DC, Morgan SL, Geels WJ, Henry KL, Conner W, Hensrud DD, Thompson G, Weinsier RL. 1996. Metabolic complications of total parenteral nutrition: Effects of a nutrition support service. *J Parenter Enteral Nutr* 20:206–210.

Christie ML, Sack DM, Pomposelli J, Horst D. 1985. Enriched branched-chain amino acid formula versus a casein-based supplement in the treatment of cirrhosis. *J Parenter Enteral Nutr* 9:671–678.

Compher C, Colaizzo T. 1992. Staffing patterns in hospital clinical dietetics and nutrition support: A survey conducted by the Dietitians in Nutrition Support Dietetic Practice Group. *J Am Diet Assoc* 92:807–812.

Compher CW, Colaizzo TM, Rieki S. 1989. Changes in nutrition support services between 1984 and 1986. *J Am Diet Assoc* 89:1452–1457.

Constans T, Bacq Y, Bréchot JF, Guilmot J-L, Choutet P, Lamisse F. 1992. Protein–energy malnutrition in elderly medical patients. *J Am Geriatr Soc* 40:263–268.

Cosnes J, Gendre J-P, Evard D, Le Quintrec Y. 1985. Compensatory enteral hyperalimentation for management of patients with severe short bowel syndrome. *Am J Clin Nutr* 41:1002–1009.

Dalton MJ, Schepers G, Gee JP, Alberts CC, Eckhauser FE, Kirking DM. 1984. Consultative total parenteral nutrition teams: The effect on the incidence of total parenteral nutrition-related complications. *J Parenter Enteral Nutr* 8:146–152.

Daly JM, Lieberman MD, Goldfine J, Shou J, Weintraub F, Rosato EF, Lavin P. 1992. Enteral nutrition with supplemental arginine, RNA, and omega-3 fatty acids in patients after operation: Immunologic, metabolic, and clinical outcome. *Surgery* 112:56–67.

Daly JM, Weintraub FN, Shou J, Rosato EF, Lucia M. 1995. Enteral nutrition during multimodality therapy in upper gastrointestinal cancer patients. *Ann Surg* 221:327–338.

Dark DS, Pingleton SK, Kerby GR.1985. Hypercapnia during weaning. A complication of nutritional support. *Chest* 88:141–143.

Deitch EA. 1990. The role of intestinal barrier failure and bacterial translocation in the development of systemic infection and multiple organ failure. *Arch Surg* 125:403–404.

Delmi M, Rapin C-H, Bengoa J-M, Delmas PD, Vasey H, Bonjour J-P. 1990. Dietary supplementation in elderly patients with fractured neck of the femur. *Lancet* 335:1013–1016.

Dickinson RJ, Ashton MG, Axon ATR, Smith RC, Yeung CK, Hill GL. 1980. Controlled trial of intravenous hyperalimentation and total bowel rest as an adjunct to the routine therapy of acute colitis. *Gastroenterology* 79:1199–1204.

di Costanzo J, Cano N, Martin J, Mercier RR, Lafille C, Depeuch D. 1987. Treatment of external gastrointestinal fistulas by a combination of total parenteral nutrition and somatostatin. *J Parenter Enteral Nutr* 11:465–470.

Doglietto GB, Gallitelli L, Pacelli F, Bellantone R., Malerba M, Sgadari A, Crucitti F, Protein-Sparing Therapy Study Group. 1996. Protein-sparing therapy after major abdominal surgery: Lack of clinical effects. *Ann Surg* 223:357–362.

Dubé MP, Johnson DL, Currier JS, Leedom JM. 1997. Protease inhibitor-associated hyperglycaemia. *Lancet* 350:713–714.

Dudrick SJ, Maharaj AR, McKelvey AA. 1999. Artificial nutritional support in patients with gastrointestinal fistulas. *World J Surg* 23:570–576.

Fan S-T, Lo C-M, Lai ECS, Chu K-M, Liu C-L, Wong J. 1994. Perioperative nutritional support in patients undergoing hepatectomy for hepatocellular carcinoma. *N Engl J Med* 331:1547–1552.

Faubion WC, Wesley JR, Khalidi N, Silva J. 1986. Total parenteral nutrition catheter sepsis: Impact of the team approach. *J Parenter Enteral Nutr* 10:642–645.

Feinstein EI, Blumenkrantz MJ, Healy M, Koffler A, Silberman H, Massry SG, Kopple JD. 1981. Clinical and metabolic responses to parenteral nutrition in acute renal failure. A controlled double-blind study. *Medicine* 60:124–137.

Feinstein EI, Kopple JD, Silberman H, Massry SG. 1983. Total parenteral nutrition with high or low nitrogen intakes in patients with acute renal failure. *Kidney Int Suppl* 16:S319–S323.

Fernández-Bañares F, Cabré E, Esteve-Comas M, Gassull MA. 1995. How effective is enteral nutrition in inducing clinical remission in active Crohn's disease? A meta-analysis of the randomized clinical trials. *J Parenter Enteral Nutr* 19:356–364.

Fiaccadori E, Lombardi M, Leonardi S, Rotelli CF, Tortorella G, Borghetti A. 1999. Prevalence and clinical outcome associated with preexisting malnutrition in acute renal failure: A prospective cohort study. *J Am Soc Nephrol* 10:581–593.

Friedmann JM, Jensen GL, Smiciklas-Wright H, McCamish MA. 1997. Predicting early non-elective hospital readmission in nutritionally compromised older adults. *Am J Clin Nutr* 65:1714–1720.

Garrel DR, Razi M, Larivière F, Jobin N, Naman N, Emptoz-Bonneton A, Pugeat MM. 1995. Improved clinical status and length of care with low-fat nutrition support in burn patients. *J Parenter Enteral Nutr* 19:482–491.

Geerling BJ, Badart-Smook A, Stockbrügger RW, Brummer R-JM. 1998. Comprehensive nutritional status in patients with long-standing Crohn disease currently in remission. *Am J Clin Nutr* 67:919–926.

Gianotti L, Braga M, Vignali A, Balzano G, Gianpaolo MD, Zerbi A, Bisagni P, Di Carlo V. 1997. Effect of route of delivery and formulation of postoperative nutritional support in patients undergoing major operations for malignant neoplasms. *Arch Surg* 132:1222–1229.

González-Huix F, Fernández-Bañares F, Esteve-Comas M, Abad-Lacruz A, Cabré E, Acero D, Figa M, Guilera M, Humbert P, de León R, Gassull MA. 1993. Enteral versus parenteral nutrition as adjunct therapy in acute ulcerative colitis. *Am J Gastroenterol* 88:227–232.

Gottschlich MM, Jenkins M, Warden GD, Baumer T, Havens P, Snook JT, Alexander JW. 1990. Differential effects of three enteral dietary regimens on selected outcome variables in burn patients. *J Parenter Enteral Nutr* 14:225–236.

Gouttebel MC, Saint-Aubert B, Astre C, Joyeux H. 1986. Total parenteral nutrition needs in different types of short bowel syndrome. *Dig Dis Sci* 31:718–723.

Grahm TW, Zadrozny DB, Harrington T. 1989. The benefits of early jejunal hyperalimentation in the head-injured patient. *Neurosurgery* 25:729–735.

Greenberg GR, Fleming CR, Jeejeebhoy KN, Rosenberg IH, Sales D, Tremaine WJ. 1988. Controlled trial of bowel rest and nutritional support in the management of Crohn's disease. *Gut* 29:1309–1015.

Griffiths AM, Ohlsson A, Sherman PM, Sutherland LR. 1995. Meta-analysis of enteral nutrition as a primary treatment of active Crohn's disease. *Gastroenterology* 108:1056–1067.

Grinspoon S, Corcoran C, Miller K, Miller K, Biller BMK, Askari H, Wang E, Hubbard J, Anderson EJ, Basgoz N, Heller HM, Klibanski A. 1997. Body composition and endocrine function in women with acquired immunodeficiency syndrome wasting. *J Clin Endocrinol Metab* 82:1332–1337.

Grinspoon S, Corcoran C, Rosenthal D, Stanley T, Parlman K, Costello M, Treat M, Davis S, Burrows B, Basgoz N, Klibanski A. 1999. Quantitative assessment of cross-sectional muscle area, functional status, and muscle strength in men with the acquired immunodeficiency syndrome wasting syndrome. *J Clin Endocrinol Metab* 84:201–206.

Hadfield RJ, Sinclair DG, Houldsworth PE, Evans TW. 1995. Effects of enteral and parenteral nutrition on gut mucosal permeability in the critically ill. *Am J Respir Crit Care Med* 152:1545–1548.

Hassell JT, Games AD, Shaffer B, Harkins LE. 1994. Nutrition support team management of enterally fed patients in a community hospital is cost-beneficial. *J Am Diet Assoc* 94:993–998.

Hellerstein MK, Wu K, McGrath M, Faix D, George D, Shackleton CHL, Horn W, Hoh R, Neese RA. 1996. Effects of dietary n-3 fatty acid supplementation in men with weight loss associated with the acquired immune deficiency syndrome: Relation to indices of cytokine production. *J Acquir Immune Defic Syndr Hum Retrovirol* 11:258–270.

Henry K, Melroe H, Huebsch J, Hermundson J, Levine C, Swensen L, Daley J. 1998. Severe premature coronary artery disease with protease inhibitors. *Lancet* 351:1328.

Hernandez G, Velasco N, Wainstein C, Castillo L, Bugedo G, Maiz A, Lopez F, Guzman S, Vargas C. 1999. Gut mucosal atrophy after a short enteral fasting period in critically ill patients. *J Crit Care* 14:73–77.

Herndon DN, Stein MD, Rutan TC, Abston S, Linares H. 1987. Failure of TPN supplementation to improve liver function, immunity, and mortality in thermally injured patients. *J Trauma* 27:195–204.

Heyland DK. 1998. Nutritional support in the critically ill patients. A critical review of the evidence. *Crit Care Clin* 14:423–440.

Heyland DK, MacDonald S, Keefe L, Drover JW. 1998. Total parenteral nutrition in the critically ill patient. A meta-analysis. *J Am Med Assoc* 280:2013–2019.

Heys SD, Walker LG, Smith I, Eremin O. 1999. Enteral nutritional supplementation with key nutrients in patients with critical illness and cancer: A meta-analysis of randomized controlled clinical trials. *Ann Surg* 229:467–477.

Hickey MM, Munyer TO, Salem RB, Yost RL. 1979. Parenteral nutrition utilization: Evaluation of an educational protocol and consult service. *J Parenter Enteral Nutr* 3:433–437.

Himal HS, Allard JR, Nadeau JE, Freeman JB, Maclean LD. 1974. The importance of adequate nutrition in closure of small intestinal fistulas. *Br J Surg* 61:724–726.

Hirsch S, Bunout D, de la Maza P, Iturriaga H, Petermann M, Icazar G, Ugarte, G. 1993. Controlled trial on nutrition supplementation in outpatients with symptomatic alcoholic cirrhosis. *J Parenter Enteral Nutr* 17:119–124.

Horst D, Grace ND, Conn HO, Schiff E, Schenker S, Viteri A, Law D, Atterbury CE. 1984. Comparison of dietary protein with an oral, branched chain-enriched amino acid supplement in chronic portal-systemic encephalopathy: A randomized controlled trial. *Hepatology* 4:279–287.

Houdijk AP, Rijnsburger ER, Jansen J, Wesdorp RIC, Weiss JK, MCCamish MA, Teerlink T, Meuwissen GM, Haarman HJTM, Thijs LG, Van Leeuwen PAM. 1998. Randomised trial of glutamine-enriched enteral nutrition on infectious morbidity in patients with multiple trauma. *Lancet* 352:772–776.

Howard L, Malone M. 1997. Clinical outcome of geriatric patients in the United States receiving home parenteral and enteral nutrition. *Am J Clin Nutr* 66:1364–1370.

Ikizler TA, Himmelfarb J. 1997. Nutrition in acute renal failure patients. *Adv Ren Replace Ther* 4:54–63.

Ikizler TA, Flakoll PJ, Parker RA, Hakim RM. 1994. Amino acid and albumin losses during hemodialysis. *Kidney Int* 46:830–837.

Incalzi RA, Capparella O, Gemma A, Landi F. Pagano F, Cipriani L, Carbonin P. 1998. Inadequate caloric intake: A risk factor for mortality of geriatric patients in the acute-care hospital. *Age Ageing* 27:303–310.

Jacobs DO, Melnik G, Forlaw L, Gebhardt C, Settle RG, DiSipio M, Rombeau JL. 1984. Impact of a nutritional support service on VA surgical patients. *J Am Coll Nutr* 3:311–315.

Jensen GL, Kita K, Fish J, Heydt D, Frey C. 1997. Nutrition risk screening characteristics of rural older persons: Relation to functional limitations and health care charges. *Am J Clin Nutr* 66:819–828.

Jin D, Phillips M, Byles JE. 1999. Effects of parenteral nutrition support and chemotherapy on the phasic composition of tumor cells in gastrointestinal cancer. *J Parenter Enteral Nutr* 23:237–241.

Jones MG, Bonner JL, Stitt KR. 1986. Nutrition support service: Role of the clinical dietitian. *J Am Diet Assoc* 86:68–71.

Kalfarentzos F, Kehagias J, Mead N, Kokkinis K, Gogos CA. 1997. Enteral nutrition is superior to parenteral nutrition in severe acute pancreatitis: Results of a randomized prospective trial. *Br J Surg* 84:1665–1669.

Kearns PJ, Young H, Garcia G, Blaschke T, O'Hanlon G, Rinki M, Sucher K, Gregory P. 1992. Accelerated improvement of alcoholic liver disease with enteral nutrition. *Gastroenterology* 102:200–205.

Keele AM, Bray MJ, Emery PW, Duncan HD, Silk DBA. 1997. Two phase randomised controlled clinical trial of postoperative oral dietary supplements in surgical patients. *Gut* 40:393–399.

Keys A, Brozel J, Henschel A, Mickelsen O, Taylor HL. 1950. *The Biology of Human Starvation*, Vol. 1, 2. Minneapolis: University of Minnesota Press.

Klein S, Koretz RL. 1994. Nutrition support in patients with cancer: What do the data really show? *Nutr Clin Pract* 9:91–100.

Klein S, Simes J, Blackburn GL. 1986. Total parenteral nutrition and cancer trials. *Cancer* 58:1378–1386.

Klein S, Kinney J, Jeejeebhoy K, Alpers D, Hellerstein M, Murray M, Twomey P. 1997. Nutrition support in clinical practice: Review of published data and recommendations for future research directions. Summary of a conference sponsored by the National Institutes of Health, American Society for Parenteral and Enteral Nutrition, and American Society for Clinical Nutrition. *Am J Clin Nutr* 66:683–706.

Kotler DP, Fogleman L, Tierney AR. 1998. Comparison of total parenteral nutrition and an oral, semielemental diet on body composition, physical function, and nutrition-related costs in patients with malabsorption due to acquired immunodeficiency syndrome. *J Parenter Enteral Nutr* 22:120–126.

Kudsk KA, Croce MA, Fabian TC, Minard G,Tolley EA, Poret HA, Kuhl MR, Brown RO. 1992. Enteral versus parenteral feeding. Effects on septic morbidity after blunt and penetrating abdominal trauma. *Ann Surg* 215:503–511.

Kudsk KA, Minard G, Croce MA, Brown RO, Lowrey TS, Pritchard FE, Dickerson RN. 1996. A randomized trial of isonitrogenous enteral diets after severe trauma. An immune-enhancing diet reduces septic complications. *Ann Surg* 224:531–543.

Lautz HU, Selberg O, Körber J, Bürger M, Müller MJ. 1992. Protein–calorie malnutrition in liver cirrhosis. *Clin Investig* 70:478–486.

Lees J. 1997. Total parenteral nutrition for patients receiving antineoplastic therapy at a regional oncology unit: A two-year study. *Eur J Cancer Care* 6:182–185.

Lennard-Jones JE. 1990. Oral rehydration solutions in short bowel syndrome. *Clin Ther* 12S:129–137.

Leonard CD, Luke RG, Siegel RR. 1975. Parenteral essential amino acids in acute renal failure. *Urology* 6:154–157.

Liljedahl SO, Larsson J, Schildt B, Vinnars E. 1982. Metabolic studies in severe burns. Clinical features, routine biochemical analyses, nitrogen balance and metabolic rate. *Acta Chir Scand* 148:393–400.

Lipman TO. 1998. Grains or veins: Is enteral nutrition really better than parenteral nutrition? A look at the evidence. *J Parenter Enteral Nutr* 22:167–182.

Lochs H, Egger-Schodl M, Potzi R, Kappel C, Schuh R. 1984. Enteral feeding—an alternative to parenteral feeding in the treatment of Crohn disease? *Leber Magen Darm* 14:64–67.

MacBurney M, Young LS, Ziegler TR, Wilmore DW. 1994. A cost-evaluation of glutamine-supplemented parenteral nutrition in adult bone marrow transplant patients. *J Am Diet Assoc* 94:1263–1266.

Marinella MA, Markert RJ. 1998. Admission serum albumin level and length of hospitalization in elderly patients. *South Med J* 91:851–854.

Maurer J, Weinbaum F, Turner J, Brady T, Pistone B, D'Addario V, Lun W, Ghazali B. 1996. Reducing the inappropriate use of parenteral nutrition in an acute care teaching hospital. *J Parenter Enteral Nutr* 20:272–274.

McClave SA, Greene LM, Snider HL, Makk LJK, Cheadle WG, Owens NA, Dukes LG, Goldsmith LJ. 1997. Comparison of the safety of early enteral vs parenteral nutrition in mild acute pancreatitis. *J Parenter Enteral Nutr* 21:14–20.

McGeer AJ, Detsky AS, O'Rourke KO. 1990. Parenteral nutrition in cancer patients undergoing chemotherapy: A meta-analysis. *Nutrition* 6:223–240.

McIntyre PB, Powell-Tuck J, Wood SR, Lennard-Jones JE, Lerebours E, Hecketsweiler P, Galmiche J-P, Colin R. 1986. Controlled trial of bowel rest in the treatment of severe acute colitis. *Gut* 27:481–485.

Meguid MM, Campos AC. 1996. Nutritional management of patients with gastrointestinal fistulas. *Surg Clin North Am* 76:1035–1080.

Mehta RL. 1994. Therapeutic alternatives to renal replacement for critically ill patients in acute renal failure. *Semin Nephrol* 14:64–82.

Melchior JC, Chastang C, Gelas P, Carbonnel F, Zazzo J-F, Boulier A, Cosnes J, Boulétreau, Messing B. 1996. Efficacy of 2-month total parenteral nutrition in AIDS patients: A controlled randomized prospective trial. *AIDS* 10:379–384.

Mendenhall CL, Anderson S, Weesner RE, Goldberg SJ, Crolic KA. 1984. Protein–calorie malnutrition associated with alcoholic hepatitis. Veterans Administration Cooperative Study Group on Alcoholic Hepatitis. *Am J Med* 76:211–222.

Michel H, Bories P, Aubin JP, Pomier-Layrargues G, Bauret P, Bellet-Herman H. 1985. Treatment of acute hepatic encephalopathy in cirrhotics with a branched-chain amino acids enriched versus a conventional amino acids mixture. A controlled study of 70 patients. *Liver* 5:282–289.

Minard G, Kudsk KA. 1998. Nutritional support and infection: Does the route matter? *World J Surg* 22:213–219.

Mirtallo JM, Schneider PJ, Mavko K, Ruberg RL, Fabri PJ. 1982. A comparison of essential and general amino acid infusions in the nutritional support of patients with compromised renal function. *J Parenter Enteral Nutr* 6:109–113.

Mizock BA. 1999. Nutritional support in hepatic encephalopathy. *Nutrition* 15:220–228.

Moore EE, Jones TN. 1986. Benefits of immediate jejunostomy feeding after major abdominal trauma—a prospective, randomized study. *J Trauma* 26:874–881.

Moore FA, Moore EE. 1996. The benefits of enteric feeding. *Adv Surg* 30:141–154.

Moore FA, Moore EE, Jones TN, McCroskey BL, Peterson VM. 1989. TEN versus TPN following major abdominal trauma—reduced septic morbidity. *J Trauma* 29:916–922.

Moore FA, Feliciano DV, Andrassy RJ, McArdle AH, Booth FVM, Morgenstein-Wagner TB, Kellum JM, Welling RE, Moore EE. 1992. Early enteral feeding, compared with parenteral, reduces postoperative septic complications. The results of a meta-analysis. *Ann Surg* 216:172–183.

Moore FA, Moore EE, Kudsk KA, Brown RO, Bower RH, Koruda MJ, Baker CC, Barbul A. 1994. Clinical benefits of an immune-enhancing diet for early postinjury enteral feeding. *J Trauma* 37:607–615.

Morlion BJ, Stehle P, Wachtler P, Siedhoff H-P, Köller, König W, Fürst P, Puchstein C. 1998. Total parenteral nutrition with glutamine dipeptide after major abdominal surgery: A randomized, double-blind, controlled study. *Ann Surg* 227:302–308.

Mowé M, Bøhmer T. 1991. The prevalence of undiagnosed protein–calorie undernutrition in a population of hospitalized elderly patients. *J Am Geriatr Soc* 39:1089–1092.

Mowé M, Bøhmer T, Kindt E. 1994. Reduced nutritional status in an elderly population (>70 y) is probable before disease and possibly contributes to the development of disease. *Am J Clin Nutr* 59:317–324.

Mulder POM, Bouman JG, Gietema JA, Van Rijsbergen H, Mulder NH, Van der Geest S, De Vries EGE. 1989. Hyperalimentation in autologous bone marrow transplantation for solid tumors. Comparison of total parenteral versus partial parenteral plus enteral nutrition. *Cancer* 64:2045–2052.

Müller JM, Brenner U, Dienst C, Pichlmaier H. 1982. Preoperative parenteral feeding in patients with gastrointestinal carcinoma. *Lancet* 8263:68–71.

Muscaritoli M, Conversano L, Torelli GF, Arcese W, Capria S, Cangiano C, Falcone C, Fanelli FR. 1998. Clinical and metabolic effects of different parenteral nutrition regimens in patients undergoing allogeneic bone marrow transplantation. *Transplantation* 66:610–616.

Nasrallah SM, Galambos JT. 1980. Aminoacid therapy of alcoholic hepatitis. *Lancet* 8207:1276–1277.

Naveau S, Pelletier G, Poynard T, Attali P, Poitrine A, Buffet C, Etienne J-P, Chaput J-C. 1986. A randomized clinical trial of supplementary parenteral nutrition in jaundiced alcoholic cirrhotic patients. *Hepatology* 6:270–274.

Naylor CD, O'Rourke K, Detsky AS, Baker JP. 1989. Parenteral nutrition with branched-chain amino acids in hepatic encephalopathy. A meta-analysis. *Gastroenterology* 97:1033–1042.

Nehme AE. 1980. Nutritional support of the hospitalized patient. The team concept. *J Am Med Assoc* 243:1906–1908.

Nightingale JMD, Lennard-Jones JE, Walker ER, Farthing MJG. 1990. Jejunal efflux in short bowel syndrome. *Lancet* 336:765–768.

Norton JA, Ott LG, McClain C, Adams L, Dempsey RJ, Haack D, Tibbs PA, Young B. 1988. Intolerance to enteral feeding in the brain-injured patient. *J Neurosurg* 68:62–66.

O'Brien DD, Hodges RE, Day AT, Waxman KS, Rebello T. 1986. Recommendations of nutrition support team promote cost containment. *J Parenter Enteral Nutr* 10:300–302.

Olree K, Skipper A. 1997. The role of nutrition support dietitians as viewed by chief clinical and nutrition support dietitians: Implications for training. *J Am Diet Assoc* 97:1255–1260.

Pichard C, Sudre P, Karsegard V, Yerly S, Slosman DO, Delley V, Perrin L, Hirschel B, Swiss HIV Cohort Study. 1998. A randomized double-blind controlled study of 6 months of oral nutritional supplementation with arginine and omega-3 fatty acids in HIV-infected patients. *AIDS* 12:53–63.

Pillar B, Perry S. 1990. Evaluating total parenteral nutrition: Final report and statement of the Technology Assessment and Practice Guidelines Forum. *Nutrition* 6:314–318.

Powers DA, Brown RO, Cowan GS Jr, Luther RW, Sutherland DA, Drexler PG. 1986. Nutritional support team vs nonteam management of enteral nutritional support in a Veterans Administration Medical Center teaching hospital. *J Parenter Enteral Nutr* 10:635–638.

Purdum PP III, Kirby DF. 1991. Short-bowel syndrome: A review of the role of nutrition support. *J Parenter Enteral Nutr* 15:93–101.

Rabeneck L, Palmer A, Knowles JB, Seidehamel RJ, Harris CL, Merkel KL, Risser, JMH, Akrabawi SS. 1998. A randomized controlled trial evaluating nutrition counseling with or without oral supplementation in malnourished HIV-infected patients. *J Am Diet Assoc* 98:434–438.

Rapp RP, Young B, Twyman D, Bivins BA, Haack D, Tibbs PA, Bean JR. 1983. The favorable effect of early parenteral feeding on survival in head-injured patients. *J Neurosurg* 58:906–912.

Rivera S, Briggs W, Qian D, Sattler FR. 1998. Levels of HIV RNA are quantitatively related to prior weight loss in HIV-associated wasting. *J Acquir Immune Defic Syndr Hum Retrovirol* 17:411–418.

Rose D, Yarborough MF, Canizaro PC, Lowry SF. 1986. One hundred and fourteen fistulas of the gastrointestinal tract treated with total parenteral nutrition. *Surg Gynecol Obstet* 163:345–350.

Ryan JA Jr, Abel RM, Abbott WM, Hopkins CC, Chesney TM, Colley R, Phillips K, Fischer JE. 1974. Catheter complications in total parenteral nutrition. A prospective study of 200 consecutive patients. *N Engl J Med* 290:757–761.

Samlowski WE, Wiebke G, McMurry M, Mori M, Ward JH. 1998. Effects of total parental nutrition (TPN) during high-dose interleukin-2 treatment for metastatic cancer. *J Immunother* 21:65–74.

Sanders RA, Sheldon GF. 1976. Septic complications of total parenteral nutrition. A five year experience. *Am J Surg* 132:214–220.

Sandström R, Drott C, Hyltander A, Arfvidsson B, Scherstén T, Wickström I, Lunkholm K. 1993. The effect of postoperative intravenous feeding (TPN) on outcome following major surgery evaluated in a randomized study. *Ann Surg* 217:185–195.

Sax HC, Warner BW, Talamini MA, Hamilton FN, Bell RH Jr, Fischer JE, Bower RH. 1987. Early total parenteral nutrition in acute pancreatitis: Lack of beneficial effects. *Am J Surg* 153:117–124.

Schloerb PR, Amare M. 1993. Total parenteral nutrition with glutamine in bone marrow transplantation and other clinical applications (a randomized, double-blind study). *J Parenter Enteral Nutr* 17:407–413.

Schloerb PR, Skikne BS. 1999. Oral and parenteral glutamine in bone marrow transplantation: A randomized, double-blind study. *J Parenter Enteral Nutr* 23:117–122.

Schürch M-A, Rizzoli R, Slosman D, Vadas L, Vergnaud P, Bonjour J-P. 1998. Protein supplements increase serum insulin-like growth factor-I levels and attenuate proximal femur bone loss in patients with recent hip fracture. A randomized, double-blind, placebo-controlled trial. *Ann Intern Med* 128:801–809.

Senkal M, Mumme A, Eickhoff U, Geier B, Späth G, Wulfert D, Joosten U, Frei A, Kemen M. 1997. Early postoperative enteral immunonutrition: Clinical outcome and cost-comparison analysis in surgical patients. *Crit Care Med* 25:1489–1496.

Sikora SS, Ribeiro U, Kane JM III, Landreneau RJ, Lembersky B, Posner MC. 1998. Role of nutrition support during induction chemoradiation therapy in esophageal cancer. *J Parenter Enteral Nutr* 22:18–21.

Skipper A, Young M, Rotman N, Nagl H. 1994. Physician's implementation of dietitians' recommendations: A study of the effectiveness of dietitians. *J Am Diet Assoc* 94:45–49.

Soeters PB, Ebeid AM, Fischer JE. 1979. Review of 404 patients with gastrointestinal fistulas. Impact of parenteral nutrition. *Ann Surg* 190:189–202.

Solomon SM, Kirby DF. 1990. The refeeding syndrome: A review. *J Parenter Enteral Nutr* 14:90–97.

Souba WW. 1997. Nutritional support. *N Engl J Med* 336:41–48.

Stack JA, Bell SJ, Burke PA, Forse RA. 1996. High-energy, high-protein, oral, liquid, nutrition supplementation in patients with HIV infection: Effect on weight status in relation to incidence of secondary infection. *J Am Diet Assoc* 96:337–341.

Sullivan DH. 1992. Risk factors for early hospital readmission in a select population of geriatric rehabilitation patients: The significance of nutritional status. *J Am Geriatr Soc* 40:792–798.

Sullivan DH, Moriarty MS, Chernoff R, Lipschitz DA. 1989. Patterns of care: An analysis of the quality of nutritional care routinely provided to elderly hospitalized veterans. *J Parenter Enteral Nutr* 13:249–254.

Sullivan DH, Nelson CL, Bopp MM, Puskarich-May CL, Walls RC. 1998. Nightly enteral nutrition support of elderly hip fracture patients: A phase I trial. *J Am Coll Nutr* 17:155–161.

Sullivan DH, Sun S, Walls RC. 1999. Protein–energy undernutrition among elderly hospitalized patients: A prospective study. *J Am Med Assoc* 281:2013–2019.

Süttmann U, Ockenga J, Schneider H, Selberg O, Schlesinger A, Gallati H, Wolfram G, Deicher H, Müller MJ. 1996. Weight gain and increased concentrations of receptor proteins for tumor necrosis factor after patients with symptomatic HIV infection received fortified nutrition support. *J Am Diet Assoc* 96:565–569.

Szeluga DJ, Stuart RK, Brookmeyer R, Utermohlen V, Santos GW. 1987. Nutritional support of bone marrow transplant recipients: A prospective, randomized clinical trial comparing total parenteral nutrition to an enteral feeding program. *Cancer Res* 47:3309–3316.

Traeger SM, Williams GB, Milliren G, Young DS, Fisher M, Haug MT III. 1986. Total parenteral nutrition by a nutrition support team: Improved quality of care. *J Parenter Enteral Nutr* 10:408–412.

Trallori G, Palli D, Saieva C, Bardazzi G, Bonanomi AG, d'Albasio G, Galli M, Vannozzi G, Milla M, Tarantino O, Renai F, Messori A, Amorosi A, Pacini F, Morettini A. 1996. A population-based study of inflammatory bowel disease in Florence over 15 years (1978–92). *Scand J Gastroenterol* 31:892–899.

Trujillo EB, Young LS, Chertow GM, Randall S, Clemons T, Jacobs DO, Robinson MK. 1999. Metabolic and monetary costs of avoidable parenteral nutrition use. *J Parenter Enteral Nutr* 23:109–113.

Turner H, Muuranainen N, Terrell C, Graeber C, Kotler D. 1994. Nutritional status and the quality of life. Presented at: The Tenth International Conference on AIDS. Abstract Book, 215 Abstract 431 B, Yokohama, Japan.

VA TPN (Veterans Affairs Total Parenteral Nutrition) Cooperative Study Group. 1991. Perioperative total parenteral nutrition in surgical patients. *N Engl J Med* 325:525–532.

Wachtler P, König W, Senkal M, Kemen M, Köller M. 1997. Influence of a total parenteral nutrition enriched with omega-3 fatty acids on leukotriene synthesis of peripheral leukocytes and systemic cytokine levels in patients with major surgery. *J Trauma* 42:191–198.

Wade JE. 1977. Role of a clinical dietitian specialist on a nutrition support service. *J Am Diet Assoc* 70:185–189.

Weinsier RL, Krumdieck CL. 1981. Death resulting from overzealous total parenteral nutrition: The refeeding syndrome revisited. *Am J Clin Nutr* 34:393–399.

Weisdorf SA, Lysne J, Wind D, Haake RJ, Sharp HL, Goldman A, Schissel K, McGlave PB, Ramsay NK, Kersey JH. 1987. Positive effect of prophylactic total parenteral nutrition on long-term outcome of bone marrow transplantation. *Transplantation* 43:833–838.

Wheeler DA, Gibert CL, Launer CA, Muurahainen N, Elion RA, Abrams DI, Bartsch GE, The Terry Beirn Communicty Programs for Clinical Research on AIDS. 1998. Weight loss as a predictor of survival and disease progression in HIV infection. *J Acquir Immune Defic Syndr Hum Retrovirol* 18:80–85.

Wilson IB, Cleary PD. 1997. Clinical predictors of declines in physical functioning in persons with AIDS: Results of a longitudinal study. *J Acquir Immune Defic Syndr Hum Retrovirol* 16:343–349.

Windsor AC, Kanwar S, Li AG, Guthrie JA, Spark JI, Welsh F, Guillou PJ, Reynolds JV. 1998. Compared with parenteral nutrition, enteral feeding attenuates the acute phase response and improves disease severity in acute pancreatitis. *Gut* 42:431–435.

Wolfson M, Jones MR, Kopple JD. 1982. Amino acid losses during hemodialysis with infusion of amino acids and glucose. *Kidney Int* 21:500–506.

Wright RA, Adler EC. 1990. Peripheral parenteral nutrition is no better than enteral nutrition in acute exacerbation of Crohn's disease: A prospective trial. *J Clin Gastroenterol* 12:396–399.

Wyncoll DL. 1999. The management of severe acute necrotising pancreatitis: An evidence-based review of the literature. *Intensive Care Med* 25:146–156.

Zaloga GP. 1998. Immune-enhancing enteral diets: Where's the beef? *Crit Care Med* 26:1143–1146.

Ziegler TR, Young LS, Benfell K, Scheltinga M, Hortos K, Bye R, Morrow FD, Jacobs DO, Smith RJ, Antin JH, Wilmore DW. 1992. Clinical and metabolic efficacy of glutamine-supplemented parenteral nutrition after bone marrow transplantation. A randomized, double-blind, controlled study. *Ann Intern Med* 116:821–828.

11

Nutrition Services in Ambulatory Care Settings

In the past decade, significant changes have occurred in health care that have influenced where and how care is delivered. Medicare's prospective payment system in acute care settings and the growth of managed care have contributed to a shift in provision of services to the ambulatory care setting. From 1987 to 1997 there was a 68 percent increase in outpatient visits (AHA, 1999). This shift in care has not been accompanied by a similar transfer of reimbursement monies, especially for nutrition and other self-management interventions.

In addition to the shift of health care to the ambulatory setting, there has also been an increased emphasis on primary, secondary, and tertiary prevention of disease. *Primary prevention* addresses the promotion of life-style changes when there are no risk factors and no apparent disease. *Secondary prevention* focuses on early identification and prompt treatment of disease, and promotes life-style changes that favorably affect known risk factors. *Tertiary prevention* emphasizes reduction in impairment or disability and prevention of disease progression following diagnosis (USPSTF, 1995). Nutrition services in ambulatory settings play a role in all three areas of prevention.

REIMBURSEMENT FOR NUTRITION THERAPY IN AMBULATORY CARE

At the present time, Medicare Part B covers medical and other health services which are *incident to* a primary care provider's services. *Incident to* refers to services specifically related to the medical care that is being provided by the physician at the time of the encounter. While Medicare Part B does not specifically cover or exclude payment for nutrition services, because regional carriers have the discretion to reimburse for nutrition services which are deemed reasonable and medically necessary, there are widespread inconsistencies and reimbursement is frequently denied. For patients who are enrolled in Medicare Part C (Medicare + Choice) it is up to the individual plan as to whether or not nutrition service is a covered benefit.

Under Medicare Part B, in order to be covered as an *incident to* service, the service must be provided by the physician or an employee of the physician, physician group practice, ambulatory surgical clinic, ambulatory clinic, or rural health clinic. If the service is provided by an employee of the above providers, it must be directly supervised by the billing physician. A nutrition professional, such as a dietitian, providing nutrition services is not authorized to submit requests for payment separately. Since dietitians are rarely employees of physician practices or ambulatory clinics, the lack of specific coverage for outpatient nutrition services is a significant barrier to nutrition therapy.

In 1996, the U.S. Preventive Services Task Force (USPSTF, 1996) recommended that "clinicians who lack the time or skills to perform a complete dietary history, to address potential barriers to changes in eating habits, and to offer specific guidance on meal planning and food selection and preparation, should either have patients seen by other trained providers in the office or clinic or should refer patients to a registered dietitian or qualified nutritionist for further counseling." However, O'Keefe and colleagues (1991) reported that less than 25 percent of physicians routinely referred patients to a dietitian and only 10 percent had a dietitian available for dietary counseling. Most physicians or physician groups do not have sufficient funding in administrative budgets, office space, or enough patients requiring nutrition therapy to support hiring a dietitian as part of their office staff.

As part of the Balanced Budget Act of 1997, reimbursement for diabetes self-management is now a covered benefit for Medicare beneficiaries (see chapter 6). Currently, the proposed regulations for diabetes self-management developed by the Health Care Financing Administration require that a registered dietitian and certified diabetes educator participate in the diabetes education program and that programs are accredited by the American Diabetes Association. Although the final regulations will not be released until early 2000, the proposed regulations include ten visits during the first year of diagnosis and one visit annually thereafter.

Medicare reimbursement for ambulatory care moves to a prospective payment system (PPS) with the Ambulatory Payment Classification system beginning in January 2000. This system provides hospital outpatient departments both opportunities and risks similar to those experienced when the PPS was implemented in acute care, short-stay hospitals (Duncan, 1999). It is unclear how this will impact services in the ambulatory setting (Lake, 1998). In the acute care setting there was adequate support for nutrition professionals prior to implementation of the PPS. However, support for the nutrition professional in the ambulatory setting is presently inconsistent and inadequate.

ACCREDITATION STANDARDS FOR THE AMBULATORY SETTING

The Joint Commission on Accreditation of Healthcare Organizations (JCAHO) accredits ambulatory facilities (free-standing ambulatory clinics) under separate guidelines from those used in hospital-based outpatient services. Hospital-based outpatient services are surveyed using hospital standards that include requirements for nutrition screening, assessment, and therapy provided by a qualified dietitian (JCAHO, 1999a). For ambulatory facilities, requirements specify that nutritional status must be assessed when warranted and dietary needs, including the provision of nutrition therapy, must be met when appropriate (JCAHO, 1999b). These standards state that a "nutritionist or other qualified individual" is to be involved in the assessment and documentation of patient needs (JCAHO, 1999b). JCAHO identifies the "dietitian or nutritionist" as the primary provider of specific nutrition services.

The National Committee for Quality Assurance (NCQA) surveys and ranks managed care organizations, including those who provide services under Medicare Part C. NCQA uses the Health Plan Employer Data and Information Set in its evaluation process. The key systems and processes that make up the health plan are evaluated, including how well the plan provides services to keep its members healthy or manage chronic disease. Current outcome measures related to nutrition therapy include lipid levels, HbA_{1c} levels, and the provision of education for individuals with diabetes. Outcome measures selected for further development include documentation of calcium intake in women and the provision of benefits for individuals who are overweight. Access to health care providers is also measured. While a nutrition professional is currently not included in the "access to health care provider" measure as mentioned above, several outcome measures in which nutrition intervention can have an impact are tracked and measured (NCQA, 1999).

NUTRITION SERVICES IN AMBULATORY SETTINGS

Primary Prevention

The U.S. Dietary Guidelines suggest numerous dietary goals to aid in the prevention of chronic disease. Several studies have evaluated the impact of resulting dietary changes. The San Diego Medicare Preventive Health Project evaluated health behavior change 1 year after an intervention that included a nutrition component. The study found significant positive changes in the participants' nutrition-related behaviors, most notably in the reduction of fat consumption (e.g., red meat, gravy, butter, fried foods) and increased fiber intake (Mayer et al., 1994). In addition, the Women's Health Initiative, which includes women ages 49 to 79, is an ongoing study that focuses on assisting participants in following a low-fat diet with increased fruits, vegetables, and grains. Overall, research that links general preventive counseling to health habit change and its corresponding alterations in the development of chronic disease is limited.

Nutrition services in ambulatory settings should include screening to identify individuals who need nutrition intervention and triaging to the most appropriate professional for care. Intervention can include basic nutrition education for disease prevention or more complex nutrition therapy. Nutrition services may be provided in physicians' offices, health maintenance organizations, outpatient departments, primary care centers, health clinics, or the private offices of a nutrition professional. The format for the encounter can be individual or group. It may occur as part of the routine medical visit or as an in-depth assessment and intervention by a nutrition professional. Information may also be provided using written materials, videoconferencing, or computer and Internet programs.

There are several major trends related to the role of nutrition and prevention in the ambulatory care setting: the increased use of dietary supplements among older individuals, changes in knowledge about how properties of foods enhance health, technological advances in communication (e.g., television and the Internet), a growing interest in complementary and alternative therapies, and the related burgeoning market for nutritional and botanical products. The older person can be particularly vulnerable to claims made about health and nutrition. Elders are often coping with the effects of chronic disease and its treatment. They may also be living on limited incomes, be socially isolated, and be unable to evaluate the accuracy of information provided by marketing materials, television advertising, and the Internet. These problems are compounded by the lack, in many cases, of strong evidence to support effectiveness, safety, potential interaction of supplements with medications, and cost-effectiveness of alternative medicine therapies.

Vitamin and Mineral Supplementation

Estimates of the numbers of elderly individuals taking vitamin and mineral supplements are as high as 55 percent (Ervin et al., 1999). With the increased marketing and varying potency of supplements on the market, elders need assistance to evaluate their current and prospective supplementation needs. As the new dietary reference intakes are being developed (IOM, 1997), tolerable upper intake levels are also being defined. This information should help consumers and professionals interpret safe levels of intake. While vitamin and mineral supplementation can help round out nutrient intake, it is recommended that health professionals continue to stress the importance of a well-balanced diet.

Functional Foods, Botanicals, and Alternative Medicine

More than 30 percent of Americans sought treatment from complementary and alternative providers in 1992 (Eisenberg et al., 1993). Many of the complementary and alternative medicine regimens include botanicals or nutrient supplements. In 1997, U.S. sales of botanicals and related remedies reached $3.24 billion (Johnston, 1997), which represents a growing share of the sale of dietary supplements. Eisenberg and coworkers (1998) estimated that 15 million adults took prescription medications concurrently with botanicals or related remedies. Data pertaining to the adverse effects of botanicals and related remedies alone or in combination with prescription medications are either limited or nonexistent. Since many individuals view botanicals and dietary supplements as food items, their use is often identified in the course of a comprehensive nutrition assessment.

The role of food in enhancing health has also emerged with the concept of "functional foods" and "functional food components." Functional foods have been defined as foods that may provide a benefit beyond basic nutrition. Functional food components have similarly been defined as nutritive and non-nutritive compounds found in food that are thought to reduce the risk of disease or promote health (IFIC, 1998). Another popular term that is emerging is "nutraceutical." It has been defined as a substance that provides medical or health benefits, including the prevention and treatment of disease, and may be considered a food or part of food (Mahan and Escott-Stump, 1996). Consumers need assistance in interpreting these new terms and their claims, as well as determining the value in relation to their own nutritional needs.

Limited research is available that evaluates the potential health benefits of nutrition-related complementary and alternative medicine for conditions such as Alzheimer's disease (Le Bars et al., 1997; Oken et al., 1998;

Sano et al., 1997; Zaman et al., 1992), osteoarthritis (Morreale et al., 1996; Pujalte et al., 1980), atherosclerotic vascular disease (Silagy and Neil, 1994; Tyler, 1993; Warshafsky et al., 1993), and cancer (Lersch et al., 1992). Further research is needed to determine efficacy for health benefits. Also, elderly consumers need assistance in translating research findings into meaningful lifestyle change.

Basic Nutrition Education

Almost all members of the health care team can and should play a role in providing various components of nutrition care. Table 11.1 summarizes the roles of many health care providers in the provision of nutrition services. Traditionally, primary care physicians and nurses have screened patients and provided basic nutrition information. *Basic nutrition education* is characterized as either a group or an individual interaction based on sound nutrition principles and is generally considered primary prevention. However, reinforcement of dietary changes required for secondary and tertiary prevention in certain conditions may also be accomplished through basic nutrition education. The education may consist of information about the importance of nutrition in relation to risk factors or known disease conditions. The role of each provider can be enhanced by using evidence-based practice guidelines and protocols to help identify patients who need nutrition care and provide information that improves quality-of-life outcomes (Wagner et al., 1996).

Nutrition Therapy

Nutrition therapy is characterized by an in-depth assessment of pertinent medical, dietary, anthropometric, and lifestyle data and is provided following a referral from a physician. The therapy is relevant to specific disease states or conditions and includes an individualized diet prescription. Nutrition therapy usually involves in-depth counseling that takes 30 to 60 minutes, depending on the number of conditions and the complexity of the diet prescription. It also includes some form of follow-up care to monitor changes, reinforce new food choices and eating behaviors, adapt to social and cultural norms, and provide feedback to the patient regarding clinical outcomes.

Nutrition therapy has been shown to be effective in the management and treatment of many chronic conditions that affect Medicare beneficiaries, including dyslipidemia, hypertension, heart failure, diabetes, and chronic renal insufficiency (see chapters 5–7). As such, nutrition therapy usually focuses on secondary or tertiary prevention.

Medicare beneficiaries undergoing cancer treatment (chemotherapy,

TABLE 11.1 Roles of Various Providers in Nutrition Care in Ambulatory Settings

Provider	Role
Primary care physician or nurse practitioner or certified nurse midwife	• Screens, initial assessment of nutritional status • Comprehensive physical assessment • Orders appropriate lab tests • Diagnosis, basic nutrition information • Provides needed biochemical and physical assessment and other data to registered dietitian on referral as defined in nutrition therapy protocols • Limits or restricts activity of patients or modifies target ranges in protocols as needed • Educates patients on food–drug interaction
Registered nurse	• Screens, requests nutrition consult per screening protocol • Provides basic nutrition information • Educates patient on food–drug interactions • Reinforces nutrition therapy principles in collaboration with registered dietitian
Registered dietitian	• Develops or implements nutrition screening tools • Provides in-service education to non-nutrition staff regarding screening, assessment, and nutrition therapy • Provides comprehensive nutrition assessment • Provides nutrition therapy and self-management training in food and nutrient modification to treat medical conditions or diagnosis • Educates patients on food–drug interactions • Makes evidence-based recommendations to patients about use of nutrient supplements, liquid dietary supplements, botanicals, etc. • Refers patients to community services, food resources (e.g., food stamps, food pantries, home delivered meals) • Collaborates or coordinates services with inpatient, long-term care, home care, and referring providers
Social worker	• Identifies patients in need of nutrition information or intervention • Collaborates with registered dietitian to plan for care in the continuum • Assists patients in obtaining needed food resources (e.g., food stamps, food pantries, home-delivered meals, Medicaid prior approval for nutritional supplements)
Psychologist or LCSW	• Identifies patients in need of nutrition information or intervention • Collaborates in behavioral group interventions

SOURCE: Adapted from Cambridge Health Alliance (1999).

radiation, or surgical intervention) may also benefit from nutrition therapy aimed at controlling side effects or improving food intake. During nutrition therapy sessions, other nutrition concerns of interest to the patient can be addressed. This may be particularly important for the older individual who is undernourished or who has questions related to vitamin and mineral supplements, liquid dietary supplements, botanicals, functional foods, or other alternative forms of care.

EFFECTIVENESS OF NUTRITION THERAPY IN AMBULATORY SETTINGS

Decreased length of stay and increased acuity levels in acute care settings have strengthened the argument that nutrition counseling is best conducted outside the hospital setting (Laramee, 1996). For education to be effective, patients must be "ready to learn." Hospitalized patients are generally too ill to participate in self-management education.

Dietary behavior changes have been identified as the most difficult component of diabetes and other chronic disease self-management programs (Lockwood et al., 1986). Food practices are an important aspect of culture and lifestyle, and unlike cigarette smoking, alcohol, or other drugs, individuals with food addictions cannot opt for avoidance. Food options are an unavoidable choice to be made multiple times each day. To effect long-term changes in food-related behaviors, adequate time and conditions conducive to the counseling process are needed.

The ambulatory setting affords the clinician time to build a relationship with the patient, which can be an essential component of guiding patients to make long-term behavior changes. Several authors have explored the skills and techniques needed for optimal self-management. Successful educational programs go beyond just providing information. They use frequent positive reinforcement, a combination of group and individual interactions, practical demonstrations and participant practice, and active participation in decision making by patients (Beck et al., 1997; Lorig et al., 1999; Prohaska, 1998). Elders are often avid learners and able to make lifestyle changes, especially when there is peer or spouse support (Clement, 1995). Appropriate self-management activities are often most effective when the older person can link symptoms of the disease with health behaviors such as diet (Prohaska and Glasser, 1994).

Some studies have looked at the effectiveness of the dietitian's counseling skills. Stetson and colleagues (1992) videotaped sessions with dietitians and concluded that interpersonal skills were good but dietitians needed supplemental training to improve teaching and adherence promotion skills. The skills identified for improvement were presentation skills, active patient involvement, assessment evaluation, feedback, formulation of a behavioral plan, negotiation and accountability, and behavioral techniques (Stetson et al., 1992). Gilboy (1994) reported a survey of 508 dietitians and found that those in outpatient or ambulatory settings used more compliance-enhancing skills, had greater self-efficacy, and had higher levels of outcome efficacy than did inpatient dietitians. For dietitians working in the outpatient setting, a greater number of counseling and follow-up sessions correlated with the best compliance-enhancing practices (Gilboy, 1994).

FUTURE AREAS OF RESEARCH

The committee found limited research documenting the efficacy of nutrition therapy focused solely on primary prevention. Further research is needed to evaluate effectiveness of nutrition therapy in assisting the consumer to appropriately select food, dietary supplements, fortified or functional foods, and nutrition-related complementary and alternative medicine therapies that are consistent with the U.S. Dietary Guidelines. In addition, research comparing the effectiveness of nutrition therapy in the acute care versus ambulatory settings in producing lasting and meaningful behavior change is lacking. Research is also needed to evaluate the effectiveness of various methods of delivering nutrition therapy and contributions of various healthcare team members.

SUMMARY

Health care trends, such as a shortened length of stay in acute care facilities, have appropriately shifted the bulk of nutrition education and nutrition therapy to the ambulatory setting. Nutrition therapy provided in the ambulatory setting is thought to better meet patients' learning needs and produce meaningful long-term, nutrition-related behavior change. Currently, Medicare coverage for nutrition therapy in ambulatory settings is at best inconsistent, but most often, nonexistent.

Consumers' interest in and the availability of dietary supplements, botanicals, alternative medicine, and functional foods have increased and a myriad of marketing mechanisms have been aimed at the consumer. Individuals evaluating products need guidance from trained nutrition professionals in interpreting the complexity of mixed messages and scientific findings. Elderly individuals in particular may need advice on the efficacy of products as well as the safety of integrating them with medications.

Basic nutrition education for the primary prevention of chronic disease in the elderly should continue to be provided by a variety of health care professionals within the context of routine preventive health. There is little evidence to support replacing such basic nutrition education by nutrition therapy focused solely on primary prevention or that the basic nutrition education should be provided by a nutrition professional. Prevention topics are routinely included in all sessions of nutrition therapy regardless of the diagnoses leading to the referral.

In contrast, there is reasonable evidence documenting the efficacy of nutrition therapy for the treatment and management (secondary and tertiary prevention) of many conditions that are common among Medicare beneficiaries. Since a majority of Medicare beneficiaries 65 years of age or older will have a diagnosis supporting a referral of nutrition therapy, the primary prevention issues would likely be addressed as part of the nutrition therapy for those diagnoses.

RECOMMENDATIONS

- For dyslipidemia, hypertension, heart failure, diabetes, and renal disease, available evidence (reviewed in chapters 5–7) supports a role for nutrition therapy in the routine management of these conditions for the Medicare population. For this reason it is recommended that nutrition therapy be considered a covered benefit for Medicare beneficiaries in the ambulatory setting.

- Nutrition education is also important in the primary prevention of chronic disease. However, a variety of health care professionals such as physicians, nurses, and pharmacists should and do provide nutrition education in the context of routine preventive health visits or patient encounters. These encounters, however, should not constitute a separate covered visit, but rather be considered incident to medical care or the nutrition therapy being provided.

- In order to eliminate a barrier to access for nutrition therapy, nutrition professionals should be considered eligible as qualified providers who receive direct Medicare reimbursement.

REFERENCES

AHA (American Hospital Association). 1999. *Hospital Statistics: The AHA Profile of United States Hospitals. Historical Trends.* Chicago, Ill.: AHA.

Beck A, Scott J, Williams P, Robertson B, Jackson D, Gade G, Cowan P. 1997. A randomized trial of group outpatient visits for chronically ill older HMO members: The cooperative health care clinic. *J Am Geriatr Soc* 45:543–549.

Cambridge Health Alliance. 1999. *Ambulatory Nutrition, Policy and Procedures—Practice Guidelines.* Cambridge, Mass.: Cambridge Health Alliance.

Clement S. 1995. Diabetes self-management education. *Diabetes Care* 18:1204–1214.

Duncan D. 1999. Preparing for Medicare's APC System. *Healthcare Finan Mgmt* 53:40–45.

Eisenberg DM, Kessler RC, Foster C, Norlock FE, Calkins DR, Delbanco TL. 1993. Unconventional medicine in the United States. Prevalence, costs, and patterns of use. *N Engl J Med* 328:246–252.

Eisenberg DM, Davis RB, Ettner SL, Appel S, Wilkey S, Von Rompay M, Kessler RC. 1998. Trends in alternative medicine use in the United States, 1990–1997: Results of a follow-up national survey. *J Am Med Assoc* 280:1569–1575.

Ervin RB, Wright JD, Kennedy-Stephenson J. 1999. Use of dietary supplements in the United States, 1988–94. National Center for Health Statistics. *Vital Health Stat* 11:1–14.

Gilboy MBR. 1994. Multiple factors affect dietitians' counseling practices for high blood cholesterol. *J Am Diet Assoc* 94:1278–1283.

IFIC (International Food Information Council). 1998. Antioxidants: Working toward a definition. *Food Insight*. Washington, D.C.: IFIC.

IOM (Institute of Medicine). 1997. *Dietary Reference Intakes for Calcium, Phosphorus, Magnesium, Vitamin D, and Fluoride*. Washington, D.C.: National Academy Press.

JCAHO. (Joint Commission on Accreditation of Healthcare Organizations). 1999a. *Comprehensive Accreditation Manual for Hospitals. Update 1 Feb 1999, Update 3 Aug 1997*. Oakbrook Terrace, Ill.: JCAHO.

JCAHO (Joint Commission on Accreditation of Healthcare Organizations) 1999b. *1998–99 Comprehensive Accreditation Manual for Ambulatory Care (CAMAC)*. Oakbrook Terrace, Ill.: JCAHO.

Johnston BA. 1997. One-third of nation's adults use herbal remedies. *HerbalGram* 40:49.

Lake T. 1998. Current trends in health plan payment methods for the facility costs of outpatient care. *J Health Care Finance* 25:1–8.

Laramee SH. 1996. Nutrition services in managed care: New paradigms for dietitians. *J Am Diet Assoc* 96:335–336.

Le Bars PL, Katz MM, Berman N, Itil TM, Freedman AM, Schatzberg AF. 1997. A placebo-controlled, double-blind, randomized trial of an extract of Ginkgo biloba for dementia. *J Am Med Assoc* 278:1327–1332.

Lersch C, Zeuner M, Bauer A, Bauer A, Siemens M, Hart R, Drescher M, Flink U, Dancygier II, Classen M. 1992. Nonspecific immunostimulation with low doses of cyclophosphamide (LDCY), thymostimulin, and echinacea purpurea extracts (echinacin) in patients with far advanced colorectal cancers: Preliminary results. *Cancer Invest* 10:343–348.

Lockwood D, Frey ML, Gladish NA, Hiss RG. 1986. The biggest problem in diabetes. *Diabetes Educ* 12:30–33.

Lorig KR, Sobel DS, Stewart AL, Brown BW, Bandura A, Ritter P, Gonzalez VM, Laurent DD, Homan HR. 1999. Evidence suggesting that a chronic disease self-management program can improve health status while reducing hospitalization. A randomized trial. *Med Care* 37:5–14.

Mahan LK, Escott-Stump S. 1996. *Food, Nutrition & Diet Therapy*. Philadelphia, Pa.: WB Saunders Company.

Mayer JA, Jermanovich A, Wright BL, Elder JP, Drew JA, Williams SJ. 1994. Changes in health behaviors of older adults: The San Diego Medicare Preventive Health Project. *Prev Med* 23:127–133.

Morreale P, Manopulo R, Galati M, Boccanera L, Saponati G, Bocchi L. 1996. Comparison of the antiinflammatory efficacy of chondroitin sulfate and diclofenac sodium in patients with knee osteoarthritis. *J Rheumatol* 123:1385–1391.

NCQA (National Committee for Quality Assurance). 1999. HEDIS. Available at: http://www.ncqa.org/pages/policy/hedis/hedis.htm. Accessed September 1999.

O'Keefe CE, Hahn DF, Betts NM. 1991. Physicians' perspectives on cholesterol and heart disease. *J Am Diet Assoc* 91:189–192.

Oken BS, Storzbach DM, Kaye JA. 1998. The efficacy of ginkgo biloba on cognitive function in Alzheimer disease. *Arch Neurol* 55:1409–1415.

Prohaska T. 1998. The research basis for the design and implementation of self-care programs. Pp. 62–84 in Ory MG, DeFriese GH, eds. *Self-Care in Later Life: Research, Program, and Policy Issues.* New York: Springer.

Prohaska TR, Glasser M. 1994. Older adult health behavior change in response to symptom experiences. *Advan Med Sociol* 4:141–161.

Pujalte JM, Llavore EP, Ylescupidez FR. 1980. Double-blind clinical evaluation of oral glucosamine sulphate in the basic treatment of osteoarthrosis. *Curr Med Res Opin* 7:110–114.

Sano M, Ernesto C, Thomas RG, Klauber MR, Schaffer K, Grundman M, Woodbury P, Growdon J, Cotman CW, Pfeiffer E, Schneider LS, Thal LJ. 1997. A controlled trial of selegiline, alpha-tocopherol, or both as treatment for Alzheimer's disease. *N Engl J Med* 336:1216–1222.

Silagy CA, Neil HA. 1994. A meta-analysis of the effect of garlic on blood pressure. *J Hypertens* 12:463–468.

Stetson BA, Pichert JW, Roach RR, Lorenz RA, Boswell EJ, Schlundt DG. 1992. Registered dietitians' teaching and adherence promotion skills during routine patient education. *Patient Educ Couns* 19:273–280.

Tyler VE. 1993. *The Honest Herbal. A Sensible Guide to the Use of Herbs and Related Remedies,* 3rd Ed. New York: Pharmaceuticals Products Press.

USPSTF (U.S. Preventive Services Task Force). 1995. *Guide to Clinical Preventive Servies, 2nd Ed. Report of the U.S. Preventive Services Task Force.* Washington, D.C.: U.S. Department of Health and Human Services, Office of Public Health, Office of Health Promotion and Disease Prevention.

Wagner EH, Austin BT, Von Korff M. 1996. Organizing care for patients with chronic illness. *Milbank Quart* 74:511–544.

Warshafsky S, Kamer RS, Sivak SL. 1993. Effect of garlic on total serum cholesterol. A meta-analysis. *Ann Intern Med* 119:599–605.

Zaman Z, Roche S, Fielden P, Frost PG, Niriella DC, Cayley AC. 1992. Plasma concentrations of vitamins A and E and carotenoids in Alzheimer's disease. *Age Ageing* 21:91–94.

12
Nutrition Services in Post-Acute, Long-Term Care and in Community-Based Programs

Previous chapters have described the strength of evidence supporting the relationship between nutritional status and morbidity, the provision of nutrition therapy for certain chronic diseases, and the nutrition services provided in ambulatory and acute care. This chapter addresses the nutrition services and food assistance programs needed in post-acute care, long-term care, and in community-based programs. The following programs are discussed:

- *Post-acute care*
  - Skilled nursing facilities (SNF) or hospital-based sub-acute units
  - Home health agencies (HHA)
- *Long-term care*
  - Institutions
  - Programs of All Inclusive Care for the Elderly (PACE)
- *Food assistance for elders in the community*
  - Congregate feeding and home delivered meals.

During the last decade, the most rapid growth in Medicare costs has occurred in the area of post-acute care (Clark, 1998; Freedman, 1999; Jackson and Doty, 1998; Liu et al., 1999; NCHS, 1999). Many forces have fueled this growth, including the change to a capitated, prospective payment system (PPS) in acute care, legal actions by patients who were denied care in SNF and HHA programs, the shift to more aggressive reimbursement strategies by Medicare providers, and (to a smaller extent) changing demographic, economic, and sociological characteristics of the elderly population in the United States.

EMERGING TRENDS

Both federally funded programs and private payers are evaluating innovative ways to provide services across the continuum of care while attempting to use the least expensive and least intensive care that is appropriate (Cohen, 1998). Examples of such innovation include privately funded social health maintenance organizations (SHMOs) and programs of all inclusive care for the elderly (PACE). SHMOs are demonstration projects that combine community care services and short-term nursing home care with Medicare's basic services. PACE is a new Medicare benefit; these programs accept the risk of providing all forms of care needed by nursing home-eligible clients for a capitated Medicare fee. When possible, these services are provided while recipients remain in their homes (HCFA, 1998).

Another trend is that traditional nursing homes are expanding "up" to include more complex services, such as subacute care, and "down" to provide less complex services, such as home care and assisted living (Evashwick et al., 1998; Lehrman and Shore, 1998). However, the largest number of elders are still being cared for by informal caregivers such as family and friends (AoA, 1998; Cutler and Sheiner, 1993).

Both federally and privately funded health insurance plans are moving from a fee-for-service system to a partially or fully capitated (PPS) in all areas of care, including skilled nursing, home care, and outpatient services.

Future trends will be affected by longer lifespans and the desire of older people to remain independent as long as possible (Economics and Statistics Administration, 1995; Hawes et al., 1999; Manard and Cameron, 1997). Increased longevity has significant cost implications. The precise impact on Medicare expenditures is unknown and depends on evolving Medicare policies and social practices, changing medical technology, and the prevalent morbidities within the older population.

As health care shifts from acute care to community and home-based programs, provided by a mix of health professionals, paraprofessionals, and informal caregivers, effective nutrition services and food assistance programs are likely to become especially important. However, the present system of including nutrition services in overall administrative costs, rather than direct reimbursement, creates a financial disincentive to address the nutrition problems of older people. If nutritional status and food security diminish as a result of this inattention, the older person may develop subsequent illnesses that require more acute and expensive care

(Cornoni-Huntley et al., 1991; Frisoni et al., 1995; Gray-Donald, 1995; Mowé et al., 1994).

SKILLED NURSING FACILITIES AND NURSING HOMES

Skilled nursing facilities (SNF) are defined as health facilities that provide the following basic services: 24-hour inpatient care that includes medical, nursing, dietary, and pharmaceutical services, and an activity program. Other services such as rehabilitation and social work, not regularly needed by all residents, may be contracted (CFR, 1998). Many SNFs provide subacute care or have special units for dementia, rehabilitation, and human immunodeficiency virus/acquired immune deficiency syndrome. Residents in these special care units often have more complex nutrition needs. SNFs are usually part of a free-standing nursing home that provides long-term care for chronically ill, frail elders. There may also be SNF units in acute care facilities.

Medicare Funding

Medicare covers 100 days of SNF care per benefit period, but it must follow a 3-day hospital stay; days 21 through 100 are subject to a copayment by supplemental insurance or by the patient.[1] Until 1998, SNFs received retrospective, cost-based reimbursement. Medicare began the transition to a PPS in 1998, and phase-in is expected to be completed by 2001. This system is based on encounter with the patient rather than on an episode, such as an admission for a specific diagnosis as in acute care facilities. In the PPS system, SNFs are paid an all-inclusive, predetermined, federal per diem rate regardless of actual costs of patient care. The rate is adjusted for the SNF's case mix, based on resource use; the case mix components that affect costs are nursing and rehabilitation use. Billing for Part A along with the services that were covered under Medicare Part B in the past, such as contracted services with rehabilitation personnel, are consolidated. Other Part B services, such as physicians' care, are still billed separately (Congressional Research Service, 1998; House Ways and Means Committee, 1996).

When a person no longer needs skilled nursing care, she or he may continue to reside in a nursing home for chronic care. In this case, Medicare payments for Part B-covered services (except physicians' services) are made directly to the nursing facility, whether the services are pro-

---

[1]A "benefit period" lasts for 60 consecutive days; it commences on the first day of admission to a hospital and ends on discharge from the SNF. Benefit periods can be renewed.

vided by an employee of the nursing home or by an outside person who contracts with the nursing home. The rest of the costs of nursing care are borne by the patient, supplemental insurance, or Medicaid.

In both the old retrospective payment system and the new PPS system, nutrition services are considered part of the per diem rate and not reimbursed directly, as are rehabilitation services. Use of a dietitian is mandated by both licensing and accreditation standards (CFR, 1998; JCAHO, 1998a). However, as SNFs face more financial risk with the new PPS, there is increased potential for cost containment of basic services (Grimaldi, 1999).

Need for Nutrition Services and the Role of the Nutrition Professional

Even though SNFs and nursing homes are required to have a dietitian, the amount of time dietitians actually spend in these facilities varies. The time budgeted for a dietitian in a facility often depends on state requirements, the severity of patients' conditions, nutrition interventions needed, results of previous licensing and accrediting surveys, and economic factors within the SNF and the community. State requirements for licensing of SNFs include the minimum level of dietitian coverage; although it varies, 8 hours per month is not uncommon. Little can be accomplished when nutrition problems are identified at this level of service. When a dietitian works part-time, there must be a full-time person in the facility to provide daily oversight of the food and nutrition services. This is usually a certified dietary manager.

Identifying Nutrition Problems

In 1986, the Institute of Medicine (IOM) Study on Nursing Home Regulation (IOM, 1986) recommended the use of a uniform, comprehensive and outcome-oriented assessment procedure for nursing home residents. The Omnibus Budget Reconciliation Act (OBRA) of 1987 enacted many of the IOM recommendations, including the requirement that all Medicare and Medicaid-certified nursing facilities implement the recommended assessment instrument. This is now part of the statutory and regulatory requirements for long-term care facilities (CFR, 1998; USC, 1998).

The Resident Assessment Instrument (RAI) was developed and validated at the Hebrew Rehabilitation Center for the Aged in Boston under a contract with the Health Care Financing Administration (HCFA) (Hawes et al., 1995; Morris et al., 1990) and updated to its present form, version 2.0, in 1995 (Allen, 1997). The RAI includes standardized procedures and forms for collecting data (Minimum Data Set [MDS]). Certain conditions trigger further assessment, based on standard Resident Assessment Protocols (RAP). The final step is to develop a comprehensive resident care plan based on the MDS and RAP information.

The following aspects of nutritional care are evaluated in the MDS: oral problems, height and weight, weight change, nutrition problems (altered taste, hunger, uneaten meals), approaches to nutritional care (nutrition support, mechanically altered food, therapeutic diets), and food intake. In addition, other aspects of care that affect or are affected by nutrition are also evaluated: dental care, skin condition, and hydration. There are specific RAPs for nutritional status, feeding tubes, dehydration/fluid maintenance, dental care, and pressure ulcers that provide guidelines for the clinician's assessment, treatment, and evaluation.

Existing research provides mixed reports on the success of the RAI. Some reports indicate improvement in the identification of and intervention for nutrition problems in the nursing home (Blaum et al., 1997; Rantz et al., 1999), whereas others report continued problems. In 1998, the Senate heard testimony regarding the persistence of nutrition problems in California nursing homes, despite the federal regulations requiring assessment, intervention, and monitoring (GAO, 1998). Because of the complexity of the RAI screening and planning process, documentation and the actual care of nursing home residents may not be linked (Rantz et al., 1999). In one descriptive observational study (Kayser-Jones et al., 1997), dietary intake as recorded by the certified nursing assistant (CNA) was significantly different from actual food consumption; in some cases the CNA was observed recording food intake data before the resident actually ate a meal or consistently recording an intake of more than 75 percent, irrespective of the resident's actual consumption (less than 75 percent food intake is the trigger on the RAP for further evaluation for poor food intake).

Nutrition Problems in Nursing Homes

Pressure Sores

The relationship between nutrient intake and pressure sores illustrates the complexity of nutrition research in the older nursing home resident. Advanced age, chronic disease, multiple and varying levels of treatment, poor nutrient intake, immobility, and cognitive impairment all contribute to unclear conclusions in studies. In all nutrition studies, three aspects have to be addressed: (1) the contribution of undernutrition to morbidity and mortality, (2) how the disease or condition alters nutrient and energy needs, and (3) the role of nutrition intervention in reversing the disease or condition.

Does Undernutrition Contribute to the Development of Pressure Sores? Undernutrition is a frequently cited risk factor for the development, presence, and inadequate healing of pressure sores (Finucane, 1995). The prevalence of pressure sores among frail, bedridden patients may be as high as 20 percent (Barbenel et al., 1977), and treatment of these wounds can prolong hospital stay and consume considerable health care resources.

Data linking recognized measures of nutritional status with pressure sores in the acute, rehabilitation, or chronic care settings are limited. Observational studies with older people have yielded mixed findings. Poor nutrient intake has been related to the development of pressure sores (Bergstrom and Braden, 1992; Berlowitz and Wilking, 1989) or to their failure to respond to treatment (Allman et al., 1986; Gorse and Messner, 1987). However, an association with nutrient intake has not been consistently observed. Sullivan and Walls (1994) studied 350 geriatric rehabilitation patients prospectively. Twenty-six percent developed complications, including 42 pressure sores of Grade II or higher. There was no association between average daily nutrient intake and these complications.

Are Nutrient Needs Altered in Those with Pressure Ulcers? Breslow and coworkers (1991) described observations of 26 nursing home residents who received tube feedings. Most of the patients were immobile, incontinent, and mentally impaired. The needs and nutrient intake of 14 people who had pressure sores were compared to those who did not. Those with pressure sores were slightly older and had lower body mass indices than those who did not have sores. The investigators concluded that those with pressure sores had higher nutrient requirements than those who did not, based on the energy and protein needed to gain weight or restore serum proteins to normal levels. They also concluded that energy and nutrient needs were being underestimated in patients who had pressure sores.

Does Nutrition Intervention Play a Part in Healing Pressure Sores? There have been few prospective, controlled trials studying the role of nutrition intervention as an independent variable in the prevention or treatment of pressure sores. Myers and colleagues (1990) randomized patients with pressure sores either to usual care or to special nutrition support consisting of nutrition assessment and prescribed intervention. Even though subjects in the intervention arm were excluded from analysis if they did not receive prescribed energy intake and supplements, the intervention was ineffective in improving pressure sore status. Breslow and coworkers

(1993) studied the effect of dietary protein on the healing of pressure sores in malnourished patients. They found that pressure sores healed in those patients receiving a high protein intake (24 percent of total kilocalories) and adequate kilocalories to prevent weight loss. However, their results were confounded by small sample size, nonrandom assignment to groups, and other forms of treatment. A more recent trial by Hartgrink and colleagues (1998) contrasted pressure sore outcomes in 129 hip fracture patients randomized to receive either nocturnal tube feedings or no supplemental feedings. They excluded patients with pressure sores of Grade II or higher on admission. In the treatment group, only 40 percent of subjects tolerated placement of a nasogastric feeding tube for more than 1 week and 26 percent of the subjects for more than 2 weeks. The subjects randomized to the tube feeding group had a greater overall energy and protein intake, but no significant differences in serum albumin levels or the development and severity of pressure sores at 1 and 2 weeks were found. There was also no impact on the development or severity of pressure sores in the subset of subjects who actually received the tube feeding.

There are multiple causes of pressure sores, but poor nutritional status is probably a contributing factor. Energy and nutrient requirements seem to be increased in patients with pressure sores. Although it follows that nutrition intervention should have an effect on reversing pressure sores, confounding variables such as an inadequate understanding of the nutrient and energy needs in this condition, problems with study design, and inadequate research methods do not permit this conclusion. More research is needed to develop better methods for assessing nutrition status, as well as the relationship between nutrient intake and the development and reversal of pressure sores.

Hydration

Inadequate fluid intake among nursing home residents has been reported in a number of studies and can lead to increased morbidity and hospitalizations (Chidester and Spangler, 1997; Gaspar, 1999; Kayser-Jones et al., 1999). Ensuring adequate water intake is particularly important because elders often have a decreased sense of thirst. They may also be dependent on caregivers for help in consuming liquids and food. A nursing protocol has recently been published that helps identify and address dehydration (Mentes and The Iowa Veterans Affairs Nursing Research Consortium, 1998). The American Dietetic Association has also developed a nutrition protocol that describes assessment and intervention strategies (Vogelzang, 1999).

Dysphagia

A substantial number of nursing home residents have problems with dysphagia, which if not addressed may result in aspiration pneumonia and undernutrition. This condition illustrates the interdependence of the nutrition professional and speech pathologists, occupational therapists, nurses, and physicians in providing appropriate nutrition care to the nursing home resident. In one study (Kayser-Jones and Pengilly, 1999), a bedside swallowing evaluation was done: 45 out of 82 nursing home residents were found to have some degree of dysphagia, yet only 10 of these 45 residents had been referred to a speech pathologist or occupational therapist for a previous evaluation. Once dysphagia is recognized, aspects of feeding such as positioning the resident during meals, consistency of foods, size of bites, and feeding techniques can be altered. Groher and McKaig (1995) studied 740 nursing home residents. They found that 36 percent were on mechanically altered diets. Following an evaluation for dysphagia, it was determined that almost all of these residents could tolerate diets at a higher level than they were receiving. For example, the majority of residents receiving tube feedings or pureed foods could tolerate mechanically soft diets.

Undernutrition

Chapter 4 describes commonly used markers and syndromes of undernutrition. Some of the important issues from that chapter are repeated here. In a review of studies evaluating nutritional intake in chronically institutionalized older people, 5 to 18 percent of nursing home residents had energy intakes below need (Rudman et al., 1989). Twenty-six percent met the MDS criterion for poor oral intake. A more recent study reported that 9 percent of nursing home residents met the MDS criterion for hunger (Blaum et al., 1997).

Weight loss has been shown to predict mortality in older people (French et al., 1999; Losonczy et al., 1995; Wallace et al., 1995; White et al., 1998). However, it is a relatively insensitive predictor in nursing homes because food intake may decrease several weeks before routine weight measurements (often monthly) are taken. Low serum albumin levels have been reported to predict mortality in residents of long-term care facilities (Abbasi and Rudman, 1993; Henderson et al., 1992; Rudman et al., 1987; Woo et al., 1989). Using the first National Health and Nutrition Examination Survey (NHANES) data, 14 risk factors were identified that were related to a low serum albumin (Reuben et al., 1997). People with six or more of these factors had an odds ratio of 6.44 of having a serum albumin level less than 3.8 g/dL. Among these factors were being 65 or more years old, having conditions that interfered with eating, being edentulous or having poor dentition, having little or no exercise, and having a low sodium diet prescription. All of these factors are common in nursing home residents.

Nutrition Interventions in Nursing Homes

Use of Modified Diets

Diets that are overly restricted in sodium and fat or do not contain familiar foods may result in a decrease in food intake and weight loss (Buckler et al., 1994). The American Dietetic Association has taken the position that there should be careful assessment of patient needs prior to using modified diets (ADA, 1998b). This assessment should include medical, psychosocial, and quality-of-life issues. Menus and dining experiences should accommodate food preferences, preserve residents' dignity, and emphasize their joy in eating (ADA, 1998a). A liberalized diet, with only moderate changes in sodium, fat, and sugar, has been shown to meet the majority of nursing home residents' needs (Aldrich and Massey, 1999).

Feeding Nursing Home Residents

Many nursing home residents have physical or cognitive impairments that affect their ability to feed themselves. Observational studies, which include both qualitative and quantitative methods, describe the effects of feeding-related care on the intake of nursing home residents (Porter et al., 1999; Steele et al., 1997). When family and nursing home staff demonstrated positive, caring feeding techniques, residents' food intake often improved or did not worsen. Other residents observed, however, failed to receive the needed help with feeding. In some cases, cognitively impaired residents were fed forcibly in violation of best-practice care. Studies have also reported inadequate nutrient intake (Porter et al., 1999) and inappropriate vitamin and mineral supplementation (Porter et al., 1999; Rudman et al., 1995) in nursing home residents.

Use of Liquid Dietary Supplements

Liquid dietary supplements are frequently prescribed when food intake is poor. The role of these supplements in the nutritional care of nursing home residents is not well understood. Retrospective studies, as well as prospective controlled trials, have shown that liquid supplements resulted in improvements in nutrient intake, weight, and some serum markers (Elmståhl and Steen, 1987; Johnson et al., 1993; Turic et al., 1998). However, other descriptive studies which have included observation of the actual feeding practices in nursing homes reported that supplements were sometimes ordered inappropriately and, when ordered, were not consumed by the resident all of the time. Frail residents did not always receive help opening containers, other patients and staff members consumed supplements, or supplements were consumed in place of meals (Kayser-Jones et al., 1998; Porter et al., 1999). It remains unclear as to what role liquid supplements play in the nutritional care of the long-term care resident.

Use of Tube Feedings

The 1987 OBRA regulations and guidelines state that a comprehensive assessment of a patient's ability to eat must be done before tube feedings are used. The facility must also document that it is unable to maintain or improve the resident's nutrition status through oral intake. The regulations also recognize the patient's autonomy to refuse tube feeding (Thomas et al., 1998).

Tube feedings have been shown to benefit some nursing home residents (Morley and Silver, 1995). There was shortened rehabilitation time and/or decreased morbidity and mortality in residents who received supplementary tube feedings following femoral neck fractures and chronic pulmonary disease (Bastow et al., 1983; Delmi et al., 1990; Whittaker et al., 1990).

Although short-term use of tube feeding that addresses specific reversible feeding problems may be appropriate, it is questionable if long-term tube feeding in the old, severely demented resident is appropriate (Mitchell et al., 1997, 1998; Peck et al., 1990). It is important that residents, their families, and a multi-disciplinary team, including the nutrition professional, consider the outcome and consequences prior to initiation of tube feedings.

Reasons for Problems

Many factors affect food intake in the elderly nursing home resident. Changes in taste and smell, the effects of chronic disease and multiple medications, depression, and a decreased basal metabolic rate and activity all may cause a decreased appetite and desire to eat (Abbasi and Rudman, 1994). Some studies have shown that investigation into causes of poor food intake is disorganized. Even when nurses and dietitians alerted physicians to feeding and weight problems, the physician seldom investigated the causes, such as swallowing disorders, poor oral health, anorexia, or depression (Johnson et al., 1993; Kayser-Jones et al., 1997, 1998).

Elders may also experience problems related to chewing and swallowing, manual dexterity, and altered cognition that make them dependent on others for feeding. However, staffing levels and skills may affect the quality of feeding assistance received. There are often too few CNAs to help with feeding, especially at the evening meal. There are also not enough registered nurses and dietitians to oversee and train CNAs about appropriate feeding techniques and to ensure the maintenance of a pleasant dining environment (Kayser-Jones and Schell, 1997; Porter et al., 1999).

Licensing agencies need to develop more effective oversight with respect to feeding, supervision of staff, and other nutrition-related issues. In response to Senate hearings on California nursing homes (GAO, 1998), HCFA has drafted investigative protocols to better evaluate the outcome of care related to pressure sores, weight loss, hydration, and dining and food service, including the way CNAs and others are trained and supervised in feeding nursing home residents. The American Dietetic Association has also responded by developing risk assessment tools (ADA, 1998a; Vogelzang, 1999).

HOME HEALTH AGENCIES

HHAs are defined as private or public organizations that provide or arrange for the provision of skilled nursing services to people who are unable to leave their temporary or permanent place of residence. According to the National Association of Home Care, there are more than 20,000 providers of home care services to some 8 million people who require services for acute illness, long-term health conditions, permanent disability, or terminal illness. Medicare certifies approximately half of the home care programs (NAHC, 1999).

Unlike skilled nursing facilities, Medicare does not require a 3-day acute care stay prior to coverage of home health care services. HHAs are required to provide preventive treatment and rehabilitative services for the specific problems related to the physician's referral. The treatment provided through HHAs must be consistent with standards of practice for the discipline involved and the person providing the care must be registered, licensed, or certified to provide the service (CFR, 1998).

Medicare Funding

Medicare beneficiaries pay nothing out-of-pocket for covered home health visits. Medicare currently reimburses HHAs on an interim payment system (IPS), although a PPS is currently under development. A 4-year transition to the PPS system of reimbursement began in late 1999. The appropriate unit of service and the number, type, and duration of visits will be determined. Per-beneficiary limits will be calculated from cost-reporting periods ending in fiscal year 1994 and updated by home health market-based surveys (Berke, 1998; *Caring*, 1998; St. Pierre, 1999).

The current IPS system is a retrospective cost-based system. Per-visit cost limits are determined separately for each type of covered home health service, such as skilled nursing, rehabilitation services, social services, and home health aide services. The services of a nutrition professional are not covered.

Medicare currently pays for some aspects of home parenteral and enteral nutrition. In order to obtain Medicare reimbursement, the patient must be unable to meet nutritional requirements using an oral diet for more than 90 days. For parenteral nutrition support, the patient must have a nonfunctioning gastrointestinal (GI) tract due to interruption in continuity or impairment in absorptive capacity. For enteral nutrition support, there must be a disruption in the ability to ingest oral foods or impairment of the upper GI tract, which interrupts the transport of food to the small intestine (Giglione, 1988; Goff, 1998).

Coverage regulations for enteral and parenteral nutrition are under the Prosthetic Devices section of Medicare. This section, which covers such things as pacemakers, braces, and artificial limbs, also defines reimbursement for home nutrition support. The assumption in placing nutrition support in this section is that it is a prosthetic device for a dysfunctional GI tract. For this reason, Medicare does not cover nutrition support if it is provided to a patient who has a functioning GI tract (e.g., intradialytic nutrition support in end-stage renal disease). Nutrition support is also not covered for the patients with significant nutritional needs, but who will be able to eat within the 90-day time period. Medicare covers solutions and equipment, but not the consultation by a nutrition professional needed for the assessment of energy and nutrient needs, implementation, and monitoring of the effects treatment on nutritional status (Goff, 1998).

Need for Nutrition Services in Home Health Agencies

Health statistics show that more than 2.4 million Medicare beneficiaries received home care services in 1996. Half had chronic diseases that are normally treated with diet (NCHS, 1999). Others report that patients who receive home care services have a high prevalence of malnutrition and need some type of nutrition services (Rebovich et al., 1990).

Malnutrition can be a risk for early nonelective hospital readmission. In one study of 92 nutritionally compromised Medicare beneficiaries, those with weight loss and failure of serum albumin levels to improve during the first month after hospitalization were at higher risk of hospital readmission than those who maintained or increased their postdischarge weight or improved their serum albumin levels (Friedmann et al., 1997).

Some evidence indicates that nutrition intervention can reduce the prevalence of undernutrition in home care populations. In a study of 417 free-living rural elders, 68 were found on screening to have undernutrition. Six months after nutrition intervention was provided as part of a comprehensive medical and social program, 38 percent were no longer at nutrition risk (Klein et al., 1997).

Many home health patients require nutrition counseling for a modified diet. A survey in the Chicago area found that more than 35 percent of patients 65 years or older were admitted to HHAs on a modified diet. After review of medical records by a dietitian, an additional 10 to 15 percent were found to need modified diets or to have their diet prescription changed (Gaffney and Singer, 1985).

Overly restricted diets may lead to low dietary intake and weight loss in older people (ADA, 1998b). For this reason it is important that a nutrition professional evaluate actual intake and make recommendations to patients and their families that address only the most important medical issues. These recommendations must be sensitive to customary food patterns, meet nutritional needs, and prevent a decrease in food intake.

Patients in the care of HHAs also require monitoring of enteral and parenteral nutrition. In 1992, it was estimated that as many as 40,000 Medicare patients received parenteral nutrition and 152,000 received enteral nutrition at home (Howard et al., 1995). Thus nutritional care of Medicare patients at home to appropriately monitor and evaluate the nutritional needs are significant.

The Nutrition Professional in Home Health Agencies

There is no mention of a nutrition professional in the Code of Federal Regulations for HHAs, either in the sections related to personnel or to conditions of participation (CFR, 1998). The Joint Commission on Accreditation of Healthcare Organizations (JCAHO) standards for HHAs require that each patient be evaluated for nutrition risk, and if nutrition problems are related to the reason for HHA referral, the program must provide the services (JCAHO, 1998b). However, most examples given in the JCAHO standards imply that health care providers other than a nutrition professional would provide these services. This is most likely related to the omission of the nutrition professional from HCFA regulations.

A small proportion of nutrition professionals work in home health settings. The most recent survey of work sites for dietitians (Bryk and Soto, 1999) indicates that only 399 (1.4 percent of the respondents) listed their primary employment in home health care. This small number becomes even more modest given a report that dietitians in the home care industry work a limited number of hours (Arensberg and Schiller, 1996). This potential work force shortage is greater for dietitians credentialed as entry-level nutrition support practitioners. Responses from 1,237 certified nutrition support dietitians revealed that 53 percent spent no time in home health, and only 61 practitioners (approximately 5 percent) were employed full-time in HHAs (Professional Testing Corporation, 1997).

The practice of the dietitian in home care has been described (Arensberg and Schiller, 1996). Dietitians who worked in home care were experienced, but new to the home care environment. They worked on average less than 10 hours per week, and typically for organizations that served between 100 and 500 patients. Most dietitians made no home visits, but provided consultation to other professionals. They also provided services to the patient by telephone. When home visits were made by the dietitian, most were for patients with diabetes and cancer. Even though a substantial number of patients enrolled in home health care were receiving nutrition support, dietitians reported making at most one visit per week to these patients.

The above study found that the greatest obstacle to providing or expanding nutrition services in home care was "lack of reimbursement." The following are areas in which dietitians did not provide services but felt capable of doing so: monitoring nutrition support, conducting home visits, providing counseling for nutrition therapy, and assessing nutrition risk. In most cases, there was no separate billing to third-party payers for nutrition services. When third-party billing was initiated, only 28 percent received reimbursement and nearly half of charges submitted received 25 percent or less of the amount billed.

In another descriptive survey (Schiller et al., 1998), administrators of HHAs recognized that patients had a high prevalence of nutrition problems and that nutrition therapy was an important form of treatment. More than half of the administrators surveyed did not have, but would like, a dietitian as a nutrition consultant for nutrition assessments, the development of nutrition care plans, nutrition therapy for specific conditions, and staff training. While in most cases a nurse provided nutrition services (Schiller et al., 1998), home care nurses demonstrated a deficit in nutrition knowledge, even though they felt it was an important part of their practice (Caie-Lawrence et al., 1995). HHA administrators stated that the main deterrent to having a dietitian provide nutrition services was lack of reimbursement by third-party payers and lack of physician request (Schiller et al., 1998).

Identification of Patients Who Would Benefit from Nutrition Services

It was expected that home health services would reduce overall health care costs by decreasing the need for acute care admissions and preventing other costly interventions. However, this expectation has not been fully realized. Although HHAs provide significant benefits to acutely ill patients, these services are often used as complements of, not substitutions for, other forms of health care. There is limited evidence that home health services significantly reduce overall health care costs or reduce readmission to hospitals or nursing homes. However, it has been shown that readmissions are less likely if careful identification and specific interventions are focused on the problems that most often precipitate readmissions (Weissert et al., 1997).

For Medicare to provide reimbursement to nutrition professionals in home care settings, such services must be carefully targeted to ensure both cost-effectiveness and adequate coverage for individuals with the greatest need. The nutrition professional has to educate other health care professionals working in home health about how to give appropriate nutrition education and how to evaluate the effectiveness of nutrition interventions. Nutrition professionals should, however, provide the most complex nutrition care themselves.

One tool that may prove helpful in identifying patients with complex nutrition problems is the Outcomes Assessment and Information Set (OASIS) (Sperling and Humphrey, 1999). Home health agencies began using this in July 1999 for Medicare patients needing skilled care. OASIS includes several questions that attempt to assess nutrition status, food security, and the patient's implementation of any prescribed dietary modifications. When the patient is experiencing problems, a referral to the dietitian is recommended. At the time of this report however, to the committee's knowledge there have been no published studies validating the effectiveness of the OASIS system in identifying and addressing nutrition problems.

Who Should Receive the Services of a Nutrition Professional in the Home Health Setting?

Patients seen in the home care setting are often the most frail, undernourished group of elders in the health care system and, because they are homebound, have no ability to use nutrition services that may be available in other ambulatory settings. Box 12.1 summarizes conditions that were identified as requiring services provided by a nutrition professional. In certain instances, these services may be delivered telephonically; however, the effectiveness may depend on the socioeconomic, cultural, and educational characteristics of patients (Short and Saindon, 1998).

BOX 12.1 Conditions that Require a Nutrition Professional in the Home Setting

- Counseling about altered nutrient needs or dietary modification
- Newly diagnosed diabetes (homebound individuals should have the same benefits for diabetes self-management as those being seen in an ambulatory setting)
- Poorly controlled diabetes related to other conditions that require skilled care
- Heart failure
- Dietary modification following myocardial infarction
- Complications of cancer treatment (i.e., chemotherapy, radiation, and surgical treatment) that result in food aversions, need for consistency modifications, or altered nutrient or energy requirements
- Dysphagia
- Undernutrition—weight loss in the absence of remedial medical or psychiatric disorders
- Pre-end-stage renal failure with complex dietary modifications
- Osteoporosis or hip fracture
- Wound-healing problems

Coverage for Home or Ambulatory Enteral and Parenteral Nutrition Support Services

There is an inequity in Medicare coverage for enteral and parenteral nutrition in the home care or ambulatory setting compared to the hospital or skilled nursing setting. Although a physician, nurse, and pharmacist are typically involved in the care of the home or ambulatory patient receiving nutrition support, the nutrition professional is often absent. Medicare beneficiaries who remain on nutrition support following hospitalization or begin it in the ambulatory or home care setting are often at high risk and could benefit from the care of a nutrition professional. The nutrition professional is also knowledgeable about how and when to transition patients to other, often less costly forms of nutrition support.

In addition to the lack of consultation by a nutrition professional, many beneficiaries need home enteral or parenteral interventions that are not reimbursed by Medicare. These people may require tube feedings or parenteral interventions that are projected to last for less than 90 days; they may also be able to take some food by mouth, but not enough to meet nutrient or energy needs. Few individuals are able to pay for this therapy on their own, and the lack of reimbursement for nutrition support puts these Medicare beneficiaries at nutritional risk. People who are unable to maintain adequate nutritional status are more likely to experience adverse outcomes, including premature readmission to the hospital, functional compromise, and mortality (Sullivan, 1992).

HHAs are required to have specialized nutrition expertise in order to be Medicare certified. However, HCFA regulations do not specifically include the nutrition professional in the list of mandated participants, and there is no provision to pay for these services, other than as administrative costs. It is unclear if the costs of the services of a nutrition professional are included in these administrative costs, particularly since HCFA did not list the nutrition professional in its regulations. This oversight encourages HHAs to use other untrained professionals or to budget so little for the nutrition professional that adequate services cannot be provided. Another way that HHAs have obtained nutrition services is to request help from dietitians in hospitals or in outpatient clinics, with or without remuneration. Yet staffing in hospitals is limited by the capitated PPS and in the outpatient setting because there is no reimbursement for nutrition services.

COMMUNITY-BASED BENEFITS

Program of All-Inclusive Care for the Elderly

The Program of All-Inclusive Care for the Elderly (PACE) is a new capitated benefit for Medicare beneficiaries authorized under the Balanced Budget Act of 1997 (HCFA, 1998). PACE is modeled from the On Lok Senior Health Services program in San Francisco. Participants continue to live in their homes while receiving a comprehensive array of services. The program is delivered through services provided at adult day health centers, homes, and inpatient facilities. Elders receive all services provided by Medicare and, at a minimum, 16 other services including nutrition counseling and meals. A multidisciplinary team, which includes a dietitian, provides or coordinates the provision of services.

PACE providers receive a monthly capitated Medicare rate. Providers receive an additional monthly premium from those participants who are not also receiving Medicaid. However, there is no deductible, coinsurance, or other cost sharing. The rate is a per capita cost calculated by HCFA for reimbursement of HMOs and adjusted for frailty factors. The rate is fixed for each contract year regardless of the changes in the participant's health status (Congressional Research Service, 1998; HCFA, 1998).

Dietitians in the San Francisco-based PACE perform quarterly nutrition assessments for each client. They identify and provide for nutrition needs or coordinate provision through other community programs such as Title III–VI Elderly Nutrition Programs. Dietitians employed by PACE may be experiencing some of the same cost containment problems as those in the acute care setting (Frances Chan, R.D., On Lok Senior Health Service, San Francisco, California, personal communication, 1999).

Assisted Living

There is no common definition of Assisted Living (AL) facilities. In most cases they include some combination of housing and services in a residential environment. The programs strive to maximize individual functioning and autonomy (Gramann, 1999; Hawes et al., 1999). Some of these facilities are part of a larger complex that also provides other forms of care, such as adult day health, skilled nursing, or acute care.

A classic feature of AL is an attempt to let residents age-in-place. However, as residents age, the acuteness of their condition increases, increasing the cost as well as the potential for inappropriate or inadequate service, particularly in free-standing units (Manard and Cameron, 1997). There are no consistent national criteria for when residents should be transitioned to higher levels of care, such as skilled nursing facilities.

Most AL facilities are expensive and, therefore, serve middle- to upper-income elders. Demographic trends show the need for more affordable AL as the population ages and wants to remain independent longer.

Medicare Reimbursement

Medicare does not reimburse for this form of elder care and most likely will not in the near future. However, residents of AL complexes receive Medicare benefits in other settings, such as acute care, ambulatory care, or home health care in AL facilities. Other federally funded programs, such as congregate feeding and home-delivered meals, may also be used by residents of some AL facilities.

Role of Nutrition Services

The focus of nutrition services for residents of AL complexes should be on disease prevention and maintenance of independence. Programs should emphasize good nutrition and activity. In this setting, elders are able to use nutrition services that may be available from local outpatient clinics, HHAs, or community-based education programs, when available.

Congregate Feeding or Home Meals

The Elderly Nutrition Program (ENP) is the largest community nutrition program provided for older people in the United States. Title III of the Older Americans Act provides services for the general elderly population, and Title VI provides services to the Native American population. Both programs are administered by the Administration on Aging (AoA) of the Department of Health and Human Services. Both provide congregate feeding and home-delivered meals. The AoA provides 37 percent of the funding for congregate feeding and 23 percent for home-delivered meals. The rest of the cost is borne by state, local and private funds; donations; and volunteer time (AoA, 1998; Ponza et al., 1996).

Participants in the programs must be 60 years of age or older. Low-income groups are targeted. Many participants face moderate or high nutritional risk and have functional disabilities. Meals served must provide at least one-third of the relevant recommended dietary allowances (IOM, 1994), and the programs must employ dietitians.

In one study, the vast majority of individuals attending meal sites were at moderate (42 percent) or high risk (39 percent) of malnutrition as assessed by the Determine Your Nutritional Health Checklist (Reuben et al., 1996). In a recent comprehensive evaluation of Title III–VI programs (Ponza et al., 1996), participants had a significantly better nutrient intake than those not receiving services; programs were shown to target high-risk populations. In addition to meals, more than half of the participants received nutrition education, screening, and counseling. Programs have long waiting lists, and funding from the federal government may not be meeting the increased need for services (Ponza et al., 1996).

Most of the participants of Title III–VI programs also use Medicare-funded programs, such as acute care, ambulatory services, and home health agencies. Almost half of the referrals for Title III–VI programs come from hospitals or community-based organizations, indicating that ENPs function as part of a larger network of community systems, addressing the comprehensive long-term care needs of the elderly.

Informal Caregiving

The majority of functionally disabled elders live in the community rather than in nursing homes. More than 7 million Americans provide informal care to approximately 4.2 million functionally disabled elders each week (AoA, 1998). More than 2 million elders need help with one or more activities such as eating, cooking, and shopping (AoA, 1998). Informal care plays a significant role in preventing or delaying the need for disabled elders to use more expensive services. Elders cared for by family and friends may also use congregate feeding or home-delivered meals. When needed, they could also use nutrition services in HHAs or ambulatory care if these were available and accessible.

FUTURE AREAS OF RESEARCH

Additional research is needed on the role of liquid dietary supplements and tube feedings in maintaining adequate nutritional status in the nursing home setting. There also should be continued investigation of nutritional assessment techniques and the relationship between nutrient intake and conditions common to nursing home residents (e.g., pressure sores).

More work is needed on the development and validation of tools that would help identify people at nutritional risk who are being seen in home health agencies. Continued research on how best to communicate with homebound clients in both urban and rural areas is needed. Specific attention should be paid to the potential applications of teleconferencing, particularly when used to provide information about food and nutrition to the client who has communication problems (hearing, speech, other languages, etc.).

SUMMARY

There has been a rapid growth in the use of skilled nursing, home health, and long-term care services over the last decade. Patients receiving these services often are undernourished due to chronic disease or its treatment. It is important that there are viable nutrition services and food assistance programs in these settings. As Medicare reimbursement moves to a capitated prospective payment system, it is imperative that nutrition services are not compromised.

Much of what is known about existing services in nursing homes comes from qualitative and quantitative observational studies. It is unclear if the OBRA-mandated screening and intervention tools have improved clinical care. Specifically, substantial problems with aspects of nutrition care persist, such as the quality of the food service, feeding techniques used for impaired patients, and the use of supplements and tube feedings. Physicians do not always carefully evaluate the causes of nutrition problems prior to prescribing liquid dietary supplements or tube feedings.

Even though HHAs are required to have specialized nutrition expertise to be Medicare certified, there is no specific requirement for a nutrition professional in HCFA regulations or JCAHO standards. Staffing for nutrition professionals is often inadequate and HHAs commonly turn to dietitians in hospitals for help, with or without remuneration. Descriptive studies have concluded that there is an inadequate work force of nutrition professionals in the home care setting due in part to insufficient reimbursement for these services. Research in HHAs indicates that it is important to carefully identify patients who need services and that services should aim to prevent hospital admissions, when possible, and to restore health and function.

The new OASIS system for assessing patient needs has not been validated for its ability to identify nutrition problems. If this system proves cumbersome or insensitive, another screening system must be developed and validated. To be most cost-effective, care by the nutrition professional should be provided to those who need the most complex services. Follow-up care should be supervised by the nutrition professional, but could be provided by others going into the home. Use of the telephone and other communications technologies should be investigated, particularly when the patient and provider do not speak a common language or the patient has hearing or speech disabilities. It is unclear from the literature when and for whom this technology is most useful. Reimbursement for parenteral and enteral nutrition support in the home care setting and ambulatory setting is inadequate in the following areas:

- coverage for the nutrition professional to assess and monitor tolerance to nutrition support or to transition patients to less costly forms of nutrition intervention; and
- coverage for patients who need nutrition support for less than 90 days in order to meet energy and nutrient needs, whether or not they are eating (patients who are unable to meet nutrient and energy needs with food alone).

Other forms of care, such as PACE, AL, and informal caregiving, depend on the complementary services of other government-funded community programs, such as congregate feeding and home-delivered meals. Recent studies indicate that these programs are an effective, integral part of the government's services to the elderly, but that funding may not match need.

Older individuals in PACE, in assisted living facilities, or cared for by family and friends also need access to viable nutrition services in ambulatory care settings or through home care services. If these services are not available, there is an increased likelihood that nutrition-related disorders will not be addressed.

The lack of good food assistance and nutrition programs may lead to increased disability and to the use of more expensive services.

RECOMMENDATIONS

Skilled Nursing Facilities and Nursing Homes

• As Medicare shifts to a prospective payment system of reimbursement for skilled nursing, nutrition services must not be compromised and must be improved beyond current practice. Internal quality improvement systems and accrediting and licensing agencies must monitor for adequate feeding techniques, the quality of food service, and the satisfaction of patients and their families with these services. Endeavors aimed at new feeding techniques, which would use staff time more efficiently, must be developed and tested. Staffing must be adequate, and staff members should be well trained and professionally supervised so that nursing home residents are fed sensitively and appropriately.

• Prior to initiating supplements and nutrition support, there should be documentation by physicians that treatable causes of weight loss and poor food intake have been considered and evaluated, if appropriate.

Home Health Agencies

• Many homebound elders need nutrition services to maintain health and functional status. Patients with complex nutrition problems require the services of a nutrition professional. Others could obtain needed services from another health care professional visiting the home, with oversight by the nutrition professional. A well-designed screening system is necessary to identify those patients who most need the more complex nutrition services. The new OASIS system must be validated to ensure that it identifies patients with the greatest need. If this system proves inadequate, another system should be developed.

• Nutrition services would be most efficacious for patients who require counseling about altered energy and nutrient needs or dietary modifications. Services have to be designed so they address, at a minimum, the problems that would most likely cause hospital readmissions.

• The efficacy of nutrition intervention in chronic disease has been covered in previous chapters. The committee has identified the following conditions as being most important for nutrition intervention in the HHA setting: newly diagnosed diabetes; poorly controlled diabetes when caused by other conditions that require skilled care; heart failure; problems following cancer treatment (surgery, radiation, chemotherapy) that result in food aversions, consistency modifications, or increased nutrient or energy needs; dysphagia; undernutrition or weight loss in the absence of remedial medical or psychiatric disorders; pre-end-stage renal failure when dietary modification is complex; severe osteoporosis or hip fracture; and wound healing problems.

• When there is evidence that nutrition services should be provided, they must be required and supported financially. Present HCFA regulations do not specifically describe a role for the nutrition professional. This needs to be clarified. Anecdotal evidence indicates that nutrition professionals in other settings (e.g., hospitals) help provide services to HHAs, with or without remuneration. Those who are planning for PPS reimbursement in HHAs should consider that both staffing and compensation for nutrition services are inadequate in the present system.

Nutrition Support in the Home Care and Ambulatory Setting

• It is recommended that reimbursement be made available to the nutrition professional with specialized training in nutrition support. This person would provide consultation and follow-up as requested by a physician. Consultation would include the assessment of nutritional needs and recommendations for appropriate intervention(s) and monitoring for feeding tolerance and complications. It is specifically intended that the participating nutrition professional work with the referring physician to discontinue inappropriate interventions and facilitate the transition to oral or other feeding modalities when indicated. There is the potential for appreciable cost offsets by encouraging appropriate interventions. Inappropriate use of costly feeding interventions and complications related to their misapplication may otherwise result.

• A major gap in coverage exists for undernourished patients who need home nutrition support for less than 90 days. It is recommended that this 90-day requirement for reimbursement be reevaluated to consider the option of reimbursement for shorter-term interventions and that the intervention include appropriate consultation and approval by the nutrition professional.

All Programs

• It is important that standards and expected outcomes for essential nutrition services are well defined so that if capitated programs face potential financial risk, these services are not jeopardized.

• Medicare-funded programs and food assistance programs often serve the same clients; their services are complementary, not duplicative. Patients seen in HHAs or PACE, or cared for in assisted living facilities or by family and friends, may need community programs such as Title III–VI Elderly Nutrition Programs to provide food assistance and additional nutrition services. Adequate funding for food assistance programs is an essential part of the government's overall nutrition services for elders and may not be keeping up with need.

• It is essential that comprehensive nutrition services are provided through HHAs, outpatient clinics, and other community programs so that people living in their homes or in assisted living facilities can maintain good health and functionality as long as possible. Essential nutrition services should be provided in a way that respects the role of the informal caregiver and the independence and functionality of the patient.

REFERENCES

ADA (American Dietetic Association) 1998a. ADA responds to nursing home initiative; task force is developing nutrition care recommendations for HCFA. *J Am Diet Assoc* 98:1106.

ADA (American Dietetic Association) 1998b. Position of the American Dietetic Association: Liberalized diets for older adults in long-term care. *J Am Diet Assoc* 98:201.

Abbasi AA, Rudman D. 1993. Observations on the prevalence of protein–calories undernutrition in VA nursing homes. *J Am Geriatr Soc* 41:117–121.

Abbasi AA, Rudman D. 1994. Undernutrition in the nursing home: Prevalence, consequences, causes and prevention. *Nutr Rev* 52:113–122.

Aldrich JK, Massey LK. 1999. A liberalized geriatric diet fits most dietary prescriptions for long-term-care residents. *J Am Diet Assoc* 99:478–480.

Allen JE. 1997. *Long Term Care Facility Resident Assessment Instrument User's Manual.* New York: Springer.

Allman RM, Laprade CA, Noel LB, Walker JM, Moorer CA, Dear MR, Smith CR. 1986. Pressure sores among hospitalized patients. *Ann Intern Med* 105:337–342.

AoA (Administration on Aging). 1998. *Informal Caregiving: Compassion in Action.* Washington, D.C.: U.S. Department of Health and Human Services.

Arensberg MBF, Schiller MR. 1996. Dietitians in home care: A survey of current practice. *J Am Diet Assoc* 96:347–353.

Barbenel JC, Jordan MM, Nicol SM, Clark MO. 1977. Incidence of pressure-sores in the Greater Glasgow Health Board area. *Lancet* 8037:548–550.

Bastow MD, Rawlings J, Allison SP. 1983. Benefits of supplementary tube feeding after fractured neck of femur: A randomised controlled trial. *Br Med J* 287:1589–1592.

Bergstrom N, Braden B. 1992. A prospective study of pressure sore risk among institutionalized elderly. *J Am Geriatr Soc* 40:747–758.

Berke D. 1998. The Balanced Budget Act of 1997—what it means for home care providers and beneficiaries. *J Long Term Home Health Care* 17:2–9.

Berlowitz DR, Wilking SVB. 1989. Risk factors for pressure sores. A comparison of cross-sectional and cohort-derived data. *J Am Geriatr Soc* 37:1043–1050.

Blaum CS, O'Neill EF, Clements KM, Fries BE, Fiatarone MA. 1997. Validity of the minimum data set for assessing nutritional status in nursing home residents. *Am J Clin Nutr* 66:787–794.

Breslow RA, Hallfrisch J, Goldberg AP. 1991. Malnutrition in tubefed nursing home patients with pressure sores. *J Parenter Enteral Nutr* 15:663–668.

Breslow RA, Hallfrisch J, Guy DG, Crawley B, Goldberg AP. 1993. The importance of dietary protein in healing pressure ulcers. *J Am Geriatr Soc* 41:357–362.

Bryk JA, Soto TK. 1999. Report on the 1997 Membership Database of the American Dietetic Association. *J Am Diet Assoc* 99:102–107.

Buckler DA, Kelber ST, Goodwin JS. 1994. The use of dietary restrictions in malnourished nursing home patients. *J Am Geriatr Soc* 42:1100–1102.

Caie-Lawrence J, Peploski J, Russell JC. 1995. Training needs of home healthcare nurses. *Home Health Nurse* 13:53–61.

Caring. 1998. The Balanced Budget Act: Effects on home care beneficiaries and providers. *Caring* 17:10–12, 14, 16.

CFR (Code of Federal Regulations). 1998. Requirements for long-term care facilties. 42CFR482–484. Washington, D.C.: U.S. Government Printing Office.

Chidester JC, Spangler AA. 1997. Fluid intake in the institutionalized elderly. *J Am Diet Assoc* 97:23–30.

Clark RF. 1998. An introduction to the national long-term care surveys. Available at: http://aspe.os.dhhs.gov/daltcp/reports/nltcssu2.htm. Accessed September 7, 1999.

Cohen MA. 1998. Emerging trends in the finance and delivery of long-term care: Public and private opportunities and challenges. *Gerontologist* 38:80–89.

Congressional Research Service. 1998. *Medicare Reimbursement Policies*. Washington, D.C.: U.S. Government Printing Office.

Cornoni-Huntley JC, Harris TB, Everett DF, Albanes D, Micozzi MS, Miles TP, Feldman JJ. 1991. An overview of body weight of older persons, including the impact on mortality. The National Health and Nutrition Examination Survey I—Epidemiologic Follow-up Study. *J Clin Epidemiol* 44:743–753.

Cutler DM, Sheiner L. 1993. Policy options for long-term care. In: Wise D, ed. *Studies in the Economics of Aging*. Chicago, Ill.: University of Chicago Press.

Delmi M, Rapin C-H, Bengoa J-M, Delmas PD, Vasey H, Bonjour J-P. 1990. Dietary supplementation in elderly patients with fractured neck of the femur. *Lancet* 335:1013–1016.

Economics and Statistics Administration. 1995. Sixty-five plus in the United States. Available at: http://www.census.gov/socdemo/www/agebrief.htm. Accessed September 7, 1999.

Elmståhl S, Steen B. 1987. Hospital nutrition in geriatric long-term care medicine: II. Effects of dietary supplements. *Age Aging* 16:73–80.

Evashwick C, Meadors A, Friis R. 1998. The role of home care in integrated delivery systems. *Home Health Care Serv Q* 17:49–69.

Finucane TE. 1995. Malnutrition, tube feeding and pressure sores: Data are incomplete. *J Am Geriatr Soc* 43:447–451.

Freedman VA. 1999. Long-term admissions to home health agencies: A life table analysis. *Gerontologist* 39:16–24.

French SA, Folsom AR, Jeffery RW, Williamson DF. 1999. Prospective study of intentionality of weight loss and mortality in older women: The Iowa Women's Health Study. *Am J Epidemiol* 149:504–514.

Friedmann JM, Jensen GL, Smiciklas-Wright H, McCamish MA. 1997. Predicting early nonelective hospital readmission in nutritionally compromised older adults. *Am J Clin Nutr* 65:1714–1720.

Frisoni GB, Franzoni S, Rozzini R, Ferrucci L, Boffelli S, Trabucchi M. 1995. Food intake and mortality in the frail elderly. *J Gerontol A Biol Sci Med Sci* 50:M203–M210.

Gaffney JT, Singer GR. 1985. Diet needs of patients referred to home health. *J Am Diet Assoc* 85:198–202.

GAO (General Accounting Office). 1998. *California Nursing Homes: Care Problems Persist Despite Federal and State Oversight*. Washington D.C.: GAO.

Gaspar PM. 1999. Water intake of nursing home residents. *J Gerontol Nurs* 25:23–29.

Giglione L. 1988. Home IV therapy—who pays? *J Intraven Nurs* 11:294–296.

Goff KL. 1998. Cost and cost-benefit of enteral nutrition. *Gastrointest Endosc Clin N Am* 8:733–744.

Gorse GJ, Messner RL. 1987. Improved pressure sore healing with hydrocolloid dressings. *Arch Dermatol* 123:766–771.

Gramann D. 1999. New frontiers in integrated care. *Caring* 18:14–17.

Gray-Donald K. 1995. The frail elderly: Meeting the nutritional challenges. *J Am Diet Assoc* 95:538–540.

Grimaldi PL. 1999. New skilled nursing facility payment scheme boosts Medicare risk. *J Health Care Finance* 25:1–9.

Groher ME, McKaig TN. 1995. Dysphagia and dietary levels in skilled nursing facilities. *J Am Geriatr Soc* 43:528–532.

Hartgrink HH, Wille J, Konig P, Hermans J, Breslau PJ. 1998. Pressure sores and tube feeding in patients with a fracture of the hip: A randomized clinical trial. *Clin Nutr* 17:287–292.

Hawes C, Morris JN, Phillips CD, Mor V, Fries BE, Nonemaker S. 1995. Reliability estimates for the minimum data set for nursing home resident assessment and care screening. *Gerontologist* 35:172–178.

Hawes C, Rose M, Phillips CD. 1999. A national study of assisted living for the frail elderly: Results of a national survey of facilities. Available at: http://aspe.os.dhhs.gov/daltcp/reports/facreses.htm. Accessed September 7, 1999.

HCFA (Health Care Financing Administration). 1998. Program of All-Inclusive Care for the Elderly (PACE) history. Available at: http://www.hcfa.gov/medicaid/pace/pacegen.htm. Accessed September 7, 1999.

Henderson CT, Trumbore LS, Mobarhan S, Benya R, Miles TP. 1992. Prolonged tube feeding in long-term care: Nutritional status and clinical outcomes. *J Am Coll Nutr* 11:309–325.

House Ways and Means Committee. 1996. *1996 Green Book*. WMCP 104-14. Washington, D.C.: U.S. Government Printing Office.

Howard L, Ament M, Fleming CR, Shike M, Steiger E. 1995. Current use and clinical outcome of home parenteral and enteral nutrition therapies in the United States. *Gastroenterology* 109:355–365.

IOM (Institute of Medicine). 1986. *Improving the Quality of Care in Nursing Homes*. Washington, D.C.: National Academy Press.

IOM (Institute of Medicine) 1994. *How Should the Recommended Dietary Allowances Be Revised?* Washington, D.C.: National Academy Press.

Jackson ME, Doty P. 1998. *Analysis of Patterns of HHA and SNF Benefit Use Among Disabled and Non-Disabled Medicare Beneficiaries: 1989–1994*. Washington, D.C.: Office of Disability, Aging and Long-term Care Policy, U.S. Department of Health and Human Services.

JCAHO (Joint Commission on Accreditation of Healthcare Organizations). 1998a. 1999–2000 Comprehensive Accreditation Manual for Home Care. Oakbrook Terrace, Ill.: JCAHO.

JCAHO (Joint Commission on Accreditation of Healthcare Organizations). 1998b. 1998–1999 Comprehensive Accreditation Manual for Long-Term Care. Oakbrook Terrace, Ill.: JCAHO.

Johnson LE, Dooley PA, Gleick JB. 1993. Oral nutritional supplement use in elderly nursing home patients. *J Am Geriatr Soc* 41:947–952.

Kayser-Jones J, Pengilly K. 1999. Dysphagia among nursing home residents. *Geriatr Nurs* 20:77–82.

Kayser-Jones J, Schell ES. 1997. Staffing and the mealtime experience of nursing home residents on a special care unit. *Am J Alzh Dis* 12:67–72.

Kayser-Jones J, Schell J, Porter C, Paul S. 1997. Reliability of percentage figures used to record the dietary intake of nursing home residents. *Nurs Home Med* 5:69–76.

Kayser-Jones J, Schell ES, Porter C, Barbaccia JC, Steinbach C, Bird WF, Redford M, Pengilly K. 1998. A prospective study of the use of liquid oral dietary supplements in nursing homes. *J Am Geriatr Soc* 46:1378–1386.

Kayser-Jones J, Schell E, Porter C, Barbaccia JC, Shaw H. 1999. Factors contributing to dehydration in nursing homes: Inadequate staffing and lack of professional supervision. *J Am Geriatr Soc* 47:1187–1194.

Klein GL, Kita K, Fish J, Sinkus B, Jensen GL. 1997. Nutrition and health for older persons in rural America: A managed care model. *J Am Diet Assoc* 97:885–888.

Lehrman S, Shore KK. 1998. Hospitals' vertical integration into skilled nursing: A rational approach to controlling transaction costs. *Inquiry* 35:303–314.

Liu K, Gage B, Harvell J, Stevenson D, Brennan N. 1999. Medicare's Post-Acute Care Benefit: Background, trends, and issues to be faced. Available at: http://aspe.os.dhhs.gov/daltcp/reports/mpacb.htm. Accessed September 7, 1999.

Losonczy KG, Harris TB, Cornoni-Huntley J, Simonsick EM, Wallace RB, Cook NR, Ostfeld AM, Blazer DG. 1995. Does weight loss from middle age to old age explain inverse weight mortality relation in old age? *Am J Epidemiol* 141:312–321.

Manard BB, Cameron R. 1997. A national study of assisted living for the frail elderly. Report on in-depth interviews with developers. Available at: http://aspe.os.dhhs.gov/daltcp/reports/indepth.htm. Accessed September 7, 1999.

Mentes JC, The Iowa Veterans Affairs Nursing Research Consortium. 1998. Hydration management research-based protocol. In: Titler M, ed. *Series on Evidence-Based Practice for Older Adults.* Iowa City, Ia.: The University of Iowa College of Nursing Gerontological Nursing Interventions Research Center, Research Dissemination Core.

Mitchell SL, Kiely DK, Lipsitz LA. 1997. The risk factors and impact on survival of feeding tube placement in nursing home residents with severe cognitive impairment. *Arch Intern Med* 157:327–332.

Mitchell SL, Kiely DK, Lipsitz LA. 1998. Does artificial enteral nutrition prolong the survival of institutionalized elders with chewing and swallowing problems? *J Gerontol A Biol Sci Med Sci* 53:M207–M213.

Morley JE, Silver AJ. 1995. Nutritional issues in nursing home care. *Ann Intern Med* 123:850–859.

Morris JN, Hawes C, Fries BE, Brant EF, Phillips CD, Mor V, Katz S, Murphy K, Drugovich ML, Friedlob AS. 1990. Designing the national resident assessment instrument for nursing homes. *Gerontologist* 30:293–307.

Mowé M, Bøhmer T, Kindt E. 1994. Reduced nutritional status in an elderly population (>70 y) is probable before disease and possibly contributes to the development of disease. *Am J Clin Nutr* 59:317–324.

Myers SA, Takiguchi S, Slavish S, Rose CL. 1990. Consistent wound care and nutritional support in treatment. *Decubitus* 3:16–28.

NAHC (National Association for Home Care). Basic statistics about home care. 1999. Available at: http://www.nahc.org/consumer/hcstats.html. Accessed March 9, 2000.

NCHS (National Center for Health Statistics). 1999. Home health and hospice care. Available at: http://www.cdc.gov/nchs/fastats/homehosp.htm. Accessed July 1999.

Peck A, Cohen CE, Mulvihill MN. 1990. Long-term enteral feeding of aged demented nursing home patients. *J Am Geriatr Soc* 38:1195–1198.

Ponza M, Ohls JC, Millen BA. 1996. *Serving Elders at Risk: The Older Americans Act Nutrition Programs—National Evaluation of the Elderly Nutrition Program, 1993–1995.* Washington, D.C.: Mathetmatica Policy Research, Inc.

Porter C, Schell ES, Kayser-Jones J, Paul SM. 1999. Dynamics of nutrition care among nursing home residents who are eating poorly. *J Am Diet Assoc* 99:1444–1446.

Professional Testing Corporation. 1997. *Nutrition Support Dietitian Role Delineation Survey: Supplemental Report*. New York: Professional Testing Corporation.

Rantz MJ, Popejoy L, Zwygart-Stauffacher M, Wipke-Tevis D, Grando VT. 1999. Minimum data set and resident assessment instrument: Can using standardized assessment improve clinical practice and outcomes of care? *J Gerontol Nurs* 25:35–43.

Rebovich EJ, Mahovich P, Blair KS. 1990. Nutrition services in home care. *Caring* 9:8–12, 14.

Reuben DB, Hirsch SH, Frank JC, Maly RC, Schlesinger MS, Weintraub N, Yancey S. 1996. The Prevention for Elderly Persons (PEP) program: A model of municipal and academic partnership to meet the needs of older persons for preventive services. *J Am Geriatr Soc* 44:1394–1398.

Reuben DB, Moore AA, Damesyn M, Keeler E, Harrison GG, Greendale GA. 1997. Correlates of hypoalbuminemia in community-dwelling older persons. *Am J Clin Nutr* 66:38–45.

Rudman D, Feller AG, Nagraj HS, Jackson DL, Rudman IW, Mattson DE. 1987. Relation of serum albumin concentration to death rate in nursing home men. *J Parenter Enteral Nutr* 11:360–363.

Rudman D, Mattson DE, Feller AG, Nagraj HS. 1989. A mortality risk index for men in a Veterans Administration extended care facility. *J Parenter Enteral Nutr* 13:189–195.

Rudman D, Abbasi AA, Isaacson K, Karpiuk E. 1995. Observations on the nutrient intakes of eating-dependent nursing home residents: Underutilization of micronutrient supplements. *J Am Coll Nutr* 14:604–613.

Schiller MR, Arensberg MB, Kantor B. 1998. Administrators' perceptions of nutrition services in home health care agencies. *J Am Diet Assoc* 98:56–61.

Short LA, Saindon EH. 1998. Telehomecare rewards and risks. *Caring* 17:36–40, 42.

Sperling RL, Humphrey CJ. 1999. OASIS and OBQI: *A Guide for Education and Implementation*. Philadelphia: Lippincott.

Steele CM, Greenwood C, Ens I, Robertson C, Seidman-Carlson R. 1997. Mealtime difficulties in a home for the aged: Not just dysphagia. *Dysphagia* 12:43–50.

St. Pierre M. 1999. A look to the future. Home health PPS. *Caring* 18:16–19.

Sullivan DH. 1992. Risk factors for early hospital readmission in a select population of geriatric rehabilitation patients: The significance of nutritional status. *J Am Geriatr Soc* 40:792–798.

Sullivan DH, Walls RC. 1994. Impact of nutritional status on morbidity in a population of geriatric rehabilitation patients. *J Am Geriatr Soc* 42:471–477.

Thomas DR, Kamel H, Morley JE. 1998. Nutritional deficiencies in long-term care: Part III. OBRA regulations and administrative and legal issues. *Ann Long Term Care* 6:325–332.

Turic A, Gordon KL, Craig LD, Ataya DG, Voss AC. 1998. Nutrition supplementation enables elderly residents of long-term-care facilities to meet or exceed RDAs without displacing energy or nutrient intakes from meals. *J Am Diet Assoc* 98:1457–1459.

USC (United States Code). 1998. Hospital insurance benefits for aged and disabled. 42USC1395. Washington, D.C.: U.S. Government Printing Office

Vogelzang JL. 1999. Overview of fluid maintenance/prevention of dehydration. *J Am Diet Assoc* 99:605–611.

Wallace JI, Schwartz RS, LaCroix AZ, Uhlmann RF, Pearlman RA. 1995. Involuntary weight loss in older outpatients: Incidence and clinical significance. *J Am Geriatr Soc* 43:329–337.

Weissert WG, Lafata JE, Williams B, Weissert CS. 1997. Toward a strategy for reducing potentially avoidable hospital admissions among home care clients. *Med Care Res Rev* 54:439–455.

White H, Pieper C, Schmader K. 1998. The association of weight change and Alzheimer's disease with severity of disease and mortality: A longitudinal analysis. *J Am Geriatr Soc* 46:1223–1227.

Whittaker JS, Ryan CF, Buckley PA, Road JD. 1990. The effects of refeeding on peripheral and respiratory muscle function in malnourished chronic obstructive pulmonary disease patients. *Am Rev Respir Dis* 142:283–288.

Woo J, Chan SM, Mak YT, Swaminathan R. 1989. Biochemical predictors of short term mortality in elderly residents of chronic care institutions. *J Clin Pathol* 42:1241–1245.

Section IV

Providers and Costs of Nutrition Services

13

Providers of Nutrition Services

The congressional language that initiated this study requested not only an analysis of the extent to which nutrition services might be of benefit to Medicare beneficiaries but also "an examination of nutritional services provided by registered dietitians." The committee decided to broaden the scope and include the provision of nutrition services by other health professionals as well. In order to accomplish this, the committee systematically reviewed available evidence regarding the education and training of registered dietitians as well as other health professionals necessary to adequately provide nutrition services.

TERMS AND DEFINITIONS

In reviewing specific providers, it must be recognized that terms such as "nutritionist," "dietitian," and "nutrition professional" can have varied definitions, however all refer to professionals who practice in the field of nutrition. In 1963, the Council on Foods and Nutrition of the American Medical Association defined the field of nutrition in the following manner:

> Nutrition is the science of food, the nutrients, and other substances therein, their action, interaction, and balance in relation to health and disease and the processes by which the organism ingests, digests, absorbs, transports, utilizes, and excretes food substances. In addition, nutrition must be concerned with certain social, economic, cultural, and psychological implications of food and eating. (Council on Foods and Nutrition, 1963).

257

The practice of *dietetics/nutrition* has been defined by the American Dietetic Association (ADA, 1991) as "the integration and application of the principles derived from the sciences of nutrition, biochemistry, food, physiology, management, and behavioral and social sciences to achieve and maintain the health of individuals through the provision of nutrition care services." They have further defined *nutrition care services* to include:

- assessing the nutrition needs of individuals and groups and determining resources and constraints in the practice setting;
- establishing priorities, goals, and objectives that meet nutrition needs and are consistent with available resources and constraints;
- providing nutrition counseling in health and disease;
- developing, implementing, and managing nutrition care systems; and
- evaluating, making changes in, and maintaining appropriate standards of quality in food and nutrition care services.

Nutrition assessment is defined as "the evaluation of the nutrition needs of individuals and groups based upon appropriate biochemical, anthropometric, physical, and dietary data to determine nutrient needs and recommend appropriate nutrition intake, including parenteral and enteral nutrition." *Nutrition counseling* is defined as "advising and assisting individuals and groups on appropriate nutrition intake by integrating information from the nutrition assessment with information on food and other sources of nutrients and meal preparation consistent with cultural background and socioeconomic status" (ADA, 1991).

TIERS OF NUTRITION SERVICES

Nutrition services are provided throughout the continuum of care: in acute and ambulatory care, in skilled nursing and long-term care, in home health agencies, and in community-based nutrition programs. The committee differentiated between nutrition-related activities. Some activities are more general, such as educating individuals on basic principles of a healthy diet, screening individuals to identify needs for more complex nutrition services, and reinforcing essential aspects of counseling provided by the nutrition professional. These basic nutrition services can be provided by a multitude of health care professionals with a small amount of training in nutrition. Other nutrition services are more complex and are referred to in this document as "nutrition therapy."

Nutrition therapy is defined as including nutrition assessment, evaluation of nutrition requirements, counseling geared towards the nutrition management of specific conditions, and follow-up care as appropriate to ensure patient compliance and success of the nutrition intervention. The provision of nutrition therapy as defined here requires health professionals who have a broad base of nutrition knowledge and experience. They need to be able to define who should receive nutrition therapy, when nutrition therapy is most likely to be effective, what the specific intervention should be, and the nature of follow-up needed. For example, in the case of enteral and parenteral nutrition, specific knowledge is necessary to judge when feedings should begin and end as well as what and how much should be provided.

EDUCATION AND SKILLS NECESSARY FOR THE PROVISION OF NUTRITION THERAPY

When determining who is qualified to be a *nutrition professional*, both academic background and supervised practice or experience are required (Glanz, 1985). Nutrition professionals must have in-depth knowledge about the role of food and nutrition in the prevention, treatment, and progression of acute and chronic disease and, likewise, how disease and treatment affect food and nutrition needs. They must also have knowledge about nutrient composition and preparation of food; alternate feeding modalities; and the socioeconomic, psychological, and educational factors that affect the food and nutrition behavior of people across the lifespan. Lastly, they must have skills to translate scientific information into laymen's terms and assist individuals in gaining knowledge, self-understanding, and improved decision making and behavior change skills (Snetselaar, 1983).

In 1972, the Study Commission on Dietetics was formed at the request of the ADA and the Governing Board of the ADA Foundation. The Commission was asked to study all aspects of dietetic practice and education (Study Commission on Dietetics, 1972). The Commission evaluated knowledge necessary and sufficient for the practice of dietetics and determined that the educational background to practice dietetics needs to be in line with that of other health professionals. It requires mastering professional knowledge as well as acquiring necessary professional skills.

The knowledge base needed can be described by two areas: nutrition science and food science. Nutrition science requires components of biochemistry, biology, medicine, behavioral health, human physiology, genetics, anatomy, psychology, sociology, economics, and anthropology. Food science requires knowledge of food chemistry, food selection, food preparation, food processing, and food economics. Professional skills required for the practice of dietetics include "therapy of disease, the maintenance of health, management, teaching and communication, research and development, organization and administration" (Study Commission on Dietetics, 1972).

The Commission also highlighted continuing education as essential to the practice of dietetics. The knowledge of medicine and nutrition science are constantly expanding. Without continuing education, the professional can not meet the dynamic needs of patients. The practitioner must be a "constant learner." If not, "knowledge becomes obsolete and his/her skill less than it can be. Worse, he/she cannot even be a truly professional practitioner given that the basic characteristic of the professional is that he/she personally and continuously translates knowledge into judgment and then action" (Study Commission on Dietetics, 1972).

LICENSURE IN THE PRACTICE OF DIETETICS

For many health professionals, state licensure can be relied on to identify individuals who meet minimum knowledge and skill requirements within a particular field. In the case of the nutrition professional, requirements for licensure vary among states and in the case of some states, licensure for nutrition professionals does not yet exist. At the time of this report,

- twenty-seven states had licensure requirements that provide an explicit scope of practice for dietitians;
- thirteen states had certification that limits the use of a particular title, yet individuals who are not certified can still practice;
- one state had an entitlement law that protects the use of the title *registered dietitian*; and
- nine states had not yet passed legislation for licensure, certification, or recognition of nutrition professionals.

For additional information regarding the status of licensure in individual states, see Appendix D.

In states that have licensure or certification for a nutrition professional, the requirements vary, however the credential of a "Registered Dietitian" is commonly accepted as meeting the requirements for licensure. In addition, some states license other professionals who may, as part of their practice, provide some nutrition services.

HEALTH CARE PROFESSIONALS
SPECIALIZING IN NUTRITION

The following section describes the background of various health care professionals and their role in providing nutrition services.

Registered Dietitian

The most commonly identified credential that constitutes a qualified nutrition professional is the registered dietitian (RD; referred to as dietitian in the rest of this chapter). The Commission on Dietetic Registration (CDR) confers the RD credential on an individual who has a minimum of a bachelor's degree from a regionally accredited college, meets specific academic and clinical requirements set by the ADA, and passes a national registration examination (CDR, 1999). These academic and clinical requirements include extensive coursework and experience in nutrition sciences, including the role of nutrition in the prevention and treatment of disease; food science, including the effects of processing and preparation on nutrient composition; alternate feeding modalities; and counseling techniques needed to elicit behavior change. The Commission on Accreditation for Dietetics Education (CADE) accredits programs that provide the required academic courses and clinical experience (ADA, 1999). An overview of the academic preparation for dietitians is described in Table 13.1. A more detailed view of the knowledge, skills and competency requirements for entry-level dietitians can be found in Appendix E. All dietitians are required to maintain 75 hours of continuing education every 5 years. Beginning in 2001, requirements for continuation of registration will also include a periodic assessment of learning needs and a plan to update needed knowledge and skills (Duyff, 1999).

The dietitian is the designated professional to oversee food and nutrition services in acute and long-term care settings by both the Health Care Financing Administration (CFR, 1998) and the Joint Commission on Accreditation of Healthcare Organizations (JCAHO, 1996).

There are several types of advanced-level credentials that certify dietitians with additional training and skill level in particular areas of practice. These are the certified specialist in pediatrics, certified specialist in renal disease, certified nutrition support dietitian, and certified diabetes educator. Other health professionals can also be certified in areas of nutrition support and diabetes education and are discussed later in this chapter. Various certifications are also described in Appendix F.

Certified Nutrition Specialist

The certified nutrition specialist certification can be earned by an individual with a graduate degree (M.S. or Ph.D.) in nutrition and either 1,000 hours of supervised practice or 4,000 hours of unsupervised practice as well as passing a certification examination given by the Certification Board associated with the American College of Nutrition. Requirements for academic and clinical preparation for this credential are not as specific

TABLE 13.1 Nutrition Related Academic and Clinical Requirements for Various Health Care Professionals

Professional Group	Accrediting Body	Academic and Clinical Requirements[a]	Aspects of Practice that Include Nutrition
Acupuncturist (licensed in some states)	Accreditation Commission for Acupuncture and Oriental Medicine	May include basic nutrition.	May use botanicals in practice.
Doctor of Chiropractic (state licensure)	Council on Chiropractic Education	Some coursework on nutrition and dietetics, public health, geriatrics. Clinical experience may include psychological counseling and dietetics.	May employ the use of vitamins, food supplements, and foods for special dietary use. The use of these substances in the treatment of illness or injury must be within the scope of the practice of chiropractic.
Doctor of Medicine (MD) (state licensure)	Liaison Committee on Medical Education of the Association of American Medical Colleges	Coursework in nutrition reviewed during accreditation. May be separate course or part of other courses.	Can prescribe and provide all nutrition services.
Doctor of Naturopathic Medicine (licensed in some states)	Council on Naturopathic Medical Education	Some coursework in basic foods, dietary assessment, therapeutic diets. Courses in botanical medicine.	Diagnoses, treats, and cares for patients, using a system of practice that bases its treatment of all physiological functions and abnormal conditions on natural laws governing the body. Utilizes physiological, psychological and mechanical methods, such as air, water, heat, earth, phytotherapy (treatment by use of plants), electrotherapy, physiotherapy, minor or orificial surgery,

mechanotherapy, naturopathic corrections and manipulation, and all natural methods or modalities, together with natural medicines, natural processed foods, herbs, and natural remedies. Excludes major surgery, therapeutic use of x-ray and radium, and use of drugs, except those assimilable substances containing elements or compounds which are compounds of body tissues and are physiologically compatible to body processes for maintenance of life.

Pharmacists (state licensure)

American Council on Pharmaceutical Education

Accrediting body reviews curriculum for issues important to pharmacists. Nutrition would be one of these areas.

Oversight of manufacturing and monitoring of parenteral nutrition support. Counseling patients about drug–food and drug–nutrient interactions, particularly as they may affect drug bioavailability. Working with other health professionals to integrate pharmaceutical treatment with dietary treatment. Counseling patients about non-prescription nutrition products, such as vitamins and minerals, liquid dietary supplements, and botanicals. On nutrition support committees, they may be involved in choice of drugs and nutrition-related formularies.

Continued on next page

TABLE 13.1 Continued

Professional Group	Accrediting Body	Academic and Clinical Requirements[a]	Aspects of Practice that Include Nutrition
Physician Assistant (state licensure)	Commission on Accreditation of Allied Health Education Programs	May be included in concepts of clinical medicine and surgery.	Can prescribe and provide nutrition services that are delegated in writing by MD who is responsible for patient.
Registered Dietitian (RD) (licensed, certified or recognized in some states; registered nationally)	Commission on Accreditation of Dietetics Education	Extensive coursework in food science, nutrition science, nutrition in prevention and treatment of disease (minimum of bachelor's degree with nationally recognized standards for academic preparation). Extensive clinical experience in application of concepts of food and nutrition (minimum of 900 hours and nationally recognized standards for supervised practice).	Primary job in health care is to assess nutritional status, intervene when nutrition problems are identified and evaluate effect of intervention. Interventions include all aspects of nutrition therapy, including provision of alternate feeding modalities and counseling to prevent chronic disease, disease progression, or disease complications. The RD works in all areas of health care: acute care, outpatient clinics, skilled nursing and long-term care facilities, home health agencies, and in community-based nutrition programs.
		Accrediting body reviews curriculum for issues important to nurses. 2–3 credit hours in basic nutrition (essential nutrients,	Specific nursing diagnoses, interventions and care outcomes include nutrition (under and over-nutrition, constipation, diarrhea, fatigue, altered oral mucous membranes, self-

265

criteria for adequate diet, nutrition in health promotion, nutrition assessment, ethical, social and political considerations of nutrition care, drug/nutrient interactions, nutrition management of selected health problems. Nutrition content also integrated throughout curriculum related to health promotion, symptom management, and disease management. Basic human nutrition may be prerequisite or part of curriculum. (Cover basics of diet therapy as part of other coursework.)

feeding deficit, impaired swallowing, knowledge deficit, body image disturbance). Nursing interventions may include feeding, eating disorders management, nutrition counseling, nutrition and nutrition support monitoring, swallowing therapy, teaching about prescribed diets, tube care, weight gain and reduction assistance.

a May be expressed as outcome expectations or course requirements.

nor are the requirements for clinical preparation as rigorous as those for a dietitian.

Dietetic Technician, Registered

The dietetic technician, registered (DTR) provides support for the dietitian in all health care settings (Arena and Walters, 1997). The DTR credential is conferred by the CDR on a person who has successfully completed an associate of science degree or a bachelor's degree in dietetics that meets the requirements of the ADA and has specific clinical experience from a program that is accredited by the CADE. The DTR works under the supervision of the dietitian and may provide the following services: screening for nutrition risk, intervention for patients with less complex nutrition problems, and preventive nutrition services.

Certified Dietary Manager

The certified dietary manager (CDM) most commonly works in a skilled nursing or long-term care facility under the supervision of a dietitian, who may work part- or full-time. In the absence of the dietitian, the CDM directs food and nutrition services. A dietary manager is trained in a certificate program, usually in a community college and is certified through a credentialing exam offered by the Certifying Board for Dietary Managers.

OTHER HEALTH CARE PROFESSIONALS

Most health professionals can impart basic nutrition advice and contribute significantly to the provision of nutrition services. Many health professionals have varying amounts of academic and clinical preparation in the field of nutrition. Most, however, do not include concentrated preparation in the fields of nutrition science and food composition to be able to translate medical nutrition concepts into attainable dietary changes for the layperson. In most cases, standards are not available for nutrition education and counseling skills in the curriculum of the health care provider; therefore, it is difficult to generalize the reliability of the information provided to patients. The academic and clinical preparation in nutrition and the roles of various health professionals in providing nutrition services are described in Table 13.1.

Physicians

The physician is responsible for prescribing nutrition therapy and may also provide and bill for this service under Part B of Medicare. Physicians with advanced-level training in nutrition, including fellowships or graduate degrees, can be certified as a certified nutrition specialist by the American College of Nutrition (see Appendix F).

Patients generally consider their physician to be a highly credible source of health and dietary information (Hiddink et al., 1997); however, the debate over whether physicians have the time or the skills to provide nutrition counseling has been a long one. In a 1994 Connecticut Behavioral Risk Factor Surveillance System survey, only 29 percent of all overweight adults and fewer than half with additional cardiovascular risk factors reported receiving counseling from physicians about weight loss (Nawaz et al., 1999). A survey of 1,030 physicians reported that they felt *lack of time* and *patient compliance* were barriers to diet counseling (Kushner, 1995). This study, however, noted that dietitians had the knowledge and skills to complement the physician and proposed a physician-dietitian team.

In 1985, a report of the National Research Council described inadequacies in the curricula of medical schools and in physicians' knowledge, attitudes, and health care practices related to nutrition (NRC, 1985). Others have since described a modest growth in physicians' training in applied nutrition, but continue to acknowledge discrepancies between knowledge and actual practice (Glanz and Gilboy, 1992). Additional barriers to physicians providing nutrition services are lack of time, staff, or insurance coverage (Glanz et al., 1995).

In 1995, the U.S. Preventive Services Task Force found that "although physicians can often provide general guidelines on proper nutrition, many lack the time and skills to obtain a thorough dietary history, to address potential barriers to changes in eating habits, and to offer specific guidance on food selection" (USPSTF, 1995). In addition, the Task Force rated the quality and strength of evidence regarding the effectiveness of both primary care clinicians and specially trained educators in counseling to change dietary habits. The Task Force reported the effectiveness of counseling by a trained educator such as a dietitian as "fair" based on evidence from at least one properly randomized controlled trial. However, the Task Force found there was "insufficient" evidence to recommend for or against dietary counseling when performed by a primary care clinician, based on level III evidence. Hence, this report rates dietary counseling performed by a trained educator such as a dietitian as more effective than by a primary care clinician (see Appendix G).

Pharmacists

Pharmacists are often in a unique position to provide nutrition information to patients as part of the discharge process or in outpatient pharmacies. They can integrate pharmaceutical treatment with diet, counsel patients about drug–food interactions as they relate to drug bioavailability, and advise patients about nonprescription nutrition products. Their knowledge of genetics, molecular biology, and botany will likely be important as more products marketed as "neutraceuticals" are approved. Of more immediate relevance is the role of the pharmacist as an important member of the nutrition support team (Allwood et al., 1996; Brown et al., 1997; Driscoll, 1996; Lee, 1996).

Registered Nurses

The registered nurse coordinates patient care, works with the dietitian and other health care team members to identify nutrition problems, and reinforces the importance of nutrition interventions. The registered nurse may also provide less complex nutrition care, such as counseling on preventing chewing and swallowing difficulties or contributing to the nutritional assessment. Most baccalaureate and some hospital diploma and associate degree nursing programs require a 2- to 3-credit hour basic nutrition course, which is usually taught by a dietitian or nurse. Nutrition content is also integrated throughout the curriculum in these programs. The baccalaureate nurse is prepared for a broader, more independent role related to patient education and patient care management, such as nurse case manager. Nurses can be certified as a Certified Nutrition Support Nurse by the National Board of Nutrition Support Certification, associated with the American Society of Parenteral and Enteral Nutrition.

Advanced practice nurses (e.g., clinical nurse specialists and nurse practitioners) are registered nurses who are prepared at the graduate degree level. Clinical nurse specialists in gerontology and geriatric nurse practitioners specialize in the care of older adults. Among their clinical roles, they may conduct nutritional assessments of older adults in community or other settings; order therapeutic diets under standard protocols; counsel older patients on prescribed or healthy diets; and manage high blood pressure, diabetes, and other nutrition-related chronic problems, either independently or in collaboration with a physician or dietitian. Advanced practice nurses attain advanced nutrition knowledge and skill through graduate level coursework and clinical experiences.

Depending upon their level of preparation, experience, and practice area, research indicates that nurses have variable amounts of nutrition knowledge. Wilt and colleagues (1990) studied the knowledge, attitudes,

treatment practices, and health behaviors of nurses regarding blood cholesterol and cardiovascular disease in a stratified, random sample of 206
registered nurses. While the nurses were convinced regarding the importance of diet in reducing heart disease risk, many had substantial knowledge gaps and were not adequately prepared to counsel patients regarding diet and medication therapy for hyperlipidemia. In another study,
Mullen and colleagues (1988) surveyed a group of allied health professionals and found that dietitians had higher self-efficacy scores than certified nurse midwives, physician assistants, and dental hygienists for counseling about fat consumption. However, Peiss and colleagues (1995)
compared the effect of information provided by physicians and nurses
versus a dietitian on patient knowledge of coronary risk factors and diet.
While physicians and nurses spent significantly less time than dietitians
in nutrition counseling, all study participants benefited from the coronary
risk reduction information, whether it was provided by physicians and
nurses or dietitians.

Multidisciplinary Team Approach

Although physicians, nurses, pharmacists, or other health professionals do not always have the knowledge of nutrition and food science that a
dietitian has, each profession brings unique skills to the provision of nutrition care. Several examples of interdisciplinary teams have been described in this report. In the nursing home, the evaluation and management of dysphagia require a combined effort by the occupational therapist
or speech pathologist and the physician, nurse, and dietitian. In the Modification of Diet in Renal Disease trial, the best results were obtained when
a team of physicians, dietitians, nurses, and patients reviewed laboratory
values in relation to the diet and tailored the dietary approach to fit patients' lifestyles (Gillis et al., 1995). In diabetes management, a team composed of a physician, nurse, and dietitian is the most effective in working
with patients to make changes in diet, medications, activity, and other
aspects of lifestyle (see chapter 6). The provision of nutrition support is
optimally managed by a multidisciplinary team consisting of a physician,
dietitian, pharmacist, and nurse who work together to recommend, ini-
tiate, and monitor enteral or parenteral forms of nutrition (see chapter 10).
Advanced training and certification in the area of nutrition support
or diabetes education is available for physicians, pharmacists, and nurses.
These certifications, among other things, indicate that the professional
has a greater knowledge and skill level in nutrition, as it relates to
the particular field, and can serve as an excellent role extender for the
dietitian.
Other health care professionals, such as acupuncturists and doctors of

chiropractic or naturopathic medicine, may have training in nutrition and consider nutrition to be part of their scope of practice. Nutrition interventions may involve advising about healthy lifestyles, including diet and the use of botanicals or other dietary supplements. It is important that recommendations for the use of botanicals and dietary supplements are supported by peer-reviewed, published, randomized, controlled trails.

WHO IS QUALIFIED TO PROVIDE BASIC NUTRITION EDUCATION OR ADVICE?

Basic nutrition education can be provided by a number of different professionals in the course of health care. It can occur during individual consultation with patients or in a group setting. This type of interaction has been defined (Murphy, 1989) as any activity intended to encourage patients to improve their dietary habits. Information is basic, can be provided verbally or in writing, and may include the importance of nutrition in relation to risk factors or known disease conditions. Recommendations should be based on sound nutrition principles, such as those specified by the Dietary Guidelines for Americans (USDA and DHHS, 1995) or the U.S. Preventive Services Task Force (USPSTF, 1995).

A basic nutrition education encounter usually lasts from 1 or 2 minutes up to about 15 minutes (Peiss et al., 1995) and is often incident to normal medical care. An example would be the counseling that could take place for osteoporosis prevention. Simple questions could be asked about the intake of calcium-rich foods, advice can be given about culturally specific foods that might be added to the diet, and, if appropriate, the physician or nurse may recommend calcium and vitamin D supplementation. However, if a patient has other chronic diseases that required more complex nutrition intervention, advice about calcium and vitamin D intake could be incorporated into the overall consultation provided by the nutrition professional.

In addition to basic nutrition information, it is important that each health professional reinforce the importance of nutrition therapy prior to counseling with a nutrition professional and again at any follow-up visit. Since patients perceive physicians to be highly credible sources of information, their reinforcement is an important aspect of dietary compliance.

Nutrition advice needs to be based on sound scientific principles and should be accompanied by simple practical suggestions on how to incorporate changes into the diet. It is important that the nutrition professional be active in updating other professionals' knowledge and skills in nutrition.

WHO IS QUALIFIED TO PROVIDE NUTRITION THERAPY?

The dietitian has strong academic and clinical training in nutrition science, food science, nutrient composition of foods, and behavior change related to food intake. This health professional is also the most knowledgeable about strengths and limitations of methods used to determine nutrient composition of foods and dietary intake. Dietitians are a resource for other members of the health care team about nutrient needs and lifestyle factors revealed during diet-counseling sessions. The dietitian is the main advocate for nutrition therapy in the overall care plan and understands how nutrition therapy relates to other forms of treatment. The dietitian or another health professional with comparable academic and clinical training should provide the more advanced level of nutrition services referred to as "nutrition therapy."

SUMMARY

Many health care providers have some education in nutrition. However the registered dietitian has the greatest amount of academic and clinical training in nutrition and food science. Basic nutrition education and advice can be provided by most health care providers, but should reflect sound evidence in the literature. The nutrition professional should be involved in educating other health professionals regarding nutrition interventions and practical suggestions for dietary change that he/she can use to educate patients. With appropriate training, all health professionals should be involved in reinforcing the concepts of nutrition therapy provided by the nutrition professional.

The registered dietitian is currently the single identifiable group of health care professionals with the standardized education, clinical training, continuing education, and national credentialing requirements necessary to provide nutrition therapy.

The importance of the interdisciplinary team is recognized. Each health professional brings a unique role to the provision of nutrition services. Multidisciplinary teams have been shown to be particularly effective in the management of chronic renal failure, diabetes, dysphagia, and the delivery of nutrition support.

RECOMMENDATIONS

• Basic nutrition education can be provided by most health professionals. It should be evidence-based and include practical suggestions for change. The nutrition professional should be involved in educating other members of the health care team regarding nutrition interventions and practical aspects of nutrition care. Additional time has been added to cost estimates for the nutrition professional in home and ambulatory care to provide consultation to other health professionals. It is not recommended that basic nutrition education be a separate reimbursable charge.

• More complex nutrition services, referred to in this report as nutrition therapy, should be provided by a nutrition professional and be a covered benefit for Medicare beneficiaries. The registered dietitian is currently the single identifiable group of health professionals qualified to provide nutrition therapy. It is recognized that other health care professionals in particular fields may be qualified to provide nutrition therapy and should be considered on an individual basis as a reimbursable provider.

REFERENCES

ADA (American Dietetic Association). 1991. ADA policy statement on licensure. *J Am Diet Assoc* 91:985.

ADA (American Dietetic Association) 1999. Commission on Accreditation for Dietetics. Available at: http://www.eatright.org/caade/. Accessed August 10, 1999.

Allwood MC, Hardy G, Sizer T. 1996. Roles and functions of the pharmacist in the nutrition support team. *Nutrition* 12:63–64.

Arena J, Walters P. 1997. Do you know what a dietetic technician can do? A focus on clinical technicians and their expanded roles and responsibilities. *J Am Diet Assoc* 97:S139–S141.

Brown RO, Dickerson RN, Hak EB, Matthews JB, Hak LJ. 1997. Impact of a pharmacist-based consult service on nutritional rehabilitation of nonambulatory patients with severe developmental disabilities. *Pharmacotherapy* 17:796–800.

CDR (Commission on Dietetic Registration). 1999. Registered dietition (RD) certification. Available at: http://www.cdrnet.org/certifications/rddtr/rdindex.htm. Accessed May 15, 1999.

CFR (Code of Federal Regulations). 1998. Requirements for long-term care facilities. 42CFR482–483. Washington, D.C.: U.S. Government Printing Office.

Council on Foods and Nutrition. 1963. Nutrition teaching in medical schools. *J Am Med Assoc* 183:995–997.

Driscoll DF. 1996. Roles and functions of the hospital pharmacist on the nutrition support team. *Nutrition* 12:138–139.

Duyff RL. 1999. The value of lifelong learning: Key element in professional career development. *J Am Diet Assoc* 99:538–543.

Gillis BP, Caggiula AW, Chiavacci AT, Coyne T, Doroshenko L, Milas C, Nowalk MP, Scherch LK. 1995. Nutrition intervention program of the Modification of Diet in Renal Disease Study: A self-management approach. *J Am Diet Assoc* 95:1288–1294.

Glanz K. 1985. Nutrition education for risk factor reduction and patient education: A review. *Prev Med* 14:721–752.

Glanz K, Gilboy MB. 1992. Physicians, preventive care, and applied nutrition: Selected literature. *Acad Med* 67:776–781.

Glanz K, Tziraki C, Albright CL, Fernandes J. 1995. Nutrition assessment and counseling practices: Attitudes and interests of primary care physicians. *J Gen Intern Med* 10:89–92.

Hiddink GJ, Hautvast JGAJ, van Woerkum CMJ, Fieren CJ, van't Hof MA. 1997. Consumers' expectations about nutrition guidance: The importance of primary care physicians. *Am J Clin Nutr* 65:1974S–1979S.

JCAHO (Joint Commission on Accreditation of Healthcare Organizations). 1996. *Comprehensive Accreditation Manual for Hospitals. The Official Handbook.* Oakbrook Terrace, Ill.: JCAHO.

Kushner RF. 1995. Barriers to providing nutrition counseling by physicians: A survey of primary care practitioners. *Prev Med* 24:546–552.

Lee HS. 1996. Roles and functions of the hospital pharmacist on the nutrition support team. *Nutrition* 12:140.

Mullen PD, Holcomb JD, Fasser CE. 1988. Selected allied health professionals' self-confidence in health promotion counseling skills and interest in continuing education programs. *J Allied Health* 17:123–133.

Murphy PS. 1989. Effect of nutrition education on nutrition counseling practices of family physicians. *Acad Med* 64:98–102.

Nawaz H, Adams ML, Katz DL. 1999. Weight loss counseling by health care providers. *Am J Publ Health* 89:764–767.

NRC (National Research Council). 1985. *Nutrition Education in U.S. Medical Schools.* Washington, D.C.: National Academy Press.

Peioo B, Kurleto B, Rubenfire M. 1995. Physicians and nurses can be effective educators in coronary risk reduction. *J Gen Intern Med* 10:77–81.

Snetselaar LG. 1983. *Nutrition Counseling Skills: Assessment, Treatment, and Evaluation.* Rockville, Md.: Aspen Systems.

Study Commission on Dietetics. 1972. The education of future dietitians. Pp. 55–60 in: *The Profession of Dietetics: The Report.* Chicago, Ill.: American Dietetic Association.

USDA (U.S. Department of Agriculture) and DHHS (U.S. Department of Health and Human Services). 1995. *Dietary Guidelines for Americans,* 4th ed. Washington, D.C.: U.S. Government Printing Office,

USPSTF (U.S. Preventive Services Task Force). 1995. *Guide to Clinical Preventive Services, 2nd ed. Report of the U.S. Preventive Services Task Force.* Washington, D.C.: U.S. Department of Health and Human Services, Office of Public Health, Office of Health Promotion and Disease Prevention

Wilt S, Hubbard A, Thomas A. 1990. Knowledge, attitudes, treatment practices and health behaviors of nurses regarding blood cholesterol and cardiovascular disease. *Prev Med* 19:466–475.

14

Economic Policy Analysis

In 1998, Medicare spent $211 billion providing medical care and related services to almost 40 million beneficiaries. Given these costs, economic analysis is essential to the proper targeting of quality health services that can have an important impact on the health and well-being of Medicare beneficiaries. Therefore, while the costs of particular services are themselves important, they also exert an important influence on the ability of Medicare to provide beneficiaries other important services. No less important, costs also can have important legislative implications, given congressional spending rules designed to balance health care expenditures with competing social needs. Therefore, it is critical that proposed changes to Medicare's provision of nutrition services be carefully scrutinized and subjected to rigorous economic analysis.

Economic analysis addresses three separate instances of provision of nutrition services: (1) new services that will require reimbursement, (2) services that are now nominally covered which may require some modification of current reimbursement to ensure appropriate care, and (3) areas in which no changes in actual practice should occur; however if the reimbursement system changes there may be attempts to obtain additional reimbursement without cause. The purpose of this chapter is to provide cost estimates for the first of these three categories, although recommendations certainly reflect all three aspects of coverage.

With regard to new nutrition services, this category of service is not included in current Medicare coverage and thus is evaluated in this analysis as mainly Part B outpatient services for nutrition therapy. In some cases, nutrition services are currently covered. However, it is unclear if the type and intensity of nutrition care is consistent with best practice recommendations as indicated by current protocols. For example, prospective payments for renal dialysis continue to include a nutrition component. However, the type and intensity of nutrition care decreased by 21.9 percent between 1982 and 1987. Data are not available to reflect changes since that time. Recently enacted coverage includes important new benefits for diabetes self-management (HCFA, 1999). However, registered dietitians and other nutrition professionals are not directly reimbursable under these new proposed regulations.

Inpatient enteral and parenteral nutrition services are included as part of the hospital prospective payment. For this reason, the committee has not analyzed the economic impact of associated recommendations. However, adherence to best-practice recommendations may create economic burdens for providers that should be considered within Medicare reimbursement and prospective payment policies. In the area of home health, prospective payment systems currently being instituted will be based on current costs. Existing research highlights several ways in which home-bound patients who would be covered under home health care are underserved, and where additional resources may be needed.

EVALUATION METHODOLOGIES

Several criteria have been proposed to evaluate the economic merits of expanded coverage for nutrition services. From a federal budgetary perspective, the simplest criterion is to compute the estimated impact of expanded coverage to overall Medicare expenditures. Congressional mandates require such calculations over a 5-year period to meet overall guidelines designed to constrain the growth of Medicare spending.

Given recent growth in Medicare costs, an analysis of likely expenditures is essential to policy analysis of coverage for nutrition therapy. However, the likely costs of such an expansion must be based on current data. Predicted Medicare expenditures for covered nutrition therapy services require uncertain forecasts of likely patient demands for nutrition services. Existing data suggest that only a small minority of Medicare patients with conditions potentially benefiting from nutrition therapy actually receive these services. The estimates presented below are therefore based on the assumption that the costs (and benefits) of nutrition therapy reflect previously observed patterns of patient service use.

The impact of nutrition services on overall Medicare expenditures is even more difficult to forecast given important interactions between nutrition therapy and other program costs. Expanded Medicare coverage for nutrition therapy is likely to avert clinically significant numbers of strokes and other adverse outcomes. The ability of nutrition therapy to avert costly acute care episodes is a major benefit associated with these services. Ironically, however, such benefits can have an ambiguous impact on overall expenditures. Health promotion interventions can, in principle, increase Medicare costs by prolonging longevity which can increase future health care expenditures.

Because nutrition therapy provides tangible patient benefits, it is financially and socially prudent to provide these services if they are cost neutral or cost saving—that is if coverage for nutrition therapy does not increase overall Medicare expenditures. In part because some interventions are cost saving, policymakers and the public often evaluate preventive services based on the ability of such interventions to save public funds. In practice, however, few preventive services are cost saving by this measure (Russell, 1986). It is therefore important to emphasize that no principle of policy analysis or economic theory demands that preventive services satisfy this strict criterion. Medicare-reimbursed medical procedures are evaluated on the basis of safety, clinical efficacy, and (increasingly) cost-effectiveness (Warner and Warner, 1993). Optimal resource allocation requires comparable evaluation of proposed nutrition therapy expenditures with competing uses of the same funds. Even if nutrition services result in positive net costs to the Medicare program, these may still be justified public expenditures if they produce sufficiently improved health.

Cost–Benefit Analysis

From the standpoint of economic theory, the most exhaustive and satisfactory way to evaluate these benefits is to perform cost–benefit analysis for specific clinical settings and diagnoses in which nutrition services might be Medicare reimbursed (Drummond et al., 1997). In principle, the policy analyst should compare the net economic costs of policy with the full array of social benefits brought about by the intervention. This requires the health care analyst to assign monetary values to the range of economic, social, and health outcomes attributable to nutrition services. These valuations might be computed from the social perspective or from the perspective of Medicare payers and patients (see Drummond et al., 1997 and chapter 7 for examples and further work).

When feasible, a full cost–benefit analysis provides the most compelling justification for proposed policy intervention. The net social benefits of nutrition services could then be compared with the net social benefits of alternative uses of the same funds. In practice, however, cost–benefit analysis is often infeasible in real policy settings. Although approaches such as contingent valuation exist to assign monetized values to outcomes (Johansson, 1995), such estimates are either controversial or unavailable for most outcomes pertinent to the present study. Other promising methods link self-assessed improvements in standardized health measures to pertinent economic outcomes to improve social valuation of quality-of-life improvements associated with clinical intervention (Kaplan et al., 1998).

Cost-Effectiveness and Cost-Utility Analyses

Two closely-linked alternative approaches are cost-effectiveness analysis (CEA) and cost-utility analysis (CUA) of specific services (Gold et al., 1996). CEA and CUA both seek to rank different interventions intended to improve health or extend life. CEA is most useful to rank interventions that promote similar or identical health outcomes. CUA is most helpful to compare interventions that may produce quite different improvements in health outcomes. A common application of CUA is the comparison of competing efforts to save or prolong human life. Most recently, 500 prominent public health interventions were evaluated using estimated costs per quality-adjusted life year (QALY) (Tengs et al., 1995). The median cost of $42,000 per QALY was estimated for interventions widely accepted by policymakers and the public to prolong human life.

Direct CEA or CUA of proposed nutrition services is beyond the scope of this report. Pertinent existing research is identified along with several diagnoses in which nutrition therapy appears especially efficacious and cost-effective. However, the recommendations are based on the known clinical efficacy and effectiveness of nutrition interventions, and are made in light of existing policy analyses of proposed coverage for nutrition therapy.

COST ESTIMATES

To assist policymakers and other stakeholders, and to gauge the approximate budgetary impact of its recommendations, likely Medicare reimbursement costs associated with proposed coverage for nutrition services were evaluated for the period of January 1, 2000 to December 31, 2004. While fully explained in this chapter, a summary of underlying assumptions is included in Appendix H. The committee used five steps to obtain these cost estimates:

1. Nationally representative data were used to estimate disease prevalence in the Medicare population. These data were augmented with administrative data for specific subpopulations when necessary.
2. Professionally accepted treatment protocols were used to deter-

mine what might constitute the level of covered nutrition therapy for various disease entities upon initial diagnosis and during subsequent years for follow-up nutrition therapy.

3. Usual and customary professional charges were used to estimate unit costs.

4. Research data from existing health care populations were used to estimate likely patient demand for covered services.

5. Cost estimates were adjusted in accordance with Congressional Budget Office scoring procedures to estimate the gross impact of proposed expanded nutrition coverage on Medicare expenditures.

This chapter also describes the potential for economically significant adverse health outcomes that could be delayed or averted through nutrition services. These estimates are useful for policy development because they indicate the direct costs of potential coverage of nutrition services and important cost avoidance likely to flow from these health interventions. These estimates should not, however, be interpreted as explicit Medicare budget forecasts. Budget forecasts require detailed actuarial analysis of specific reimbursement structures and specific patterns of patient utilization that are beyond the scope of this report.

This analysis follows a four-step process to estimate the economic magnitude of such effects:

1. Clinical efficacy data summarized in earlier chapters were used to estimate the linkage between improved nutrition status and reduction in adverse outcomes.

2. Peer reviewed research or committee clinical judgments were used to evaluate the contribution of nutrition services to improved nutrition status.

3. Published research accounts were used to link changes in intermediary variables to reduced incidence of adverse outcomes. For example, in the case of coronary heart disease (CHD) outcomes, data from the Framingham Heart Study were used to compute both underlying disease risk and the relative risk reduction likely to result from dietary intervention (Wilson et al., 1998). For patients with diabetes mellitus, cost data from an observational study (Gilmer et al., 1997) were employed because this study provided more detailed cost results with comorbid conditions.

4. Medicare reimbursement data were used to estimate Medicare charges associated with averted adverse health events. Accurate estimates of the fiscal impact of these adverse events for the Medicare program require detailed actuarial analysis beyond the scope of this study. Therefore "net Medicare costs" that incorporate the health benefits of nutrition services were not explicitly computed.

Estimation of Direct Charges for Nutrition Therapy

Several data sources were employed to estimate reimbursement costs for nutrition therapy.

Disease Prevalence

Medicare expenditures for expanded nutrition coverage depend upon the prevalence of pertinent diagnosed conditions within the Medicare population. Because almost 90 percent of Medicare recipients are over the age of 65, the bulk of the analysis focused on this patient group. As described in previous chapters, Medicare expenditures for nutrition therapy are likely to be concentrated within several prominent diagnoses in which dietary intake and individualized nutritional advice play important clinical roles: diabetes, dyslipidemia, hypertension, heart failure, and renal disease.

Data from the Third National Examination Health and Nutrition Survey (1988–1994) (NHANES III) were used to estimate the prevalence of diabetes, hypertension, dyslipidemia, and renal disease among Americans 65 years and older (NCHS, 1997). NHANES is a weighted, stratified survey of non-institutionalized respondents. A statistical analysis of these data, using standard survey methods to account for the stratified design of the NHANES survey, was performed.[1] For selected conditions such as heart failure or end-stage renal disease, Medicare administrative data was used. The small but important group of individuals 65 years and over receiving home care services are implicitly included within the NHANES group.

Data are more limited regarding the important group of disabled Medicare beneficiaries under 65 years of age and for recipients at least 65 years of age who have less prevalent conditions that potentially require nutritional intervention. For example, human immunodeficiency virus-infected Medicare recipients might require nutrition therapy for specific conditions arising from that disease.

For purposes of cost estimation, the committee assumed that of the remaining Medicare beneficiaries who either do not have one of the nutrition-related diagnoses indicated or are under the age of 65, 25 percent would be eligible for one annual nutrition therapy session. Patient demand for covered services are assumed similar to the scenarios for hypertension and hyperlipidemia for purposes of cost calculations.

---

[1]Dr. Tate Erlinger, Johns Hopkins University, personal communication, 1999. Analysis performed as requested by the committee.

TABLE 14.1 Prevalence of Selected Conditions Among National Health and Nutrition Examination Survey Respondents 65 Years of Age and Older

Diagnosis	Estimated Prevalence in Population (%)	Estimated Number of Medicare Beneficiaries in 2000 (million)	Data Source
Single diagnosis			
HTN[a] only	20.5	7.26	NHANES III
↑LDL[b] only	19.8	7.01	NHANES III
DM[c] only	1.1	0.39	NHANES III
Renal disease[d]	0.6	0.21	NHANES III
Heart failure	2	0.74[e]	Discharge data for all Medicare Patients
Combination diagnoses			
HTN & ↑ LDL	37.1	13.1	NHANES III
HTN & ↑ LDL & DM	3.3	1.17	NHANES III
DM & HTN	3.0	1.06	NHANES III
DM and ↑ LDL	1.9	0.67	NHANES III
No HTN or DM or ↑LDL	13.3	4.71	NHANES III

[a] HTN = hypertension.
[b] ↑LDL = elevated plasma low-density lipoproteins >130 mg/dL.
[c] DM = diabetes mellitus.
[d] Renal disease = serum creatinine >2.5 g/dL for women and >3.0 g/dL for men.
[e] Annual hospital discharges.

Table 14.1 shows the prevalence of selected diagnoses among NHANES respondents who were at least 65 years old. As shown, most Medicare beneficiaries have comorbidities with substantial implications for clinical practice and Medicare costs. Eighty-six percent of individuals within this age group are estimated to have at least one diagnosed condition that potentially requires nutrition intervention. Data are less readily available regarding the 12 percent of Medicare recipients who are less than 65 years old and eligible for reasons of disability. At a minimum, Table 14.1 implies that at least 75 percent of all Medicare beneficiaries have at least one identified ailment potentially requiring nutrition intervention.

Estimated Medicare Population Changes

The estimated population of current and new Medicare beneficiaries is based upon forecasts provided by the Office of the Actuary, Health Care Financing Administration. Some treatment protocols mandate relatively intense nutritional assessment, counseling, and treatment for newly-diagnosed patients, followed by less-intensive maintenance therapy for previously-diagnosed individuals. It is therefore important to distinguish the incidence and prevalence of treated conditions within the Medicare population.

For purposes of cost estimation, it is assumed that all Medicare beneficiaries would be entitled to one service bundle intended for newly diagnosed patients, with a smaller amount of nutrition therapy in subsequent years. In each subsequent year, the number of newly diagnosed patients is assumed equal to the number of new Medicare beneficiaries multiplied by observed prevalence as summarized in Table 14.1.

This calculation makes three important approximations given the lack of more precise data regarding Medicare beneficiaries. First, it presumes that the incidence and detection of selected diagnoses will change slowly over time among Medicare recipients. Second, it presumes that recipients with specific conditions requiring maintenance therapy have a similar mean lifespan to the overall Medicare population. Third, it presumes that new (or newly-diagnosed) Medicare beneficiaries will not have received comparable services in a non-Medicare health plan and will be entitled to the full initial bundle of services. This conservative methodology would overstate Medicare costs if a large proportion of new beneficiaries do not require such intense initial services. This might be the case if the new Medicare beneficiaries had received nutrition therapy from their previous health plan.

Estimation of Nutrition Services Utilization

Patients with specific conditions are likely to receive nutrition therapy given the proposed expansion in Medicare coverage. The number and type of covered visits and the accompanying costs are influenced by Medicare policies, by the pattern of services offered by qualified providers, and by patient demand for covered services.

Reimbursement Rates

The average cost of typical nutrition services was estimated using data from previous economic studies. From the Medicare budgetary perspective, the three principal components of these costs are wage and nonwage compensation for dietitians, medical supplies, equipment and operating costs, and associated expenses such as rent, utilities, and office supplies. For the purpose of cost estimates, these services are assumed to be provided in an individualized setting, although in some cases the option of group sessions was explored. Forecasts are adjusted to rise with inflation at an expected rate of 3 percent per year.

Per-session costs of nutrition therapy were estimated using data published by the Health Care Financing Administration (HCFA, 1999). In the case of diabetes self-management, HCFA (1999) recently published detailed estimates in computing proposed payments. HCFA estimated an adjusted cost of $55.41 for individualized treatment by a registered nurse or registered dietitian, and $32.62 for group sessions based on an average of ten patients.

To provide conservative estimates of likely program costs, individualized counseling sessions were used as the foundation of the resulting cost estimates given here. Because the relative efficacy and cost-effectiveness of group counseling depends upon specific diagnoses and patient groups, selected provision of group sessions may allow lower program costs.

Medicare Cost Adjustment Factors

To explore federal budgetary implications, 5-year budgetary forecasts were computed to estimate gross costs—that is the direct reimbursement costs—borne by the Medicare program of proposed nutrition therapy coverage over the 5-year period from January 1, 2000 to December 31, 2004. All estimates have been adjusted to account for 20 percent patient copayments for Medicare services. For the 65 years and older population, estimates were further adjusted to reflect 25 percent associated changes in Part B Medicare premiums following standard Congressional Budget Office practice.

Several important benefits associated with expanded nutrition coverage such as reduced incidence of coronary heart disease were also explored. These data illustrate the clinical and policy importance of improved nutrition. As described below, explicit cost offsets based upon this analysis were not computed. Accurate calculation of the fiscal consequences of life-improving and life-extending nutrition therapies requires detailed actuarial analysis beyond the scope of the current study.

Practice Patterns for Nutrition Therapy

For some diagnoses such as diabetes, clinical protocols and Medicare policies distinguish between nutrition therapy for newly diagnosed patients and maintenance therapy for individuals who were previously diagnosed. In these cases, it is assumed that all Medicare beneficiaries would be entitled to one bundle of services intended for newly diagnosed patients, with subsequent coverage for maintenance therapy.

Likely patterns of nutrition therapy were estimated using clinical practice guidelines proposed by the American Dietetic Association (ADA, 1998) and expert clinical judgment. These guidelines provide a pertinent Medicare model because they reflect the consensus of dietetic professionals. Moreover, these guidelines are already used by some insurers to design reimbursement policies (Blue Cross/Blue Shield of Massachusetts, TUFTS Health Plan, Blue Cross/Blue Shield of North Dakota). In specific cases, these guidelines were modified for this analysis to reflect best-practice clinical judgment or to capture prevailing practice patterns that differed from available guidelines.

An important complication arose because most Medicare recipients have comorbidities that may require different kinds of nutrition intervention. Among NHANES III respondents, 88 percent of individuals at least 65 years of age with diagnosed diabetes also experienced hypertension or hyperlipidemia. Because the appropriate therapeutic response is not clear in nonclinical survey data, and because the same nutrition therapy session may address multiple concerns, reasonable approximation was required.

After deliberation, clinicians involved with this analysis approximated these requirements by computing the number of visits associated with the most intense diagnosis and then including at least one additional annual visit for each comorbid condition. These recommendations are used solely for the purposes of cost estimation and are not intended to convey recommended care.

Patient Demand

Patient demand for nutrition therapy is perhaps the most important unknown factor in projecting the costs (and the benefits) of expanded coverage. Existing studies suggest that most Medicare beneficiaries with pertinent conditions will not utilize nutrition services, even when these services are fully reimbursed. No study has evaluated patient demand for nutrition services in a national representative population that is fully comparable to Medicare. However, the two most pertinent studies found that less than 20 percent of eligible patients received any covered nutrition services within the 45- or 60-month time period studied.

Utilization of covered nutrition services by Medicare health maintenance organization (HMO) patients in the Group Health Cooperative of Puget Sound were examined. Sheils and coworkers (1999) determined that 13.7 percent of patients with diabetes, 5.3 percent of patients with cardiovascular disease, and 15 percent of patients with renal disease were seen at least once by a dietitian in a 5-year period. A replication of this study within a military population indicated that 19.7 percent of patients with diabetes, 9.7 percent of patients with cardiovascular disease, and 20.3 percent of those with renal disease were seen at least once in a nutrition clinic within a 45-month period (1.5 visits per 5 years) (ADA, 1999). In both studies, the average number of visits per patient was far below the number of visits used in this cost estimate (seven to nine visits in a 5-year period) (see Table 14.2).

Whether these patterns accurately reflect patient preferences or reflect other system barriers is not known. These data may overestimate or underestimate patient demand for nutrition services within a national, predominantly fee-for-service Medicare environment. Broad coverage may stimulate patient demand and may also stimulate more aggressive provider marketing of nutrition services. Alternatively, the overall Medicare population may be less motivated to seek nutrition services than the military or Group Health beneficiaries previously studied. Finally, epidemiological developments such as the increased prevalence of obesity (Mokdad et al., 1999) may have unexpected implications for the use of nutrition services.

Given uncertain utilization of nutrition therapy, a baseline scenario analysis based upon the best available data was augmented with a high-use and a low-use scenario designed to illustrate the range of uncertainty that underlies these results. Appendix H gives a specific example of the methodology used. Within each scenario, patients who receive nutrition therapy are assumed to receive services that match protocol guidelines for nutrition therapy. When such guidelines were unavailable, clinical judgment was applied to estimate likely patterns of service use.

The *baseline scenario* represents the best estimate of likely patient utilization of nutrition therapy within each diagnostic category explored. Table 14.2 indicates the assumed guidelines and patient utilization for each diagnosis. Estimated patient utilization in initial and subsequent years is chosen to be consistent with the research literature or adjusted to more closely match more recently published nutrition therapy guidelines.

The *low utilization scenario* describes possible expenditures if patient utilization falls below expected levels. This scenario is especially pertinent if medical care providers are slow to adjust to the new benefit or if patients perceive little incremental benefit to receipt of nutrition services.

In contrast, the *high utilization scenario* describes possible expenditures if utilization exceeds expected levels. Given existing pressure on Medicare finances, this scenario is most worrisome to Medicare budget analysts, and may arise due to unexpectedly strong patient preferences for nutrition services, due to unintended financial incentives for increased use, or due to other factors.

Table 14.2 displays utilization assumptions and associated costs for all three scenarios. The table includes both Medicare reimbursements and payments by individual patients. Non-Medicare-covered costs such as lost work time to obtain nutrition services and the cost (or savings) of food or nutrition supplements are not included in these figures. These ancillary costs to patients would be important in a broader economic analysis.

After adjusting for both copayments and premium increases, the Medicare estimated direct reimbursement cost of nutrition therapy for selected conditions is $1.069 billion for the period January 1, 2000 to December 31, 2004. This estimate is somewhat lower than those provided by Sheils and colleagues (1999) in the Group Health study. More important, the corresponding low-utilization and high-utilization scenarios indicate the uncertainty associated with these projections. The low-utilization scenario yields estimated direct Medicare expenditures of $740 million, while the high-utilization estimate yields a comparable figure of $1.97 billion.

Nutrition Therapy Reimbursement Assumptions By Diagnosis

Cardiovascular Disease

Reimbursements are based upon three initial nutrition therapy sessions for newly diagnosed patients, with one session each subsequent year. It is assumed that all Medicare recipients with hypertension and CHD are entitled to three initial sessions. Sensitivity analysis was based on the upper limit shown in the Sheils and coworkers (1999) Group Health study for persons with cardiovascular diagnoses. These authors observed 154 nutrition therapy sessions per 1,000 patients per year.

The low-utilization scenario was computed using observed patterns within the Department of Defense (DOD) sample (ADA, 1999), which included an observed utilization rate of 79 per 1,000 patients per year. (See Appendix H for explanation of utilization rate calculations.) Utilization rates among patients with hypertension were assumed to be lower than other diagnoses because hypertension is less likely to produce explicit symptoms leading individuals to seek care.

Diabetes

For purposes of cost estimation, it is assumed that patients receive three initial nutrition therapy sessions per year for newly diagnosed diabetes, with one additional annual session per year beyond what would otherwise be covered as part of the new diabetes self-management benefit, which includes a nutrition component conducted by a registered

TABLE 14.2 Estimated Direct Medicare Costs of Nutrition Therapy
Treatment for Selected Conditions for 2000 to 2004

Diagnosis or Condition	Assumed Guideline for Proposed Nutrition Therapy Visits per Year[a]		Assumed Utilization in Low-Cost Scenario (%)	Estimated Medicare Nutrition Therapy Reimbursement Costs in Low-Cost Scenario[b] ($ million)
	In Year of Diagnosis	Subsequent Years		
Single Diagnosis				
↑LDL[c] only	3	1	5	124
HTN[d] only	3	1	5	138
Heart failure	3	1	10	28
DM[e] only	3	1	12	18
Renal disease[f]	3	1	7	10
Combination Diagnoses				
HTN & ↑ LDL	4	1	5	269
DM & HTN	5	1	12	63
DM & ↑ LDL	5	1	12	40
HTN & ↑ LDL & DM	6	1	12	78
Eligible patients with none of the above conditions[g]	1	1	5	106
Medicare portion of estimated charges[h]				$873 million
Adjusted Medicare portion after corresponding premium increase[i]				$740 million

[a] Based on Medical Nutrition Therapy Across the Continuum of Care protocols (ADA, 1998) and expert clinical judgment.

[b] Based on 35.4 million beneficiaries, estimated cost per nutrition session is $55.41 (HCFA, 1999).

[c] ↑LDL = low-density lipoprotein >130 mg/dL.

[d] HTN = hypertension.

[e] DM = diabetes mellitus

Assumed Utilization in Baseline Scenario (%)	Estimated Medicare Nutrition Therapy Reimbursement Costs in Baseline Scenario ($ million)	Assumed Utilization in High Scenario (%)	Estimated Medicare Nutrition Therapy Reimbursement Costs in High-Cost Scenario ($ million)
8	198	16	396
8	221	16	442
15	42	20	56
21	31	30	45
12	17	30	36
8	431	16	861
21	111	30	158
21	70	30	100
21	136	30	194
8	169	16	338
	$1.43 billion		$2.63 billion
	$1.07 billion		$1.97 billion

f Renal disease = serum creatinine >2.5 g/dL for women and >3.0 g/dL for men.
g Includes disabled under 65 years-of-age patients. See text.
h Assumed 20% Medicare copayment for nutrition therapy.
i Assuming that Medicare Part B premiums will increase to recover 25% of associated increase in Medicare costs.

dietitian (HCFA, 1999). Patient utilization in the baseline scenario is modeled using observed data from two recent studies. A rate of 464 sessions per 1,000 eligible patient-years were reported within the Group Health population (Sheils et al., 1999) and a rate of 193 per 1,000 patient-years was observed among military recipients (ADA, 1999). These rates were used to calibrate the baseline range. A range of plausible values for the high-utilization and low-utilization scenarios were chosen that, in the committee's clinical judgment, captured the reasonable range of patient use of nutrition services.

Renal Disease

Reimbursements for nutrition therapy for pre-end-stage renal disease are estimated based on three initial nutrition therapy sessions, with one additional annual session per year. The baseline scenario is based upon the two available studies, which yielded 519 sessions per 1,000 patient-years for the Group Health population (Sheils et al., 1999) and 197 sessions per 1,000 in the military population studied (ADA, 1999). As with diabetes, a range of plausible values for the high-utilization and low-utilization scenarios were chosen that, in the committee's clinical judgment, captured the reasonable range of patient use of nutrition services.

Osteoporosis

A nutrition visit is not warranted at the present time for a diagnosis of osteoporosis. However, in some patients with special needs or food practices (e.g., cultural and religious factors, vegetarian diets or food allergies), it may be warranted when referred by a physician. There is strong evidence regarding the cost-effectiveness, and potential cost savings, of treating individuals diagnosed with osteoporosis with calcium and vitamin D supplements.

Comorbidities

The presence of multiple conditions and diagnoses must somehow be considered in the analysis because many Medicare recipients have comorbidities requiring specific nutrition intervention. Within the NHANES III data set, more than 90 percent of those individuals 65 years and over with diabetes also experienced hypertension or hyperlipidemia. Because the appropriate therapeutic response is unclear in nonmedical survey data, and because the same nutrition intervention may address multiple concerns, a reasonable approximation was used to address comorbidity concerns. In particular, patients are assumed to need the maximum recommended number of visits for the most nutrition-intensive diagnosis. Patients are then assumed to have one additional annual visit for each listed comorbid condition. As above, these estimates are used solely for the purpose of cost estimation and are not intended to convey a standard of recommended care.

Provider Incentives

Another source of cost uncertainty stems from the specific design of Medicare coverage of nutrition services. The level and detailed implementation of coverage and provider payment are likely to influence provider supply and patient demand for these services. Reimbursement policies create complex incentives for bundling or unbundling of existing services, incentives that can have a great impact on resulting expenditure. For example, if physicians alter billing by submitting claims for nutrition therapy based on the assumption that basic in-office nutrition education qualifies as nutrition therapy, then the expanded coverage for nutrition services might generate unexpected costs (as is discussed in chapter 1, Table 1.1). These basic education components of standard medical care should not receive additional reimbursement under expanded coverage.

Because of such complexities, the content of reimbursable nutrition services and the required qualifications of providers will greatly influence subsequent costs. For the same reasons, administrative oversight of nutrition services in general outpatient settings, renal dialysis centers, and other settings is important to the proper targeting of services.

ECONOMICALLY SIGNIFICANT AVERTED COSTS

Direct reimbursements provide the simplest estimate of Medicare costs. However, these estimates do not capture the full budgetary implications of coverage for nutrition services because they neglect important cost savings and also expenditures likely to result from improved nutritional status. Reasonable clinical evidence has been discussed in previous chapters to demonstrate that nutrition therapy can reduce the complications of diabetes, hip fracture, renal failure, and other adverse events that would otherwise require costly acute services. Nutrition therapy may also allow hypertensive patients to reduce utilization of prescription drugs. Improved coverage for nutrition therapy may also result in some offsetting reduction in outpatient physician use. All of these possibilities suggest that estimated direct charges likely overstate the net impact on Medicare costs.

Given the role of nutrition therapy in the prevention and management of chronic diseases and conditions, some researchers and policymakers suggest that expanded nutrition services for Medicare beneficiaries will generate significant offsetting cost reductions and that such services may even be cost saving to the Medicare program (Sheils et al., 1999). Although nutrition services may generate offsetting cost savings by these means, experiences of other medical interventions such as home health care, medical devices, and renal dialysis suggest the inherent difficulty of forecasting the budget impact of policy innovations. For example, nutrition therapy may increase lifespan, which has an ambiguous impact on resulting Medicare costs. Although many preventive services improve health status, primary and secondary preventive services are rarely cost saving. In specific settings, vaccination and some other primary interventions have reduced medical costs (Russell, 1994).

For most diagnoses, limited reliable data exist to estimate the overall economic effect of nutrition intervention. Given evidence of treatment effectiveness for highly prevalent conditions in the Medicare population, it is believed that expanded eligibility will improve population health. Such improved health status is likely to produce important economic benefits for the Medicare program, although existing data do not permit reliable estimates of these effects. Previous experience highlights the inherent difficulty of projecting Medicare costs, as well as the potential perils associated with over-optimistic estimated cost savings associated with new services (Weissert, 1985).

Experience also highlights several problems in extrapolating promising results from specific populations into convincing evidence for broader patient groups. Nutrition therapy is generally provided within a multidisciplinary and multimodality treatment plan. Identifying the specific contribution of nutrition therapy to improved health outcomes is therefore difficult. Best-practice clinical trials on selected patients can overstate the range of plausible program benefits because these efforts are difficult to replicate in large-scale practices serving the full patient population (Rossi and Freeman, 1995). Moreover, benefits that are valuable from a social perspective may have paradoxical effects for specific budgets. Life-extending interventions may have strong net social benefits and may be extremely cost-effective by standard criteria while increasing Medicare program costs. Finally, it is inappropriate to assume additive averted costs or social benefits within a population of individuals who typically have multiple diagnoses and comorbidities.

Cost Savings Documented in the Group Health Study

In part because of the significant methodological concerns mentioned above, little evidence was available to evaluate the cost savings associated with a population-wide provision of nutrition services. The most pertinent study uses data from the Group Health Cooperative of Puget Sound to explore the likely cost of nutrition services for the full Medicare population (Sheils et al., 1999). Because Group Health covers dietitian services as a supplemental Medicare benefit, this patient group provides useful data to examine the likely impact of expanded eligibility throughout the Medicare population.

Sheils and colleagues (1999) found that the receipt of dietitian services was associated with reduced inpatient admissions and physician office visits for patients with diabetes and cardiovascular diagnoses. In particular, these authors found that dietitian services were associated with a 9.5 percent reduction in hospital admissions for patients with diabetes and an 8.6 percent reduction in hospital admissions for patients with cardiovascular disease. Estimated reductions in physician visits were even greater for these diagnoses, from 16.9 percent to 23.5 percent. Because of the large savings associated with these diagnoses, Sheils and colleagues estimated that coverage of either dietitian services for diabetes alone, or coverage for diabetes and cardiovascular disease, would be cost saving from the perspective of the Medicare program as a whole (see Table 14.3).

Although dietitian coverage for diabetes and cardiovascular disease for all Medicare recipients was estimated (Sheils et al., 1999) to cost $2.308 billion over the 7 year period, the same services were estimated to yield an estimated $2.363 in cost savings, producing negative estimates of net costs. The majority of estimated cost savings would accrue to Medicare Part A due to reduced inpatient hospitalization costs. Coverage for all

TABLE 14.3 Estimated Gross and Net Costs of Nutrition Therapy Coverage Based on Data from Group Health Cooperative of Puget Sound

1998–2004 Projected Costs	Dietitian Coverage for all Medicare Beneficiaries ($ billion)	Dietitian Coverage for Diabetes Only ($ billion)	Dietitian Coverage for Diabetes and Cardiovascular Disease ($ billion)
Benefit cost	2.732	1.371	2.308
Savings	2.363	1.578	2.363
Net costs	0.370	−0.208	−0.055
Part A	−1.248	−0.720	−1.248
Part B	1.617	0.512	1.193

SOURCE: Sheils et al. (1999).

Medicare beneficiaries was estimated to have a gross cost of $2.73 billion, and a positive net cost of $370 million.

These results suggest the promise of nutrition therapy in producing significant reductions in costs. However, three features of this study suggest caution in applying these findings to the full Medicare population.

First, Group Health patients and providers may be unrepresentative of the broader population of Medicare patients and providers. Group Health may include higher-quality providers or more health-conscious consumers than are typical in the broader Medicare population, although a similar study of usage by active duty military, their families, retired members of the military, and their families shows similar results (ADA, 1999). As a staff-model HMO, the impact of dietitian services in Group Health may be difficult to replicate in more decentralized systems of reimbursement and care. Across a wide range of social policy and health arenas, best-practice interventions in unusual settings prove difficult to replicate on a broader scale (Currie, 1995). The generalizability of these results is therefore unclear.

Second, the underlying data reflect a strong process of patient self-selection into the receipt of nutrition care. Multiple linear regression and individual fixed-effects models are used to minimize potential biases that might arise from unobserved individual factors. For both clinical and econometric reasons, however, this specification is vulnerable to unobserved heterogeneity in the data. The underlying data include limited controls for individual variation in health status, preferences, and resources that influence subsequent health outcomes, adherence, and utilization.

Even controlling for diagnosis and other observable patient characteristics, recipients of nutrition therapy are likely to be more highly motivated than comparable patients who have the same diagnoses but do not receive nutrition therapy. Although some self-selection will occur in the Medicare population, it is not clear how this selection process will be influenced if prevailing reimbursement systems provide financial incentives for referral.

Given the resulting difficulty in estimating net impact on the *overall* Medicare budget associated with coverage of nutrition therapy, specific diagnoses for which nutrition therapy is likely to be especially cost-effective or even cost saving were examined. Clinicians and policy analysts involved identified several diagnostic categories for which well-implemented nutrition therapy would bring important and beneficial economic effects. Estimates for several diagnostic categories are discussed below.

Diabetes Mellitus

In 1997, the estimated direct costs attributed to diabetes in the United States amounted to $44 billion. Costs due to work loss, disability, and premature death are estimated to be even higher (CDC, 1998).

Diabetes provides perhaps the best-documented example of potential benefits associated with nutrition therapy. Per capita Medicare expenditures are 50 percent higher among patients with diabetes than among the overall Medicare patient group (Krop et al., 1998). Per-capita Medicare expenditure also varies greatly across the diabetic population. The most expensive 10 percent of patients with diabetes account for 56 percent of Medicare expenditures for diabetes care. The least expensive 50 percent of Medicare patients with diabetes account for only 4 percent of the same expenditures (Krop et al., 1998).

Many of the above mentioned charges are associated with complications of diabetes whose incidence has been reduced in randomized trials of intensive self-management that included nutrition therapy (Collins and Anderson, 1995; DCCT, 1995, 1996; Franz et al., 1995; Herman et al., 1997). Chapter 6 summarized pertinent clinical results. Evidence is suggestive, but less conclusive, regarding the specific contribution of registered dietitians to improved outcomes. Studies have indicated that more intensive interaction with nutrition professionals improves glycemic control compared to less intensive care (Franz et al., 1995; Sheils et al., 1999). However, the relative contributions of specific professionals within multidisciplinary health care settings is difficult to discern.

The study by Franz and collaborators (1995) provides the most informative analysis of this question. These authors compared the impact of "usual" nutrition care of one nutrition therapy visit to the impact of three visits, as recommended by practice guidelines. Both modalities resulted in improved glycemic control when compared to a control group without nutrition counseling. However, the practice guidelines (three visits) proved more cost-effective than usual care (one visit) in reducing blood glucose levels. Few prospective studies compare the efficacy and cost-effectiveness of competing nutrition therapy modalities, however studies have indicated that group-based modalities can be effective as part of intensive self-management (Heller et al., 1988).

From an economic perspective, the United Kingdom Prospective Diabetes Study (UKPDS) which involved 6,000 patients with type 2 diabetes in a randomized control trial, best demonstrates potential cost savings from intensive diabetes self-management. The study compared the benefits of intensive blood glucose control to the benefits of standard care (UKPDS Group, 1998). In this study, both the treatment group and control group received dietary advice from a dietitian. After 10 years, hemoglobin A_{1c} (HbA$_{1c}$) levels were 0.9 percentage points lower in the treatment group than in a control group receiving usual care (HbA$_{1c}$ of 7.0 percent versus 7.9 percent). The treatment group experienced clinically significant reductions in the incidence of many diabetes complications, including a 10 percent reduced incidence of diabetes-related deaths and a 25 percent reduction in microvascular end points. Such findings highlight the large potential savings to medical payers and patients associated with improved glycemic control.

Another study provides further evidence of cost-effective diabetes treatment. Comprehensive treatment of type 2 diabetes to maintain HbA$_{1c}$ at 7.2 percent reduced the cumulative incidence of blindness, end-stage renal disease, and lower-extremity amputation by 76 percent, 88 percent, and 67 percent respectively, with a life expectancy gain of 1.4 years (Herman et al., 1997). The associated estimated cost of approximately $20,000 per quality-adjusted life-year was far below standard thresholds used to evaluate life-prolonging interventions (Heller et al., 1988; Tengs et al., 1995).

The magnitude of such economic benefits is directly explored in several analyses. Most recently, Gilmer and colleagues (1997) examined the cost to health plans of poor glycemic control. Using 1993 to 1995 expenditure data, these authors employed gamma regression analysis to estimate the short-term relationship between glycemic control and medical charges for 3,017 adults (mean age 59.7 years) in a large HMO.

This analysis is noteworthy for its use of explicit controls for gender effects and for prevalent diabetes comorbidities such as hypertension. It should also be noted that Gilmer and coworkers do not include patients who died over the study period. These exclusions may understate the value of nutrition services given UKPDS data which suggest that the incidence of heart attacks and sudden death may be reduced through more intensive intervention.

Table 14.4 presents the estimated annual costs of poor glycemic control as determined by elevated HbA$_{1c}$ concentration in hypothetical 65-year-old patients with accompanying comorbidities. As shown, the incremental costs associated with poor glycemic control increase with higher HbA$_{1c}$ levels. Incremental costs are also elevated in the presence of comorbidities such as hypertension. Incremental costs of poor glycemic control appear to decline with age in this population and appeared to vary continuously, thus allowing estimates of incremental responses.

These point estimates provide one means to examine the magnitude of Medicare "cost offsets" associated with nutrition therapy for patients with diabetes. As discussed above, these numbers should not be interpreted as budget forecasts, which require detailed actuarial calculations beyond the scope of this committee report.

TABLE 14.4 Estimated Annual Costs of Poor Glycemic Control in a
Health Maintenance Organization Population (in dollars)

Condition	HbA$_{1c}$ Level		
	7–8%	8–9%	9–10%
65-Year-old-man			
Diabetes only	192.03	235.51	286.38
Diabetes and hyperlipidemia	159.76	195.94	238.26
Diabetes and hypertension	289.93	355.58	432.39
Diabetes and hyperlipidemia and hypertension	241.21	295.83	359.73
65-Year-old-woman			
Diabetes only	181.22	222.25	270.26
Diabetes and hyperlipidemia	177.51	217.71	264.74
Diabetes and hypertension	303.36	372.06	452.42
Diabetes and hyperlipidemia and hypertension	297.16	364.46	443.17

SOURCE: Computed from Gilmer et al. (1997).

Using the HbA$_{1c}$ range of 7 to 8 percent, one can estimate potential short-term savings to Medicare and patients attributable to nutrition therapy. Given that patients with diabetes have access to other self-management services in addition to nutrition therapy, it is unlikely that coverage of nutrition therapy would produce the full improvements observed in controlled trials that compare high-quality nutrition therapies to minimal standard services. Averted costs estimated here are based on the assumption that coverage of nutrition therapy would lead to an additional 0.25 percentage point reduction in HbA$_{1c}$. This appears conservative in light of clinical reports of best-practice nutrition therapy services. Table 14.4 indicates that a 1 percentage point reduction of HbA$_{1c}$ is associated with a corresponding reduction of 18 percent in costs.

Using the same coefficients as above, averted costs for Medicare beneficiaries with diabetes that can be reasonably associated with nutrition therapy can be estimated (Table 14.5). These assumptions imply large short-term benefits associated with nutrition therapy. Although nutrition therapy is not cost saving, direct medical charges are substantially offset by savings associated with the prevention of adverse health events. Within the baseline scenario, the cost of averted adverse events is estimated to be $231 million. The comparable analysis in the low-utilization and high-utilization scenarios yield analogous figures of $132 million and $330 million.

TABLE 14.5 Estimated Cost of Nutrition Therapy and Costs of Averted Adverse Outcomes in Baseline Scenario (Savings to Both Medicare and Private Patients)

Condition	Total Charges for Nutrition Therapy within Baseline Scenario[a] ($ million)	Estimated Total Cost of Averted Outcomes Attributable to Nutrition Therapy[b] ($ million)
Diabetes only	31	20
Diabetes and hyperlipidemia	70	32
Diabetes and hypertension	111	89
Diabetes and hyperlipidemia and hypertension	136	90

[a] This column shows estimated charges from the baseline scenario of Table 14.2. For comparability, total charges (including copayments) are shown.

[b] This column indicates the estimated cost of averted outcomes based upon the coefficients computed by Gilmer et al. (1997).

The long-term implications for Medicare program costs are less clear from these data. Gilmer and coworkers (1997) examined expenditures over a 3-year period and therefore did not examine important future costs, including future Medicare expenditures for marginal survivors who experience increased lifespan due to the intervention.

Osteoporosis

An estimated 10 million Americans suffer from osteoporosis, including more than 25 percent of non-Hispanic white women 65 years and over. Osteoporosis may also have significant prevalence among older men (Ebeling, 1998).

Many studies document that calcium and vitamin D supplements can slow bone loss in older adults (Bendich et al., 1999; Chapuy et al. 1992; Cummings et al. 1995; Jönsson et al., 1995). (See chapter 8 for further discussion.) From an economic perspective, this is especially important because improved or maintained bone density has been linked with reduced incidence of hip fracture in randomized trials involving older adults. For example, a group of women treated with calcium and vitamin D supplementation experienced cumulative hip fractures of 6 percent versus 13 percent in a comparable control group (Dawson-Hughes et al., 1997).

Medicare diagnosis-related group (DRG) reimbursements—a measure which includes many important medical and social costs—average

$3,900 for fractures of the femur. Preventive measures to improve calcium and vitamin D intake are therefore likely to be cost-effective among women at least 65 years old who are the principal osteoporosis patient group.

It has been estimated that osteoporosis prevention costs $30,000 per QALY (Tosteson et al., 1997). These estimates compare favorable to widely accepted public health interventions and to widely prescribed treatments to control hypertension. Nutrition supplements for osteoporosis management appear to be more cost-effective than widely cited statin drugs for control of CHD (Bendich et al., 1999; Chapuy et al., 1992; Cummings et al., 1995; Jönsson et al., 1995; Tengs et al., 1995).

Cardiovascular Diseases

Chapter 5 reviewed existing clinical evidence regarding dyslipidemia, hypertension, and heart failure. Diet plays a central role in the primary, secondary, and tertiary prevention of each form of cardiovascular disease.

Hypertension

There is extensive literature to support the cost-effectiveness of interventions for hypertension. Existing literature provides mixed support for the cost-effectiveness of nonpharmaceutical interventions in the 65 years and older population. Because older persons face competing mortality and morbidity risks, interventions for this population sometimes appear less cost-effective than preventive measures targeting younger populations (Garber et al., 1991; Johannesson, 1994; Johannesson et al., 1997). Research in Sweden by Johannesson and colleagues indicates that nonpharmaceutical interventions alone can be less cost-effective than available drug therapy (Johannesson and Fagerberg, 1992; Johannesson and Le Lorier, 1996; Johannesson et al., 1991, 1995).

Despite these limitations, nutrition therapy is associated with several economically significant improvements in hypertension management. Alone and in combination with drug therapy, reduced salt intake is associated with reduced diastolic blood pressure in older persons (see chapter 5). Evidence is more limited regarding the linkage between reduced blood pressure and reduced incidence of CHD and stroke. However, the causal linkage between improved diet and improved health outcomes is strongly supported in clinical research. Chapter 5 reviews the Trials of Nonpharmacologic Interventions in the Elderly in which registered dietitians assisted adults 65 years and older to reduce salt intake and to significantly reduce the reliance of patients upon antihypertensive medications.

Results cited in Hebert et al. (1992) suggest that reductions in diastolic blood pressure of 5 to 6 mm Hg would prevent 42 percent of strokes and 14 percent of CHD events. The effects of drug and diet appear additive; so nutrition therapy has the potential to reduce mortality, morbidity, and health care utilization even when hypertension is also addressed through drug treatment.

Table 14.6 indicates the economic implications of these patterns for the baseline scenario of 8 percent assumed utilization. It examines the short-term implications of a 1.25 mm Hg reduction in diastolic blood pressure attributable to nutrition intervention among patients with CHD who actually received nutrition therapy. This program effect is approximately one-fourth of that observed in clinical trials of intense dietary interventions (see chapter 5 section on hypertension). To allow for the possibility of lagged effects, these calculations presume a 2-year period between coverage of nutrition therapy and resulting health gains.

While nutrition therapy does not appear to be cost saving for hypertension, as it had appeared in the case of diabetes, such treatment does yield important clinical and policy effects. Although the precise magnitude of these effects is unclear given current data, Table 14.6 presents approximate estimates of potential averted strokes and CHD events among patients with simple hypertension in the baseline scenario. Assuming a 2-year time-lag in program benefits, a conservative approach is to consider only the first 3 years of clinical effects. With a direct program cost of $221 million in the baseline scenario (Table 14.2), nutrition therapy is estimated to prevent approximately 9,000 stroke hospitalizations and 7,000 hospitalizations due to CHD events (Table 14.6).

If policymakers value the direct and indirect consequences of stroke prevention at more than $25,000 per case, or if they value the direct and indirect consequences of CHD hospitalization at more than $32,000 per case, the coverage of nutrition therapy appears cost-effective compared with other life-extending interventions. Moreover, these calculations may understate the value of nutrition intervention because they do not include the impact on other health risks. It is important to note that these estimates are based only on direct DRG charges, which in all probability may substantially understate averted costs because they fail to consider accompanying outpatient care and other services funded by Medicare and by the beneficiary.

Dyslipidemia

Interventions to reduce excessive blood lipids have received extensive clinical and policy attention. The development of cholesterol-lowering medications such as pravastatin have allowed substantial reductions in low-density lipoprotein (LDL) cholesterol and have been associated with substantially reduced mortality and morbidity from cardiovascular causes (Hunninghake et al., 1993; Knopp, 1999; Shepherd et al., 1995).

Given the availability of powerful (and costly) cholesterol-reducing medication, diet is not often used alone as initial therapy for elevated cholesterol, but rather is used in combination with medication. Data suggest that diet and medication operate independently to reduce disease risk (Hunninghake et al., 1993); nutrition therapy can have a substantial impact on mortality and morbidity despite the presence of effective cholesterol-reducing drugs (McGehee et al., 1995).

The impact of cholesterol reduction on mortality and morbidity in older persons has been disputed (Garber et al., 1991; Goldman et al., 1992; Kronmal et al., 1993; Larson, 1995). However, data from the 4S and pravastatin studies demonstrate reduced cardiovascular mortality and reduced incidence of CHD events (Shepherd et al., 1995). Data reviewed in chapter 5 indicate that every 1 percent reduction in cholesterol is associated with a corresponding 2 percent reduction in the incidence of CHD.

Reduced CHD incidence is especially significant since CVD accounts for almost 50 percent of all deaths in the United States (Knopp, 1999), and heart disease accounts for approximately 17 percent of all medical spending in the United States (Cutler and McLellan, 1996; McGehee et al., 1995). Acute myocardial infarction (AMI) is the most costly and fatal aspect of heart disease. Medicare reimbursements in 1991 for AMI-related episodes averaged $14,772 (in 1991 dollars). Real expenditures for AMI-related Medicare services are estimated to have increased by 4 percent annually (all figures from Cutler and McLellan, 1996).

To gauge the potential impact of nutrition therapy coverage on the incidence of coronary heart disease, epidemiological findings from the Framingham study were used to estimate baseline risks and the approximate relative risk reduction associated with nutrition intervention (Kronmal et al., 1993; Wilson et al., 1998). The efficacy of nutrition therapy in reducing LDL levels was modeled as the principal mechanism of reduced CHD risk for patients with hypertension, diabetes mellitus, and dyslipidemia (Wilson et al., 1998). Because data are unavailable on many biological risk factors within the Medicare population, this analysis was useful to gauge the approximate health impact of coverage for nutrition therapy. A more extensive epidemiological study (ideally informed by randomized clinical trials among Medicare beneficiaries) would provide superior estimates.

Existing studies suggest that best-practice nutrition therapy can achieve a 6 percent reduction in LDL levels beyond the levels controlled by accompanying medication (see chapter 5 for a summary of this research). Broadly deployed nutrition therapy may be less effective than is

TABLE 14.6 Averted Acute-Care Episodes Associated with Nutrition Therapy Treatment for Patients with Hypertension for Baseline Scenario[a]

Estimate for Cost Offset	2000	2001	2002	2003	2004	5-Year Total
Medicare discharges due to stroke (n)	389,169	391,504	393,853	397,003	400,179	
Potential stroke patients with simple hypertension who utilize nutrition therapy assuming 8 percent utilization among covered patients (n)	31,133	31,320	31,508	31,760	32,014	
Potential strokes averted due to 1.25 mm Hg blood pressure reduction attributable to nutrition therapy (n)	2,958	2,975	2,993	3,917	3,041	
DRG[b] payment per patient for stroke (Assuming 3% increase in DRG rate per year)	$5,145	$5,299	$5,458	$5,622	$5,791	
DRG payments for stroke avoided attributable to nutrition therapy[c]	Assumed 2 year time lag	Assumed 2 year time lag	$16,144,003	$16,728,093	$17,333,315	
Discharges due to coronary heart disease (CHD) (n)	726,901	731,262	735,650	740,064	744,504	
Potential CHD patients with simple hypertension who utilize nutrition therapy assuming 8% utilization among covered patients (n)	58,152	58,501	58,852	59,205	59,560	

Potential CHD events reduced due to 1.25 mm blood pressure reduction attributable to nutrition therapy (n)	2,326	2,340	2,354	2,368	2,382	
Estimated average DRG payment per patient for coronary heart disease	$4,392	$4,524	$4,659	$4,799	$4,943	
DRG payments for CHD avoided due to nutrition therapy[c]	Assumed 2 year time lag	Assumed 2 year time lag	$10,838,322	$11,230,453	$11,636,770	
Averted costs for both stroke and CHD events[c]	Assumed 2 year time lag	Assumed 2 year time lag	$26,982,325	$27,958,545	$28,970,086	$83,910,956[d]
Medicare reimbursement charges for nutrition therapy services to hypertensive patients	$62,140,763[e]	$26,204,130	$27,114,393	$28,119,655	$29,160,815	$172,739,756[d]

[a] Baseline scenario assumes 8% utilization and a reduction in diastolic blood pressure of 1.25 mm Hg.

[b] DRG = diagnostic related group.

[c] A 3% annual increase in DRG payment rates is assumed within these calculations. Cost data were obtained by The Lewin Group, Inc. for the committee.

[d] Low Utilization Scenario of 5% is:
$52,444,347 averted costs
$107,962,345 Medicare reimbursement charges

High Cos: Utilization Scenario of 16% is:
$167,821,912 averted costs
$345,477,505 Medicare reimbursement charges

[e] Assumes all current beneficiaries with existing diagnoses receive initial nutrition therapy in first year.

TABLE 14.7 Estimated Impact of Nutrition Therapy Aimed at Reducing Elevated Low-density Lipoprotein (LDL) Cholesterol on 5-Year Incidence of Coronary Heart Disease (CHD) among Medicare Beneficiaries

	Low Utilization Scenario[a] (percent)	Estimated Reduction in CHD Events Given 3% Reduction in LDL[b]
Cardiovascular risk diagnoses		
↑LDL[c] only	5	1,690
HTN[d] only	5	1,750
DM[e] only	12	180
Combination diagnoses		
HTN & ↑LDL	5	4,857
DM & HTN	12	763
DM & ↑LDL	12	483
HTN & DM & ↑LDL	12	1,252
Potential CHD events averted due to nutrition therapy		10,975
Estimated costs associated with averted CHD events[f]		$54,249,425

[a] See text for discussion of utilization scenarios.

[b] The estimated number of averted CHD episodes is computed using regression coefficients reported by Wilson et al. (1998) using data from the Framingham study. Predicted probabilities are age-adjusted, and include an additional risk score of 1.0 to account for mean tobacco prevalence and other risk factors.

observed in best-practice clinical trial interventions. For illustrative purposes, it is therefore assumed that nutrition therapy patients achieve an average 3 percent reduction in LDL.

Table 14.7 shows the resulting estimated reduction in CHD events associated with coverage for nutrition therapy which reduces LDL levels across CHD related diagnoses (diabetes mellitus, hypertension, and dyslipidemia) for the period 2000 to 2004. As above, these calculations presume a 2-year lag between coverage and resulting health gains. Within the baseline utilization scenario, coverage for nutrition therapy is estimated to delay or avert approximately 18,000 cases of coronary heart disease over the period 2000 to 2004. Within the low-utilization scenario, coverage of nutrition therapy is estimated to delay or avert almost 11,000

Baseline Utilization Scenario[a] (percent)	Estimated Reduction in CHD Events Given 3% Reduction in LDL[b]	High Utilization Scenario[a] (percent)	Estimated Reduction in CHD Events Given 3% Reduction in LDL[b]
8	2,704	16	5,408
8	2,799	16	5,599
21	315	30	450
8	7,771	16	15,542
21	1,336	30	1,908
21	846	30	1,209
21	2,191	30	3,130
	17,962		33,246
	$88,786,166		$164,349,078

c ↑LDL = low-density lipoprotein >130.

d HTN = hypertension.

e DM = diabetes mellitus.

f Estimated at 2004 payment rate, assumed that 3% annual increase in diagnostic-related group payments between calendar year 2000 and calendar year 2004.

CHD cases, whereas within the high-utilization scenario, it is estimated to delay or avert approximately 33,000 CHD cases.

These results provide some basis for policymakers to evaluate the economic trade-offs associated with coverage for nutrition therapy. Within the baseline scenario, excluding patient coinsurance payments, Medicare's estimated reimbursement cost for expanded coverage of nutrition therapy is $1.43 billion over the same period. The accompanying estimated Medicare cost per averted CHD event is therefore approximately $80,000.[2]

---

[2] In several respects, this calculation also understates the benefits associated with coverage of nutrition therapy. For example, reductions in dyslipidemia and CHD will also reduce the incidence of stroke (Fine-Edelstein et al., 1994).

At this level of treatment effectiveness, independent of any other benefit associated with nutrition therapy, expanded coverage for nutrition therapy would be justified if policymakers value the social and medical costs of CHD at more than $80,000. Using this measure, Medicare coverage of nutrition therapy appears comparable in cost-effectiveness to population-wide education campaigns and other approaches to cholesterol reduction (Pharoah and Hollingworth, 1996; Tosteson et al., 1997).

Further evidence of the potential economic benefits associated with nutrition therapy is also provided in Table 14.7. Given reasonable assumptions regarding treatment efficacy and service use, initial estimates indicate that within the baseline scenario, the cost of averted CHD events is estimated to be $89 million. The comparable analysis in the low-utilization and high utilization scenarios yields analogous figures of $54 million and $164 million.

Heart Failure

As the most frequent cause of hospitalization among older individuals, heart failure accounts for more than 1 million hospitalizations annually. In fiscal year 1998, heart failure was the most costly single category of Medicare short-stay inpatient services. Covered charges for this DRG exceeded $7 billion (HCFA, 1998). Nutrition therapy, which includes sodium restriction and other measures, is an important component of standard care for heart failure patients. As summarized in chapter 5, nonadherence to diet or medication is associated with risk of rehospitalization. Randomized control trials document that multidisciplinary interventions that include nutrition therapy reduce rehospitalization and may even be cost saving (Rich and Nease, 1999; Rich et al., 1995). Data was unavailable to approximate contributions of nutrition therapy.

From an economic perspective, expanded coverage of nutrition therapy for patients with heart failure is especially attractive because these services are targeted to a discrete patient group that faces large and immediate health risks intimately linked with dietary factors. Given the low cost of nutrition intervention, and the high economic and social costs associated with dietary non-adherence in this patient group, expanded coverage of nutrition therapy for patients with heart failure is likely to be highly cost-effective. However, economic benefit estimates could not be prepared following the framework used in this study.

SUMMARY

• The Medicare portion of estimated charges for coverage of nutrition therapy during the 5-year period 2000 to 2004, is $1.069 billion for the baseline utilization scenario after adjusting for copayment and potential increase in premiums. The range of estimates are from $740 million for the low-utilization scenario to $1.97 billion for the high-utilization scenario. Net adjustments to overall Medicare budget estimates for offsets due to costs of averted care require more detailed actuarial calculation beyond the scope of this report. Current data are insufficient to accurately forecast the overall impact of nutrition therapy on general Medicare expenditures.

• Provider supply and patient demand for nutrition therapy are difficult to estimate. Specific features of Medicare coverage and reimbursement rates may have a strong impact on likely utilization. Current data are insufficient to predict reliably the utilization rates for a new nutrition therapy benefit.

• Few data exist to distinguish competing delivery strategies for nutrition therapy. Clinical trials to compare individual and group sessions will be helpful in improving policy knowledge in this area. All cost estimates were based on the cost of individual nutrition therapy sessions. Substantial cost savings may be possible for some services and diagnoses in which group nutrition therapy is found to be clinically effective.

• The clinical literature contains evidence that nutrition therapy reduces mortality and morbidity through reduced complications of diabetes and reduced incidence of heart failure and cardiovascular disease. Given data limitations, it is difficult to reliably estimate the budgetary implications of such averted costs for the Medicare program. However, economic benefits to the Medicare program and to its beneficiaries are likely to be significant. Given reasonable assumptions regarding treatment efficacy and service use, initial estimates indicate that averted costs due to a reduced incidence of coronary heart disease could range from $52 million to $167 million for patients with hypertension, $132 million to $330 million for patients with diabetes, or $54 million to $164 million for patients with dyslipidemia. It is not appropriate to add these estimates together since beneficiaries have overlapping diagnoses. Given the strong link between improved nutrition and critical health outcomes and the low average costs of nutrition interventions, expanded Medicare coverage for outpatient nutrition therapy is likely to be cost-effective when compared with other Medicare expenditures for patient care.

• Estimates were not made for the 5.62 million beneficiaries likely to receive nutrition therapy for other diagnosis such as chronic renal insufficiency and heart failure. Expanded coverage may be cost saving in some of these patient groups, although data are inadequate to reliably establish these patterns. Depending on implementation features, nutrition therapy may be cost saving in larger patient groups though existing data do not allow definitive analysis of these patterns.

• Some physicians and office staff are already providing basic nutrition education or advice incidental to routine office visits. These existing services should not receive additional reimbursement. It is assumed that general nutrition education and reinforcement of nutrition will be necessary as part of normal medical care as specified in the U.S. Preventive Services Task Force recommendations (USPSTF, 1995).

• Existing oversight and reimbursement systems must be scrutinized to assure adequate provision of nutrition services in acute care, dialysis centers, home care, and skilled nursing and long-term care facilities where nutrition is believed to be included in prospective payment systems. Where existing Medicare policies already provide coverage for nutrition services within overall reimbursement systems, administrative oversight is essential to ensure that high-quality nutrition services are actually delivered. In some cases, reimbursement rates may require adjustment to ensure that providers have adequate resources to deliver required services.

REFERENCES

ADA (American Dietetic Associaiton). 1998. *Medical Nutrition Therapy Across the Continuum of Care: Client Protocols*, 2nd ed. Chicago Ill.: American Dietetic Association and Morrison Health Care.

ADA (American Dietetic Association). 1999. Defense Department study confirms the value of medical nutrition therapy. *ADA Courier* 38:5.

Bendich A, Leader S, Muhuri P. 1999. Supplemental calcium for the prevention of hip fracture: Potential health-economic benefits. *Clin Ther* 21:1058–1072.

CDC (Centers for Disease Control and Prevention). 1998. *National Diabetes Fact Sheet: National Estimates and General Information on Diabetes in the United States. Revised Edition*. Atlanta, Ga.: CDC.

Chapuy MC, Arlot ME, Duboeuf F, Brun J, Crouzet B, Arnaud S, Delmas PD, Meunier PJ. 1992. Vitamin D_3 and calcium to prevent hip fractures in the elderly women. *N Engl J Med* 327:1637–1642.

Collins RW, Anderson J. 1995. Medication cost savings associated with weight loss for obese non-insulin-dependent diabetic men and women. *Prev Med* 24:369–374.

Cummings SR, Nevitt MC, Browner WS, Stone K, Fox KM, Ensrud KE, Cauley J, Black D, Vogt TM. 1995. Risk factors for hip fracture in white women. Study of Osteoporotic Fractures Research Group. *N Engl J Med* 332:767–773.

Currie J. 1995. *Welfare and the Well-Being of Children*. Newark, NJ: Harwood Academic Publishers.

Cutler DM, McLellan. 1996. *The Determinants of Technological Change in Heart Attack Treatment*. Cambridge, Mass.: National Bureau of Economic Research.

Dawson-Hughes B, Harris SS, Krall EA, Dallal GE. 1997. Effect of calcium and vitamin D supplementation on bone density in men and women 65 years of age or older. *N Engl J Med* 337:670–676.

DCCT (The Diabetes Control and Complications Trial) Research Group. 1995. Resource utilization and costs of care in the diabetes control and complications trial. *Diabetes Care* 18:1468–1478.

DCCT (The Diabetes Control and Complications Trial) Research Group. 1996. Lifetime benefits and costs of intensive therapy as practiced in the diabetes control and complications trial. *J Am Med Assoc* 276:1409–1415.

Drummond MF, O'Brien BJ, Stoddart GL, Torrance GW. 1997. *Methods for the Economic Evaluation of Health Care Programmes*, 2nd ed. New York: Oxford University Press.

Ebeling PR. 1998. Osteoporosis in men. New insights into aetiology, pathogenesis, prevention and management. *Drugs Aging* 13:421–434.

Fine-Edelstein JS, Wolf PA, O'Leary DH, Poehlman H, Belanger AJ, Kase CS, D'Agostino RB. 1994. Precursors of extracranial carotid atherosclerosis in the Framingham study. *Neurology* 44:1046–1050.

Franz MJ, Splett PL, Monk A, Barry B, McClain K, Weaver T, Upham P, Bergenstal R, Mazze R. 1995. Cost-effectiveness of medical nutrition therapy provided by dietitians for persons with non-insulin-dependent diabetes mellitus. *J Am Diet Assoc* 95:1018–1824.

Garber AM, Littenberg B, Sox HC Jr, Wagner JL, Gluck M. 1991. Costs and health consequences of cholesterol screening for asymptomatic older Americans. *Arch Intern Med* 151:1089–1095.

Gilmer TP, O'Connor PJ, Manning WG, Rush WA. 1997. The cost to health plans of poor glycemic control. *Diabetes Care* 20:1847–1853.

Gold MR, Siegel JE, Russell LB, Weinstein, MC. 1996. *Cost-Effectiveness in Health and Medicine*. New York: Oxford University Press.

Goldman L, Gordon DJ, Rifkind BM, Hulley SB, Detsky AS, Goodman DW, Kinosian B, Weinstein MC. 1992. Cost and health implications of cholesterol lowering. *Circulation* 85:1960–1968.

HCFA (Health Care Financing Administration). 1998. Medicare Provider Analysis and Review (MEDPAR) 100% inpatient file, fiscal year 1998. Available from: http://www.hcfa.gov/stats/medpar/medpar.htm. Accessed December 27, 1999.

HCFA (Health Care Financing Administration). 1999. Medicare program: Extended coverage for outpatient diabetes self-management training services. *Fed Reg* 64:6827–6852.

Hebert PR, Manson JE, Hennekens CH. 1992. Pharmacologic therapy of mild to moderate hypertension: Possible generalizability to diabetics. *J Am Soc Nephrol* 3:S135–S139.

Heller SR, Clarke P, Daly H, Davis I, McCulloch DK, Allison SP, Tattersall RB. 1988. Group education for obese patients with type 2 diabetes: Greater success at less cost. *Diabet Med* 5:552–556.

Herman WH, Dasbach EJ, Songer TJ, Eastman RC. 1997. The cost-effectiveness of intensive therapy for diabetes mellitus. *Endocrinol Metab Clin North Am* 26.679–695.

Hunninghake DB, Stein EA, Dujovne CA, Harris WS, Feldman EB, Miller VT, Tobert JA, Laskarewski PM, Quiter E, Held J, Taylor AM, Hopper S, Leonard SB, Brewer BK. 1993. The efficacy of intensive dietary therapy alone or combined with lovastatin in outpatients with hypercholesterolemia. *N Engl J Med* 328:1213–1219.

Johannesson M. 1994. The impact of age on the cost-effectiveness of hypertension treatment: An analysis of randomized drug trials. *Med Decis Making* 14:236–244.

Johannesson M, Fagerberg B. 1992. A health-economic comparison of diet and drug treatment in obese men with mild hypertension. *J Hypertens* 10:1063–1070.

Johannesson M, Le Lorier J. 1996. How to assess the economics of hypertension control programs. *J Hum Hypertens* 10:S93–S94.

Johannesson M, Åberg H, Agréus L, Borgquist L, Jönsson B. 1991. Cost-benefit analysis of non-pharmacological treatment of hypertension. *J Intern Med* 230:307–312.

Johannesson M, Agewall S, Hartford M, Hedner T, Fagerberg B. 1995. The cost-effectiveness of a cardiovascular multiple-risk-factor intervention program in treated hypertensive men. *J Intern Med* 237:19–26.

Johannesson M, Meltzer D, O'Conor RM. 1997. Incorporating future costs in medical cost-effectiveness analysis: Implications for the cost-effectiveness of the treatment of hypertension. *Med Decis Making* 17:382–389.

Johansson O. 1995. *Evaluating Health Risks: An Economic Approach*. Cambridge, U.K.: Cambridge University Press.

Jönsson B, Christiansen C, Johnell O, Hedbrandt J. 1995. Cost-effectiveness of fracture prevention in established osteoporosis. *Osteoporos Int* 5:136–142.

Kaplan RM, Ganiats TG, Sieber WJ, Anderson JP. 1998. The Quality of Well-Being Scale: Critical similarities and differences with SF-36. *Int J Qual Health Care* 10:509–520.

Knopp RH. 1999. Drug treatment of lipid disorders. *N Engl J Med* 341:498–511.

Kronmal RA, Cain KC, Ye Z, Omenn GS. 1993. Total serum cholesterol levels and mortality risk as a function of age. A report based on the Framingham data. *Arch Intern Med* 153:1065–1073.

Krop JS, Powe NR, Weller WE, Shaffer TJ, Saudek CD, Anderson GF. 1998. Patterns of expenditures and use of services among older adults with diabetes. Implications for the transition to capitated managed care. *Diabetes Care* 21:747–752.

Larson MG. 1995. Assessment of cardiovascular risk factors in the elderly: The Framingham Heart Study. *Stat Med* 14:1745–1756.

McGehee MM, Johnson EQ, Rasmussen HM, Sahyoun N, Lynch MM, Carey M, Massachusetts Dietetic Association. 1995. Benefits and costs of medical nutrition therapy by registered dietitians for patients with hypercholesterolemia. *J Am Diet Assoc* 95:1041–1043.

Mokdad, AH, Serdula MD, Dietz WH, Bowman BA, Marks JS, Kaplan JP. 1999. The spread of the obesity epidemic in the United States, 1991–1998. *J Am Med Assoc* 282:1519–1522.

NCHS (National Center for Health Statistics). 1997. *Third National Health and Nutrition Examination Survey* (Series 11, No. 1, SETS version 1.22a). [CD-ROM]. Washington, D.C.: U.S. Government Printing Office.

Pharoah PD, Hollingworth W. 1996. Cost effectiveness of lowering cholesterol concentration with statins in patients with and without pre-existing coronary heart disease: Life table method applied to health authority population. *Br Med J* 312:1443–1448.

Rich MW, Nease RF. 1999. Cost-effectiveness analysis in clinical practice: The case of heart failure. *Arch Intern Med* 159:1690–1700.

Rich MW, Beckham V, Wittenberg C, Leven CL, Freedland KE, Carney RM. 1995. A multidisciplinary intervention to prevent the readmission of elderly patients with congestive heart failure. *N Engl J Med* 333:1190–1195.

Rossi PH, Freeman, H. 1995. *Evaluation*, 5th ed. Newbury Park, Calif.: Sage Publishing.

Russell LB. 1986. *Is Prevention Better Than Cure?* Washington, D.C.: Brookings Institution.

Russell LB. 1994. *Educated Guesses: Making Policy About Medical Screening Tests*. Berkeley, Calif.: University of California Press and Milbank Memorial Fund.

Sheils JF, Rubin R, Stapleton DC. 1999. The estimated costs and savings of medical nutrition therapy: The Medicare population. *J Am Diet Assoc* 99:428–435.

Shepherd J, Cobbe SM, Ford I, Isles CG, Lorimer AR, Macfarlane PW, McKillop JH, Packard CJ. 1995. Prevention of coronary heart disease with pravastatin in men with hypercholesterolemia. *N Engl J Med* 333:1301–1307.

Tengs TO, Adams ME, Pliskin JS, Safran DG, Siegel JE, Weinstein MC, Graham JD. 1995. Five-hundred life-saving interventions and their cost-effectiveness. *Risk Anal* 15:369–390.

Tosteson AN, Weinstein MC, Hunink MG, Mittleman MA, Williams LW, Goldman PA, Goldman L. 1997. Cost-effectiveness of population wide educational approaches to reduce serum cholesterol levels. *Circulation* 95:24–30.

USPSTF (U.S. Preventive Services Task Force). 1995. *Guide to Clinical Preventive Services, 2nd ed. Report of the U.S. Preventive Services Task Force.* Washington, D.C.: U.S. Department of Health and Human Services, Office of Public Health, Office of Health Promotion and Disease Prevention.

UKPDS (UK Prospective Diabetes Study) Group. 1998. Intensive blood-glucose control with sulphonylureas or insulin compared with conventional treatment and risk of complications in patients with type 2 diabetes (UKPDS 33). *Lancet* 352:837–853.

Warner KE, Warner PA. 1993. Is an ounce of prevention worth a pound of cure? Disease prevention in health care reform. *J Ambulatory Care Manage* 16:38–49.

Weissert W. 1985. Seven reasons why it is so difficult to make community-based long-term care cost-effective. *Health Serv Res* 20:423–433.

Wilson PW, D'Agostino RB, Levy D, Belanger AM, Silbershatz H, Kannel WB. 1998. Prediction of coronary heart disease using risk factor categories. *Circulation* 97:1837–1847.

15

Overall Findings and Recommendations

Congress directed the Department of Health and Human Services to request the Institute of Medicine of The National Academy of Sciences to complete the study that resulted in this report. The preceding chapters examined, to the extent data were available, the efficacy and cost of providing nutrition services for Medicare beneficiaries across the continuum of care.

The charge to the committee was to evaluate evidence and make recommendations regarding technical and policy aspects of the provision of comprehensive nutrition services, including the following:

- coverage of nutrition services provided by registered dietitians and other health care practitioners for inpatient care of medically necessary parenteral and enteral nutrition therapy;
- coverage of nutrition services provided by registered dietitians and other health care practitioners for patients in home health and skilled nursing facility settings; and
- coverage of nutrition services provided by registered dietitians and other trained health care practitioners in individual counseling and group settings, including both primary and secondary preventive services.

For the purposes of this report, the committee considered the term "nutrition services" to consist of two levels. The first tier is *basic nutrition education or advice*, which is generally brief, informal, and typically not the focal reason for the health care encounter. The second tier of nutrition services is the provision of *nutrition therapy*, which includes the assessment of nutritional status, evaluation of nutritional needs, intervention that ranges from counseling on diet prescriptions to the provision of enteral and parenteral nutrition, and follow-up care as appropriate.

In considering the provision of nutrition services across the continuum of care, the committee focused on distinct patient care settings that included acute (inpatient) care, ambulatory (outpatient) services, home care, and long-term care. Evidence for specific diseases and conditions that commonly impact Medicare beneficiaries and for which nutrition intervention has generally been recommended was examined in depth. In addition, numerous research recommendations were made and can be found at the end of each chapter. The committee's deliberations led to the following recommendations.

MEDICARE COVERAGE OF NUTRITION THERAPY

Recommendation 1. Based on the high prevalence of individuals with conditions for which nutrition therapy was found to be of benefit, nutrition therapy, upon referral by a physician, should be a reimbursable benefit for Medicare beneficiaries.

Although few randomized clinical trials have directly examined the impact of nutrition therapy, there is consistent evidence from limited data to indicate that nutrition therapy is effective as part of a comprehensive approach to the management and treatment of the following conditions: dyslipidemia, hypertension, heart failure, diabetes, and kidney failure. Conditions evaluated for which data at this time are lacking or insufficient to support a recommendation for nutrition therapy included cancer and osteoporosis. In the case of osteoporosis, although nutrition intervention through calcium and vitamin D supplementation has clearly been found to improve health outcomes, there is a lack of available evidence to suggest that nutrition therapy, as opposed to basic nutrition education from various health care professionals, would be more effective. For cancer treatment, however, with the exception of the role of enteral and parenteral nutrition therapy, a preliminary review of the literature revealed insufficient data at this time regarding the role of nutrition therapy, specifically nutrition counseling, in the treatment of cancer and the management of its symptoms. For this reason, only evidence pertaining to enteral and parenteral nutrition therapy in the management and treatment of cancer was extensively reviewed.

Summaries of the evidence for conditions which were extensively reviewed can be found in Box 15.1. In addition, a summary of the types of evidence available for these conditions can be found in Table 15.1. It was

BOX 15.1 Summary of Evidence Supporting the Use of Nutrition Therapy in Selected Prevalent Diagnoses

Dyslipidemia Substantial evidence from observational studies and from randomized trials supports the use of nutrition therapy as a means to improve lipid profiles and thereby prevent cardiovascular disease in the elderly. Furthermore, numerous professional organizations including the American Heart Association, the National Cholesterol Education Program of the National Heart, Lung, and Blood Institute, and the Second Joint Task Force of European and Other Societies on Coronary Prevention advocate nutrition therapy as an integral part of medical therapy for persons with dyslipidemia. Recommendations for nutrition therapy extend to those individuals not on cholesterol-lowering therapy as well as persons on medications such as statins.

Hypertension Available evidence from several trials conducted in the elderly and from numerous studies conducted in other populations strongly supports nutrition-based therapy as an effective means to reduce blood pressure in older-aged persons with hypertension. At a minimum, such therapy can be an adjuvant to medication. In selected individuals, medication stepdown and potentially medication withdrawal are feasible. Nutrition therapy is recommended as part of the standard of care by the Joint National Committee on Prevention, Detection, Evaluation, and Treatment of High Blood Pressure and the National Heart, Lung, and Blood Institute Working Group report on Hypertension in the Elderly.

Heart Failure Available evidence from several small clinical trials and a few observational studies supports the use of nutrition therapy in the context of multidisciplinary programs. Such programs can prevent readmissions for heart failure, re-

beyond the scope of this report to examine all possible medical conditions for which nutrition therapy may be indicated. There are likely other conditions that were not specifically reviewed but may warrant coverage. Likewise, medical conditions which individually might not warrant nutrition therapy may well require intervention from a trained nutrition professional when these conditions occur in combination.

An underlying factor for the recommendation that coverage be included for nutrition therapy upon physician referral for any condition, including those not reviewed in this report, is that 87 percent of Medicare beneficiaries over 65 years of age have diabetes, hypertension, and/or dyslipidemia. This estimate does not include those individuals with heart failure, chronic renal insufficiency, or undernutrition. Thus, it may be administratively more efficient for the Health Care Financing Administration (HCFA) to base coverage on physician referral rather than on specific diagnoses. In addition, while physicians may not necessarily be duce subsequent length of stay, and improve functional status and quality of life. Nutrition therapy is recommended as part of the standard of care in guidelines prepared by the American College of Cardiology-American Heart Association and by the Agency for Healthcare Research and Quality.

Diabetes Available evidence from randomized clinical trials, including data in substantial numbers of individuals over the age of 65, supports the use of nutrition therapy as part of the overall multidisciplinary approach to the management of diabetes, which also includes exercise, medications, and blood glucose monitoring. Nutrition therapy is also recommended as part of the standard of care by the American Diabetes Association and the World Health Organization.

Pre-Dialysis Kidney Failure Research findings from a randomized clinical trial and two meta-analyses suggest that nutrition therapy may have a beneficial effect, over the long term, in delaying the progression of kidney disease. A National Institutes of Health consensus conference has recommended nutrition therapy as part of the management for chronic renal insufficiency.

Osteoporosis Enhanced intake of calcium and vitamin D for both the prevention and treatment of osteoporosis in the at-risk elderly population is strongly supported by a considerable body of evidence including multiple randomized controlled trials. Increased calcium and vitamin D intake is recommended as part of the standard of care by the National Osteoporosis Foundation as well as the World Health Organization. Whether or not nutrition therapy by a trained nutritional professional is needed depends on the individual's desired mode of calcium and vitamin D intake, specifically supplements versus foods, as well as other potential nutrient restrictions or unique meal planning circumstances.

trained in nutrition therapy, they are trained to gauge which conditions warrant referral to a nutrition professional, just as they are trained to recognize any other conditions which require referral for subspecialty care. Additionally, by basing nutrition therapy on referral from a physician, it will prevent self-referral for conditions for which evidence of efficacy is not available. For these reasons it is recommended to Congress that reimbursement for nutrition therapy be based on physician referral rather than on a specific medical condition.

Recommendations regarding the number of nutrition therapy visits for various conditions, other than for the necessary purpose of producing cost estimates, were not made because it is within the appropriate role of HCFA to establish reasonable limits in accordance with accepted practice.

Recommendation 2. With regard to the selection of health care professionals to provide nutrition therapy, the registered dietitian is currently the single identifiable group with standard-

TABLE 15.1 Summary of Evidence Supporting the Use of Nutrition Therapy for Medicare Beneficiaries in Specific Conditions or Diseases

Conditions[a,b]	Types of Evidence					Overall Strength of Evidence Supporting Nutrition Therapy
	Observational Studies[b]	Consensus Document	Systematic Review	Some Clinical Trial Evidence	Extensive Clinical Trial Evidence	
Dyslipidemia	✓	✓	✓		✓	Strongly supportive[c]
Hypertension	✓	✓	✓		✓	Strongly supportive[c]
Heart failure	✓	✓	✓	✓		Supportive[c]
Diabetes	✓	✓	✓		✓	Strongly supportive[c]
Pre-dialysis kidney failure	✓	✓	✓	✓		Supportive[d]
Osteoporosis[e]	✓		✓		✓	Strongly supportive[c]
Undernutrition	✓		✓	✓		Supportive[d]

[a] Conditions listed are those for which evidence supports the use of nutrition therapy.

[b] Obesity was evaluated in the context of conditions related to it (dyslipidemia, hypertension, and diabetes) rather than a separate condition.

[c] This category includes case series, case-control studies, cohort studies, and nonrandomized trials of nutrition-based therapies including nonhuman studies.

[d] From studies of the elderly as well as studies conducted in broader population age groups.

[e] Predominantly from studies in broad population age groups rather than studies in elderly.

[f] Evidence for the intake of calcium and vitamin D in the prevention and treatment of osteoporosis is strongly supportive. However, at this time it is unclear whether an equivalent and consistent intake of calcium and vitamin D can be achieved through foods as has been demonstrated in trials in which supplements were given.

ized education, clinical training, continuing education, and national credentialing requirements necessary to be directly reimbursed as a provider of nutrition therapy. However, it is recognized that other health care professionals could in the future submit evidence to be evaluated by HCFA for consideration as reimbursable providers.

The congressional language that initiated this study requested not only an analysis of the extent to which nutrition services might be of benefit to Medicare beneficiaries but also "an examination of nutritional services provided by registered dietitians..." (see chapter 13). Available evidence regarding the education and training of registered dietitians as well as other health professionals needed to adequately provide nutrition services was systematically reviewed. A summary of this information can be found in Table 13.1. The committee however, found a paucity of literature that compared the roles of specific providers of nutrition services to patient outcome or efficacy of treatment.

The committee determined that in the spectrum of health care settings and patient conditions, two tiers of nutrition services exist. The first tier is basic nutrition education and advice, which is generally provided incidental to other health services. This type of nutrition service, *nutrition education*, can generally be provided by most health care professionals who have had basic academic training in food, nutrition, and human physiology (e.g., physicians, nurses, pharmacists). The second tier of nutrition services is nutrition therapy, which involves the secondary and tertiary prevention and treatment of specific diseases or conditions.

The provision of nutrition therapy was found to require significantly more training in food and nutrition science than is commonly provided in typical medical, nursing, pharmacy, or chiropractic education curricula. Nutrition science requires components of biochemistry, biology, medicine, behavioral health, human physiology, genetics, anatomy, psychology, sociology, economics, and anthropology. Food science requires knowledge of food chemistry, food selection, food preparation, food processing, and food economics (see chapter 13). In summary, nutrition therapy involves a comprehensive working knowledge of food composition, food preparation, and nutrition and health sciences, in addition to components of behavior change. This broad knowledge base is necessary to translate complex diet prescriptions into meaningful *individualized* dietary modifications for the layperson.

The committee therefore finds that, with regard to the selection of health care professionals, the registered dietitian is currently the single identifiable group of health care professionals with standardized education, clinical training, continuing education, and national credentialing requirements necessary to be a directly reimbursable provider of nutrition therapy. This recommendation is in line with the U.S. Preventive Services Task Force rating of professionals to deliver dietary counseling which indicated that, based on available evidence, counseling performed by a trained educator such as a dietitian is more effective than by a primary care clinician (USPSTF, 1995).

It is recognized, however, that other health care professionals within certain subspecialty areas of practice may be knowledgeable in particular areas of nutrition intervention through individual training and experience and should be considered for reimbursement on a case-by-case basis. Some health professionals may be knowledgeable with regard to nutrition intervention for specific categories of patients (e.g., certified diabetes educators). These health professionals serve as excellent reinforcers of nutrition interventions and behavior modification following individualized nutrition therapy by a dietitian. While their involvement contributes to the nutritional management of diabetes, it is considered basic nutrition education and should continue to be viewed as incidental to routine medical care and not specifically reimbursable as nutrition therapy.

In addition to providing reimbursable nutrition therapy directly to clients and patients, a registered dietitian should be involved in educating other members of the health care team regarding nutrition interventions and practical aspects of nutrition care. This is of particular importance in the areas of home care, ambulatory (outpatient) care, and care given in skilled nursing and long-term care facilities, where basic nutrition advice or reinforcement of the nutrition plan will likely be provided by other health professionals.

In the congressional conference report that described the areas to be reviewed by the requested study, the effectiveness of group versus individual counseling was also identified. A lack of scientific data comparing the effectiveness of individual versus group nutrition counseling sessions was apparent. While group education can provide elderly individuals with opportunities for discussion and support, it may be a suboptimal environment for many elderly individuals with learning barriers such as vision or hearing loss. Individualized counseling can better take into account the multiple diagnoses frequently encountered in older individuals when relating dietary interventions, food preferences, life-style, and cultural factors—all of which are important factors in achieving and sustaining dietary changes. For these reasons, it was concluded that at least one session of *individualized* nutrition therapy is necessary and should be included for optimal effectiveness. However, given that learning styles vary among individuals, it may not be possible to generalize as to whether group or individual counseling is more effective in specific disease states for the remainder of the educational process.

Recommendation 3. Reimbursement for enteral and parenteral nutrition-related services in the acute care setting should be continued at the present level. A multidisciplinary approach to the provision of this care is recommended.

The provision of enteral and parenteral nutrition in the acute care setting is currently covered for Medicare beneficiaries as part of the prospective payment system. Medical conditions for which enteral and parenteral nutrition regimens may be warranted were reviewed and it was concluded that their use in preventing complications and overt malnutrition has been shown to be effective in many conditions (see Table 10.1).

The delivery and oversight of enteral and parenteral nutrition therapy is best carried out by a multidisciplinary team including a physician, pharmacist, nurse, and dietitian. Although a multidisciplinary team is optimal, a variety of formal and informal multidisciplinary models have utility, and ultimately their composition and administration should be dependent upon the institutional setting and available resources. However, the critical involvement of an individual trained in the progression of patients from enteral nutrition to solid food must be ensured.

ADMINISTRATIVE RECOMMENDATIONS REGARDING THE PROVISION OF NUTRITION SERVICES

Recommendation 4. HCFA as well as accreditation and licensing groups should reevaluate existing reimbursement systems and regulations for nutrition services along the continuum of care (acute care, ambulatory care, home care, skilled nursing and long-term care settings) to determine the adequacy of care delineated by such standards.

The committee found numerous inconsistencies with regard to regulations and reimbursement systems related to the provision of nutrition services across the continuum of care. The most pronounced inconsistency is the variation in coverage of nutrition services between the acute care inpatient setting and the ambulatory care outpatient setting. Patients are often discharged from a short-stay, acute care setting in need of nutrition therapy. However, although nutrition services are part of the bundled payment system in the acute care setting, coverage is no longer available upon discharge to the ambulatory setting. Ironically, it is the ambulatory (outpatient) setting in which patients may benefit the most from nutrition counseling. In the home care setting, weak regulations with regard to nutrition therapy result in inadequate services being provided.

HCFA relies on accrediting agencies to enforce standards of nutrition care. Although the Joint Commission on Accreditation of Healthcare Organizations (JCAHO) designates the geriatric population as a high-risk group and has emphasized nutrition in its on-site inspections during the last few years, increased attention still has to be drawn to developing and implementing standards related to the process of assessing the nutritional and functional status of elders as well as identifying and correcting inadequacies of care.

Nutrition services for Medicare beneficiaries in acute care, home care, and long-term care settings are covered largely through bundled payment systems. Reimbursement systems must be strengthened to ensure the provision of adequate nutrition care in acute care, home care, dialysis centers, and skilled nursing and long-term care facilities. It is recommended that HCFA as well as accreditation and licensing groups reevaluate all existing reimbursement systems and regulations for nutrition care in acute care, ambulatory care, home care, and long-term care settings. Several areas have been identified that should specifically be addressed and are included in the following recommendations.

Screening for Malnutrition in Acute Care Settings

Recommendation 4.1. While screening for nutrition risk in the acute care setting is crucial, the JCAHO requirement that nutrition screening be completed within 24 hours of admission is not evidence-based and may produce inaccurate and misleading results. It is recommended that validation of nutrition screening methodologies as well as the optimal timing of nutrition screening be reviewed.

Although the committee recognizes that the optimal method of identification of undernutrition in the hospitalized older patient has not been determined, the current JCAHO requirement of nutrition screening within 24 hours of admission to a hospital lacks sensitivity and specificity. Though screening within the first 24 hours of admission may help identify older persons with undernutrition prior to hospitalization, the medical instability of these patients precludes an accurate assessment of how well they will be able to meet their nutritional needs in the hospital. Undernutrition indicators, when available in this time frame, may be altered by acute illness and hence may be inaccurate. Moreover, the acute illness or procedure precipitating hospitalization may result in a transient inability to eat.

Screening within 24 hours of hospital admission, when accomplished, uses resources which may be better utilized helping elderly patients select food they can eat, helping them to eat, and monitoring food intake. In addition, with decreased lengths of stay in acute care settings, patients found to be at risk for malnutrition are often discharged before interventions to improve nutritional status can take place. The most appropriate and clinically useful method of nutritional screening of hospitalized older persons remains an unanswered question and should be a high priority for further research.

Provision of Nutrition Services in the Home Care Setting

Recommendation 4.2. The availability of nutrition services should be improved in the home health care setting. Both types of nutrition services are needed in this setting: nutrition education and nutrition therapy. A registered dietitian should be available to serve as a consultant to health professionals providing basic nutrition education and follow-up, as well as to provide nutrition therapy, when indicated, directly to Medicare beneficiaries being cared for in a home setting.

Medicare beneficiaries are often discharged from hospitals to home care settings with, or at high risk for, overt malnutrition. Yet there is currently no HCFA regulation that requires a nutrition professional to participate in the nutritional management of homebound patients. The adequate provision of services and the staffing of appropriately credentialed nutrition professionals in home care are essential for the training and education of home health nurses and nurses aides so that they may adequately provide appropriate basic nutrition screening and other services. In addition, nutrition professionals should provide nutrition therapy directly to homebound patients when indicated.

Enteral and Parenteral Nutrition in the Ambulatory Care and Home Health Care Settings

Recommendation 4.3. In ambulatory and home care settings, the regulation that excludes coverage for enteral and parenteral nutrition if the gut functions within the next 90 days needs to be reevaluated.

The committee identified a major gap in the coverage of enteral and parenteral nutrition for undernourished ambulatory and home care patients. The current regulation, which excludes coverage for enteral and parenteral nutrition unless the gut is expected to be dysfunctional for at least 90 days, needs to be reevaluated. To avoid the complications of extended semistarvation and possible rehospitalization, reimbursement for enteral or parenteral nutrition in selected Medicare beneficiaries who would otherwise be unable to eat or to assimilate adequate nutrition due to gastrointestinal dysfunction or neurological impairment for longer than 7 days, must be evaluated as a prudent, potentially cost-saving, alternative. Patients who are already malnourished or highly stressed due to infection or response to trauma may not even tolerate this duration of starvation or semistarvation.

In addition, monitoring of patients while on enteral and parenteral nutrition regimes is crucial to avoid both the under- and the overuse of this type of expensive therapy. The registered dietitian is an integral member of the multidisciplinary team and should be involved in the transition of feeding from enteral and parenteral therapies to oral or other modalities, when appropriate or indicated by the referring physician.

Nutrition Services in Skilled Nursing and Long-Term Care Facilities

Recommendation 4.4. HCFA, as well as accrediting and licensing agencies, should improve requirements and standards for food and nutrition services in skilled nursing and long-term care facilities.

As Medicare shifts to a prospective payment system for skilled nursing and long-term care facilities, the nutrition services provided must not be compromised, but should be improved beyond the current pattern of practice. Some states require that long-term care facilities employ dietitians for so little time (8 hours per month) that little can be accomplished when nutrition problems are identified. Staffing must be adequate, and staff members should be well trained and supervised by nutrition professionals so that patients are fed sensitively and appropriately. Efforts to improve quality of care should be aimed at improving staffing patterns, the quality of food services, the incorporation of appropriate feeding techniques into patient services, and the education and training of staff on feeding techniques for patients with functional limitations. Nutrition professionals should be available to educate and train nursing staff and aides on the prevention, detection, and treatment of malnutrition in elderly patients. In addition, registered dietitians, along with other members of the multidisciplinary team, should also be available for the provision and monitoring of enteral and parenteral nutrition regimes.

Research Agenda

Recommendation 4.5. Federal agencies such as the National Institute on Aging, the Agency for Healthcare Research and Quality, and HCFA should pursue a research agenda in the area of nutrition in the older person.

Throughout this study, the committee found a paucity of usable data with regard to nutritional status of the older person, particularly in the area of evaluating the success of interventions with regard to treatment of nutritionally related multiple diseases and conditions. In some instances, issues had not been studied, and in others, previously conducted research did not provide definitive answers. The committee identified numerous areas for research, which can be found in the at the end of relevant chapters of this report.

ECONOMIC POLICY ANALYSIS

Cost to the Medicare program of expanded coverage for nutrition therapy will be directly determined by the specific design of the reimbursement benefit, patient demand, and other factors. Forecasts of these costs are thus imprecise given currently available data. However, because of the comparatively low treatment costs and ancillary benefits associated with nutrition therapy, expanded coverage will improve the quality of care and is likely to be a valuable and efficient use of Medicare resources.

The committee's approach to cost estimation used generic practices consistent with the Congressional Budget Office process (e.g., not discounting estimates to present value). A more detailed description of the cost estimate process is in chapter 14. Data from other cost studies, current accepted practice guidelines, clinical studies, and Medicare cost data were used in the cost estimates. Previous studies show that from 5 to 20 percent of beneficiaries would likely use a nutrition therapy service if it were a covered benefit. The Medicare portion of estimated charges for coverage of nutrition therapy during the 5-year period 2000 to 2004 is $1.43 billion. However, due to uncertainty about the actual utilization of a nutrition therapy benefit, two additional scenarios were calculated to reflect a low utilization estimate and a high utilization estimate. The range is from $873 million (low utilization scenario) to $2.63 billion (high utilization scenario) with diagnosis specific utilization rates ranging from 5 to 30 percent. Some of these costs will be passed on to Medicare beneficiaries through associated premium increases.

Expanded coverage for nutrition therapy is likely to generate economically significant benefits to beneficiaries, and in the short term to the Medicare program itself, through reduced healthcare expenditures. Nutrition therapy, in the context of multidisciplinary care, has a potential short-term cost savings for specific populations such as those with hypertension, dyslipidemia, and diabetes. While these effects have been expressed in economic terms, detailed budget forecasts of these effects require a more extensive actuarial analysis that is beyond the scope of this study. Initial estimates for potential cost avoidance for individuals with hypertension, elevated lipids, and diabetes have been included. The estimates were provided in ranges corresponding to the utilization scenarios and are $52 million to $167 million for hypertension, $54 million to $164 million for those with elevated lipids, and $132 million to $330 million for those with diabetes. It is not appropriate to add these estimates together since beneficiaries have overlapping diagnoses patterns. Estimates were not made for the 5.62 million beneficiaries likely to receive nutrition therapy for other diagnoses such as chronic renal insufficiency and heart failure. Expanded coverage may be cost saving in these broader patient groups, although data are inadequate to reliably establish these patterns.

Whether or not expanded coverage reduces overall Medicare expenditures, it is recommended that these services be reimbursed given the reasonable evidence of improved patient outcomes associated with such care.

In addition to decreased mortality and morbidity, nutrition therapy can have an impact on quality of life in less tangible ways that cannot be measured quantitatively. Meals provide the social context for important religious and family experiences across the lifespan. Because food is central to an individual's social attachment and role, dietary problems that require significant behavior change or interfere with long-established social relationships can have a significant impact on patient well-being independent of their impact on mortality or morbidity. Nutrition therapy translates the desired treatment goals into daily life skills such as grocery shopping, food preparation, and selecting from restaurant menus. Nutrition therapy that assists homebound patients to participate in family meals may have a greater impact on subjective well-being than many other interventions that have equal impact on physical health.

CONCLUDING REMARKS

In summary, evidence exists to conclude that nutrition therapy can improve health outcomes for several conditions that are highly prevalent among Medicare beneficiaries while possibly decreasing costs to Medicare. Basic nutrition advice for healthy living and the primary prevention of disease can often be provided by a multitude of health care professionals who have had less extensive academic preparation in nutrition science and/or clinical training than a registered dietitian. This is not considered a service that should be a separately covered benefit to Medicare beneficiaries. However, the provision of nutrition therapy requires in-depth knowledge of food and nutrition science. Registered dietitians are currently the primary group of health care professionals with the necessary type of education and training to provide this level of nutrition service. It is recognized that there may be others within medical subspecialties who may have particularly strong levels of expertise and could in the future be evaluated by HCFA as a certified provider.

The committee found numerous inconsistencies in current health care regulations and standards. Agencies responsible for oversight need to reevaluate regulations associated with the provision of quality nutrition care to ensure that policies and standards are based on evidence and represent the best use of resources. In addition, reimbursement policies must be reevaluated to ensure that the nutritional needs of Medicare beneficiaries are met consistently across the continuum of care.

REFERENCE

USPSTF (U.S. Preventive Services Task Force). 1995. *Guide to Clinical Preventive Services, 2nd ed. Report of the U.S. Preventive Services Task Force*. Washington, D.C.: U.S. Department of Health and Human Services, Office of Public Health, Office of Health Promotion and Disease Prevention.

Appendixes

Appendix A

Acronyms

ACE	Angiotensin-converting enzyme
ADA	American Dietetic Association
ADL	Activity of daily living
AHA	American Hospital Association
AHRQ	Agency for Healthcare Research and Quality (formerly the Agency for Health Care Policy and Research)
AL	Assisted living
AMI	Acute myocardial infarction
AoA	Administration on Aging, Department of Health and Human Services
APC	Ambulatory payment classification
ASCVD	Atherosclerotic cardiovascular disease
BBA	Balanced Budget Act of 1997
BMD	Bone mineral density
BMI	Body mass index, weight (kg)/height (cm)^2
BMT	Bone marrow transplantation
BP	Blood pressure
CAADE	Commission on Accreditation/Approval for Dietetics Education
CAM	Complementary and alternative
CDC	Centers for Disease Control and Prevention
CDE	Certified Diabetes Educator

327

CDM	Certified Dietary Manager
CDR	Commission on Dietetic Registration
CEA	Cost-effectiveness analysis
CHD	Coronary heart disease
CI	Confidence interval
CNA	Certified Nursing Assistant
CNS	Certified Nutrition Specialist
CNSD	Certified Nutrition Support Dietitian
CPR	Customary, prevailing, and reasonable
CPT	Current procedural terminology
CSP	Certified Specialist in Pediatric Nutrition
CSR	Certified Specialist in Renal Disease
CT	Computed tomography
CUA	Cost–utility analysis
CSFII	Continuing Survey of Food Intakes by Individuals
CVD	Cardiovascular disease
DASH	Dietary Interventions to Stop Hypertension
DC	Doctor of Chiropractic
DBP	Diastolic blood pressure
DCCT	Diabetes Control and Complications Trial
DOD	Department of Defense
DRG	Diagnosis related group
DT	Dietetic Technician
DTR	Dietetic Technician, Registered
DXA	Dual-energy x-ray absorption
EBC	Evidence-based center
ECRI	Emergency Care Research Institute
ENP	Elderly nutrition program
EPC	Evidence-based practice center
EPESE	Established Populations for the Epidemiologic Studies of the Elderly
ESRD	End-stage renal disease
FADA	Fellow of the American Dietetic Association
FPG	Fasting plasma glucose
GFR	Glomerular filtration rate
GH	Growth hormone
HCFA	Health Care Financing Administration
HDL	High-density lipoprotein

HEDIS	Health plan employer data and information set
HF	Heart failure
HHA	Home health agency
HI	Hospitalization insurance
HMG-CoA	β-Hydroxy-β-methylglutarylcoenzyme A
HMO	Health maintenance organization
HRT	Hormone replacement therapy
HTN	Hypertension

IDPN	Intradialytic parenteral nutrition
IGF	Insulin-like growth factor
IL	Interleukin
IPS	Interim payment system
IU	International unit

JCAHO	Joint Commission on Accreditation of Healthcare Organizations

LBM	Lean body mass
LDL	Low-density lipoprotein

MAMC	Mid-arm muscle circumference
MDRD	Modification of Diet in Renal Disease
MDS	Minimum data set
MNA	Mini nutritional assessment
MRI	Mortality risk index

NCEP	National Cholesterol Education Program
NCQA	National Committee on Quality Assurance
NSI	Nutrition screening initiative
ND, NMD	Doctor of Naturopathic Medicine
NHANES	National Health and Nutrition Examination Survey
NHLBI	National Heart, Lung, and Blood Institute

OASIS	Outcomes Assessment and Information Set
25-(OH)D	25-Hydroxyvitamin D_3

PACE	Programs of All Inclusive Care for the Elderly
PATHS	Prevention and Treatment of Hypertension Study
PESRD	Pre-end stage renal disease
PEU	Protein–energy undernutrition
PPN	Peripheral parenteral nutrition
PPO	Preferred provider organization

PPS	Prospective payment system
PRCT	Prospective randomized clinical trial
PSO	Provider-sponsored organization
QALY	Quality-adjusted life year
RAP	Resident assessment protocol
RD	Registered Dietitian
RR	Relative risk
SBP	Systolic blood pressure
SMI	Supplementary medical insurance
SNF	Skilled nursing facility
TNF	Tumor necrosis factor
TONE	Trial of Nonpharmacologic Interventions in the Elderly
TPN	Total parenteral nutrition
TSF	Triceps skinfold thickness
UKPDS	United Kingdom Prospective Diabetes Study
VA	Department of Veterans Affairs
WHI	Women's Health Initiative

Appendix B

Glossary

Ambulatory care   In this report, ambulatory care refers to the out-patient care setting.

Cachexia   Loss of fat-free mass, especially body cell mass, with little or no weight loss. The metabolic hallmarks of cachexia are hypermetabolism and hypercatabolism, driven by inflammatory cytokine-mediated acute phase responses.

Capitation   A per-member monthly payment to a provider that covers contracted services to health management organization members and is paid in advance. A provider agrees to provide specified services for this fixed, predetermined payment for a specified length of time, regardless of how many times the member uses the services. The rate can be fixed for all members or adjusted for the age and sex of the member, based on actuarial projections of medical utilization.

Certified Diabetes Educator   An individual credentialed by the National Certification Board of Diabetes Educators. The credential requires unrestricted license or registration (e.g., RN, RD), a master's degree from a U.S. college or university in nutrition, and 2 calendar years of experience in direct diabetes patient and self-management education. Within 5 calendar years prior to the date of application, the individual must have worked a minimum of 1,000 hours in direct diabetes patient and self-management education. Must be engaged in practice of direct diabetes patient and self-management education at time of application.

Certified Dietary Manager   A professional who works together with registered dietitians to provide quality nutritional care for clients in a variety of noncommercial settings and performs a myriad of specialized tasks; many work as food service managers in a hospital, long-term care center, or other facility. Must pass a nationally recognized credentialing exam and fulfill the requirements needed to maintain certified status.

Certified Nutrition Specialist   An individual credentialed by the Certification Board for Nutrition Specialists. The credential requires an advanced degree in nutrition from a regionally accredited program. Requires at least 1,000 hours of supervised experience or 4,000 hours of unsupervised experience.

Certified Nutrition Support Dietitian   A professional who has been certified to deliver parenteral or enteral nutrition support. Certification by written examination is available through the National Board of Nutrition Support Education, Inc., to nurses, physicians, and dietitians.

Commission on Accreditation of Dietetics Education   The American Dietetic Association's accrediting agency for education programs preparing students for careers as Registered Dietitians or Dietetic Technicians, Registered.

Commission on Dietetic Registration   Credentialing agency for the American Dietetic Association. The purpose of the commission is to protect the nutritional health and welfare of the public by establishing and enforcing certification and recertification standards for the dietetics profession. Credentials are issued to individuals who meet its standards to practice in the profession.

Current procedural terminology   A system of procedure codes and descriptions published annually by the American Medical Association. This procedure coding system is accepted by almost all commercial insurance carriers and is required by Medicare and Medicaid.

Diagnosis-Related Group Program   A program in which hospital procedures are rated in terms of cost, taking into consideration the intensity of the services delivered. A standard flat rate per procedure is derived from this scale, which is paid by Medicare for its beneficiaries, regardless of the cost to the hospital to perform the procedure.

Dialysis   Dialysis involves filtering the blood to remove toxins. Two primary forms of dialysis are available to outpatients: hemodialysis, which is usually administered three times a week for several hours, and continuous ambulatory peritoneal dialysis. Continuous ambulatory peritoneal dialysis is performed by the patient who administers and then drains a dextrose-containing fluid into and out of the peritoneal space.

Dietetic technician, registered Professionals who have (1) completed a minimum of an associate degree at a U.S. regionally accredited college or university; (2) completed a dietetic technician program approved by the CAADE of the ADA; (3) successfully completed the registration examination for dietetic technicians; and (4) accrued 50 hours of approved continuing professional education every 5 years. Often work with dietitians in a variety of employment settings, including health care, business and industry, public health, food service, and research.

Disease management The process of standardizing treatment of common disorders and ensuring appropriate utilization and high-quality care at all levels by the provider. In disease management, the total management of the disease (e.g., practice guidelines and standards of care that direct clinicians) is evaluated, along with the cost of the process. Outcomes are evaluated by continuous quality improvement measures. By standardizing care, providers may reduce long-term care of patients with chronic illness.

Doctor of Chiropractic A provider of spinal and other therapeutic manipulation or adjustments. Chiropractors also utilize a variety of manual, mechanical, and electrical therapeutic modalities, and provide patient evaluation and instructions regarding disease prevention and health promotion through proper nutrition, exercise, and life-style modifications.

Doctor of Naturopathic Medicine A professional who is trained in basic medical science and conventional diagnostics, and qualified through licensing to scientifically apply natural therapeutics in the treatment of disease and restoration of health. Attends a 4-year, graduate-level naturopathic medical school and is educated in all of the same basic sciences as an M.D. but also studies holistic and nontoxic approaches to therapy with a strong emphasis on disease prevention and optimizing wellness.

Elderly Nutrition Program Title III–VI feeding, congregate feeding, and home delivered meals for the elderly.

End-stage renal disease Renal disease that is treated by dialysis.

Enteral nutrition Nutrition provided through a feeding tube into the gastrointestinal tract.

Failure to thrive A syndrome of weight loss, decreased appetite, poor nutrition, and inactivity often accompanied by dehydration, depressive symptoms, impaired immune function, and low cholesterol. Recently, some have advocated abandoning this term as a disease construct in favor of four treatable contributor domains: (1) impaired physical functioning, (2) malnutrition, (3) depression, and (4) cognitive impairment.

Fee for service   Traditional reimbursement system in which providers are paid according to the service performed. This is the system used by conventional indemnity insurers.

Fellow of the American Dietetic Association   Registered dietitian with advanced education and experience who demonstrates exceptional professional abilities and expertise; can document professional achievement; is committed to self-growth, innovation, and service to others; and serves as an exemplary professional role model.

Home health agency   An agency providing care to individuals requiring skilled home care services. Home health agencies are often Medicare certified and meet minimum federal requirements for patient care and management. Some agencies deliver a variety of home care services through physicians, nurses, therapists, social workers, and others, whereas other agencies limit their services to nursing and one or two other specialties. Home health agencies can also coordinate a caregiving team to administer services that are comprehensive for individuals who require care from more than one specialist. Personnel are assigned according to the needs of each patient; since home health agencies recruit and supervise their personnel, they assume liability for all care.

Home nutrition care provider   Clinician with expertise in nutrition support who is responsible for medical aspects of a patient's home nutrition care.

Home nutrition therapy   Nutrition therapy in the home environment.

Interim payment system   Presently being used in home care until a prospective payment system is developed.

Intradialytic parenteral nutrition   Infusion of an energy and/or amino acid mixture during dialysis treatment.

Long-term care   Services that are ordinarily provided in a skilled nursing care, intermediate care, personal care, supervisory care, or elder care facility.

Long-term care facility   Residential institution that provides extended care to individuals under the direct guidance of qualified health care providers.

Malnutrition   Any disorder of nutrition status including disorders resulting from a deficiency of nutrient intake, impaired nutrient metabolism, or overnutrition.

Managed care   A full range of health care structures and strategies that focus on decreasing fragmentation of care and increasing quality and cost-efficiency.

Micronutrient   Nutrient present and required in the body in minute quantities (e.g., vitamins, trace elements).

Nutrients   Proteins, carbohydrates, lipids, vitamins, minerals, trace elements, and water.

Nutrition screening   The process of identifying characteristics known to be associated with nutrition problems. Its purpose is to identify individuals who are nutritionally at risk for malnutrition or who are malnourished.

Nutrition services   For the purposes of this report, nutrition services consist of two tiers. The first tier of services is basic nutrition education or advice, which is generally brief, informal, and typically not the focal reason for the health care encounter. More often than not, its aim is to promote general health and/or the primary prevention of chronic diseases or conditions. The second tier of nutrition services is the provision of nutrition therapy, which includes individualized assessment of nutritional status, evaluation of nutritional needs, and intervention, which ranges from counseling on diet prescriptions to the provision of enteral and parenteral nutrition.

Nutrition therapy   The treatment of a disease or condition through the modification of nutrient or whole-food intake. Nutrition therapy encompasses the assessment of an individual's nutritional status, evaluation of nutritional needs, and interventions or counseling to achieve optimal clinical outcomes. The assessment of nutritional needs takes into consideration the individual's medical and dietary histories, as well as physical, anthropometric, and laboratory data. Nutrition therapy includes oral, enteral, and parenteral nutrition interventions and takes into consideration the cultural, socioeconomic, and food preferences of the individual.

Nutritional assessment   A comprehensive evaluation to define nutrition status, including medical history, dietary history, physical examination, anthropometric measurements, and laboratory data.

Nutritional support services or team   Multidisciplinary group of health-care professionals with expertise in nutrition who aid in the provision of nutrition support.

Obesity   Body mass index $(wt(kg)/ht(cm)^2)$ greater than 30.

Parenteral nutrition   Delivery of nutrients intravenously rather than through the gastrointestinal tract.

Post-acute care   Care in any setting beyond a short-stay, acute care hospital.

Practice guidelines   Systematically developed statement to assist practitioner and patient decisions about appropriate health care for specific circumstances. Statements suggesting the proper indications for a procedure or treatment or the proper management of specific clinical problems.

Pre-end-stage renal disease   Renal disease identified prior to dialysis or defined in terms of glomerular filtration rates of 13 to 50 ml/min/1.73 m^2.

Primary prevention   Prevention of the development of disease in a person who does not have the disease through promotion of health, including mental health, and specific protection, as in immunization, as distinguished from the prevention of complications or after effects of existing disease.

Programs of All-Inclusive Care for the Elderly   Programs that integrate acute and long-term services in an attempt to improve coordination by bridging through common financing, acute care benefits, and home- and community-based long-term care services.

Prospective payment system   A payment system under which health care providers are paid a predetermined, fixed amount for patient care. Although prospective payment rates may be related to the costs providers incur in providing services, the amount a provider is paid for a service is unrelated to the provider's actual cost of providing the specific service to a given individual.

Protein–energy undernutrition   The presence of clinical (physical signs such as wasting, low body mass index) and biochemical (albumin or other protein) evidence of insufficient intake.

Registered Dietitian (RD)   Food and nutrition expert who has met the following criteria to earn and maintain the RD credential: (1) completed a minimum of a bachelor's degree; (2) met current minimum academic requirements as approved by the CAADE; (3) completed preprofessional experience accredited or approved by the CAADE; (4) successfully completed the registration examination for dietitians; and (5) accrued 75 hours of approved continuing professional education every 5 years.

Sarcopenia   Loss of muscle mass specifically, which appears to be an age-related condition.

Secondary prevention   Prevention of recurrence of a disease in a person who has already been diagnosed with the disease.

Skilled nursing facility   An institution that primarily provides skilled nursing care and related services for residents who require medical or nursing care; rehabilitation services for the rehabilitation of injured, disabled, or sick persons; or, on a regular basis, health-related care and services to individuals who because of their mental of physical condition require care and services, above the level of room and board, which can be made available to them only through institutional facilities.

Tertiary prevention   Prevention of disability, poor quality of life, and death in persons with advanced stages of a disease.

Wasting   Unintentional loss of weight, including both fat and fat-free components. Experience in the human immunodeficiency virus epidemic suggests that wasting is driven largely by inadequate dietary intake.

Appendix C

Workshop Speakers, Organizations Contacted, and Consultants to the Committee

WORKSHOP SPEAKERS

Bess Dawson-Hughes, M.D.
Tufts University

Linda Delahanty, M.S., R.D.
Massachussets General Hospital

V. Annette Dickinson, Ph.D.
Council for Responsible Nutrition

Marion Franz, M.S., R.D.
International Diabetes Center

Samuel Klein, M.D.
Washington University School of
  Medicine

William Mitch, M.D.
Emory University

Tom Prohaska, Ph.D.
University of Chicago

Ernest Schaefer, M.D.
Tufts University

Dennis Sullivan, M.D.
University of Arkansas

Mackenzie Walser, M.D.
Johns Hopkins University

ORGANIZATIONS CONTACTED FOR RESPONSES TO COMMITTEE QUESTIONS

American Association of
Diabetes Educators

American Association of
Retired Persons
American Cancer Society

American Chiropractic Association
* American College of Health Care Administrators
American Diabetes Association
* American Dietetic Association
American Geriatric Society
American Health Foundation
American Heart Association
American Nurses Association
American Obesity Association
* American Society for Clinical Nutrition
* American Society for Enteral and Parenteral Nutrition
American Society for Nutritional Sciences
American Society of Consultant Pharmacists

Center for Food and Nutrition Policy, Georgetown University
Food and Drug Administration
* Fresenius Medical Care North America
Gerontological Society of America
Library of Congress
* National Kidney Foundation
National Osteoporosis Foundation
Nutrition Screening Initiative
Office of Dietary Supplements
Office of the Surgeon General
Partnership for Prevention
Physicians Committee for Responsible Medicine
Visiting Nurse Association of America

COMMITTEE CONSULTANTS

Rowan Chlebowski, M.D.
Division of Medical Oncology & Hematology
Harbor UCLA Medical Center

Bess Dawson-Hughes, M.D.
Calcium and Bone Metabolism Laboratory
Tufts University

The Lewin Group
Falls Church, VA

Rosanna Gibbons, M.S., R.D.
Consultant Dietitian in Home Care
Baltimore, MD

Talat Alp Ikizler, M.D.
Division of Nephrology
Vanderbilt University Medical Center

John Kostis, M.D.
University of Medicine and Dentistry of New Jersey-Robert Wood Johnson Medical School

Andrew S. Levey, M.D.
Division of Nephrology
New England Medical Center

---

* Denotes that either an oral presentation was made or written comments were received.

Appendix D

State Licensure Laws for the Practice of Dietetics (as of June 1999)

STATUTORY DEFINITIONS

- **Licensing statutes** explicitly define the scope and requirements of professional practice. It is illegal to practice a regulated profession without first obtaining a license from the state.
- **Statutory certification** limits the use of particular professional titles to persons meeting predetermined requirements, but persons not certified can still practice the profession.
- **Registration** is the least restrictive form of state regulation. In California (the only state where this statutory category is currently used), registration is an entitlement law that prohibits use of the title "dietitian" by persons not meeting state-mandated qualifications. However, unregistered persons may practice the profession. Typically, exams are not given and enforcement of the registration requirement is minimal.

PROFESSIONAL REGULATION: STATE UPDATE

Alabama (1989)[1] —licensing of dietitian-nutritionists
Arkansas (1989)—licensing of dietitians
California (1995)[1]—registration of dietitians
Connecticut (1994)—certification of dietitians
Delaware (1994)—certification of dietitian-nutritionists
District of Columbia (1986)—licensing of dietitians and nutritionists
Florida (1988)—licensing of dietitian-nutritionists and nutrition counselors

Georgia (1994)[1]—licensing of dietitians
Idaho (1994)—licensing of dietitians
Illinois (1990)—licensing of dietitians and nutrition counselors
Indiana (1994)—certification of dietitians
Iowa (1985)—licensing of dietitians
Kansas (1989)[1]—licensing of dietitians
Kentucky (1994)[1]—licensing of dietitians and certification of nutritionists
Louisiana (1987)[1]—licensing of dietitian-nutritionists
Maine (1994)[1]—licensing of dietitians and dietetic technicians
Maryland (1994)[1]—licensing of dietitians and nutritionists
Minnesota (1994)—licensing of dietitian-nutritionists
Mississippi (1994)[1]—licensing of dietitians and protection of nutritionist title
Montana (1987)[1]—licensing of nutritionists and protection of dietitian title
Nebraska (1995)[1]—licensing of medical nutrition therapist
Nevada (1995)—certification[2] of dietitians
New Mexico (1997)[1]—licensing of dietitians, nutritionists, and nutrition associates
New York (1991)—certification of dietitians and nutritionists
North Carolina (1991)—licensing of dietitians and nutritionists
North Dakota (1989)[1]—licensing of dietitians and certification[2] of nutritionists
Ohio (1986)—licensing of dietitians
Oklahoma (1984)—licensing of dietitians
Oregon (1989)—certification[2] of dietitians
Puerto Rico (1974)[1]—licensing of dietitians and nutritionists
Rhode Island (1991)[1]—licensing of dietitians and nutritionists
South Dakota (1996)—licensing of dietitian-nutritionists
Tennessee (1987)—licensing of dietitian-nutritionists
Texas (1993)[1]—certification[2] of dietitians
Utah (1996)[1]—certification of dietitians
Vermont (1993)—certification of dietitians
Virginia (1995)—certification[2] of dietitians and nutritionists
Washington (1988)—certification of dietitians and nutritionists
West Virginia (1996)—licensing of dietitians
Wisconsin (1994)—certification of dietitians

SOURCE: Reproduced with permission from the *Journal of the American Dietetic Association*. 1997. Update on state licensure laws and ADA regulatory remarks. *J Am Diet Assoc* 97:1251.

---

[1]Year amended or authorized.

[2]These laws provide the certified practitioner with a license and are termed "voluntary licensing" laws.

Appendix E

The American Dietetic Association Foundation Knowledge and Skills and Competency Requirements for Entry-Level Dietitians

Individuals interested in becoming Registered Dietitians should expect to study a wide variety of topics focusing on food, nutrition, and management. These areas are supported by the sciences: physical and biological, behavioral and social, and communication. Becoming a dietitian involves a combination of academic preparation, including a minimum of a baccalaureate degree, and a supervised practice component.

The following foundation knowledge and skill requirements are listed in the eight areas that students will focus on in the academic component of a dietetics program. Foundation learning is divided as follows: basic knowledge of a topic, working or in-depth knowledge of a topic as it applies to the profession of dietetics, and ability to demonstrate the skill at a level that can be developed further. To successfully achieve the foundation knowledge and skills, graduates must demonstrate the ability to communicate and collaborate, solve problems, and apply critical thinking skills.

These requirements may be met through separate courses, combined into one course, or as part of several courses as determined by the college or university sponsoring a program accredited or approved by the Commission on Accreditation/Approval for Dietetics Education (CAADE) of The American Dietetic Association.

FOUNDATION KNOWLEDGE AND SKILLS

Content Area	Basic Knowledge about	Working Knowledge of	Demonstrated Ability to
COMMUNICATIONS	negotiation techniques, lay and technical writing, media presentations	interpersonal communication skills, counseling theory and methods, interviewing techniques, educational theory and techniques, concepts of human and group dynamics, public speaking, educational materials development	present an educational session for a group, counsel individuals on nutrition, demonstrate a variety of documentation methods, explain a public policy position regarding dietetics, use current information technologies, work effectively as a team member
PHYSICAL AND BIOLOGICAL SCIENCES	exercise physiology	organic chemistry, biochemistry, physiology, microbiology, nutrient metabolism, patho-physiology related to nutrition care, fluid and electrolyte requirements, pharmacology: nutrient-nutrient and drug-nutrient interaction	interpret medical terminology, interpret laboratory parameters relating to nutrition, apply microbiological and chemical considerations to process controls
SOCIAL SCIENCES	public policy development	psychology, health behaviors and educational needs, economics and nutrition	
RESEARCH	research methodologies, needs assessments, outcomes based research	scientific method, quality improvement methods	interpret current research, interpret basic statistics

continued

FOUNDATION KNOWLEDGE AND SKILLS

Content Area	Basic Knowledge about	Working Knowledge of	Demonstrated Ability to
FOOD	food technology, biotechnology, culinary techniques	socio-cultural and ethnic food consumption issues and trends for various consumers, food safety and sanitation, food delivery systems, food and non-food procurement, availability of nutrition programs in the community, formulation of local, state, and national food security policy, food production systems, environmental issues related to food, role of food in promotion of a healthy lifestyle, promotion of pleasurable eating, food and nutrition laws/regulations/ policies, food availability and access for the individual, family, and community, applied sensory evaluation of food	calculate and interpret nutrient composition of foods, translate nutrition needs into menus for individuals and groups, determine recipe/formula proportions and modifications for volume food production, write specifications for food and foodservice equipment, apply food science knowledge to functions of ingredients in food, demonstrate basic food preparation and presentation skills, modify recipe/ formula for individual or group dietary needs

continued

FOUNDATION KNOWLEDGE AND SKILLS

Content Area	Basic Knowledge about	Working Knowledge of	Demonstrated Ability to
NUTRITION	alternative nutrition and herbal therapies, evolving methods of assessing health status	the influence of age, growth, and normal development on nutritional requirements; nutrition and metabolism; assessment and treatment of nutritional health risks; medical nutrition therapy, including alternative feeding modalities, chronic diseases, dental health, mental health, and eating disorders; strategies to assess need for adaptive feeding techniques and equipment; health promotion and disease prevention theories and guidelines; influence of socioeconomic, cultural, and psychological factors on food and nutrition behavior	calculate and/or define diets for common conditions, i.e., health conditions addressed by health promotion/disease prevention activities or chronic diseases of the general population, e.g., hypertension, obesity, diabetes, diverticular disease; screen individuals for nutritional risk; collect pertinent information for comprehensive nutrition assessments; determine nutrient requirements across the life span, i.e., infants through geriatrics and a diversity of people, culture, and religions; measure, calculate, and interpret body composition data; calculate enteral and parenteral nutrition formulations

continued

FOUNDATION KNOWLEDGE AND SKILLS

Content Area	Basic Knowledge about	Working Knowledge of	Demonstrated Ability to
MANAGEMENT	program planning, monitoring, and evaluation, strategic management, facility management, organizational change theory, risk management	management theories; human resource management, including labor relations; materials management; financial management, including accounting principles; quality improvement; information management; systems theory; marketing theory and techniques; diversity issues	determine costs of services/operation, prepare a budget, interpret financial data, apply marketing principles
HEALTH CARE SYSTEMS	health care policy and administration, health care delivery systems	current reimbursement issues, ethics of care	

Individuals are expected to develop competence to practice dietetics through a supervised practice component in programs accredited or approved by CAADE. Competency statements specify what every dietitian should be able to do at the beginning of his or her practice career. The core competency statements build on appropriate knowledge and skills necessary for the entry-level practitioner to perform reliably at the level indicated. One or more of the emphasis areas are added to the core competencies so that a supervised practice program can prepare graduates for identified market needs. Thus, all entry-level dietitians will have the core competencies and additional competencies according to the emphasis area(s) completed.

Core Competencies for Entry-Level Dietitians

1. Perform ethically in accordance with the values of The American Dietetic Association
2. Refer clients/patients to other dietetics professionals or disciplines when a situation is beyond one's level or area of competence
3. Participate in professional activities
4. Perform self assessment and participate in professional development
5. Participate in legislative and public policy processes as they affect food, food security, and nutrition
6. Use current technologies for information and communication activities
7. Supervise documentation of nutrition assessment and interventions
8. Provide dietetics education in supervised practice settings
9. Supervise counseling, education, and/or other interventions in health promotion/disease prevention for patients/clients needing medical nutrition therapy for common conditions, e.g., hypertension, obesity, diabetes, and diverticular disease
10. Supervise education and training for target groups
11. Develop and review educational materials for target populations
12. Participate in the use of mass media for community-based food and nutrition programs
13. Interpret and incorporate new scientific knowledge into practice
14. Supervise quality improvement, including systems and customer satisfaction, for dietetics service and/or practice
15. Develop and measure outcomes for food and nutrition services and practice
16. Participate in organizational change and planning and goal-setting processes
17. Participate in business or operating plan development
18. Supervise the collection and processing of financial data
19. Perform marketing functions
20. Participate in human resources functions
21. Participate in facility management, including equipment selection and design/redesign of work units
22. Supervise the integration of financial, human, physical, and material resources and services
23. Supervise production of food that meets nutrition guidelines, cost parameters, and consumer acceptance
24. Supervise development and/or modification of recipes/formulas

25. Supervise translation of nutrition into foods/menus for target populations
26. Supervise design of menus as indicated by the patient's/client's health status
27. Participate in· applied sensory evaluation of food and nutrition products
28. Supervise procurement, distribution, and service within delivery systems
29. Manage safety and sanitation issues related to food and nutrition
30. Supervise nutrition screening of individual patients/clients
31. Supervise nutrition assessment of individual patients/clients with common medical conditions, e.g., hypertension, obesity, diabetes, diverticular disease
32. Assess nutritional status of individual patients/clients with complex medical conditions, i.e., more complicated health conditions in select populations, e.g., renal disease, multi-system organ failure, trauma
33. Manage the normal nutrition needs of individuals across the life span, i.e., infants through geriatrics and a diversity of people, cultures, and religions
34. Design and implement nutrition care plans as indicated by the patient's/client's health status
35. Manage monitoring of patients'/clients' food and/or nutrient intake
36. Select, implement, and evaluate standard enteral and parenteral nutrition regimens, i.e., in a medically stable patient to meet nutritional requirements where recommendations/adjustments involve primarily macronutrients
37. Develop and implement transitional feeding plans, i.e., conversion from one form of nutrition support to another, e.g., total parenteral nutrition to tube feeding to oral diet
38. Coordinate and modify nutrition care activities among caregivers
39. Conduct nutrition care component of interdisciplinary team conferences to discuss patient/client treatment and discharge planning
40. Refer patients/clients to appropriate community services for general health and nutrition needs and to other primary care providers as appropriate
41. Conduct general health assessment, e.g., blood pressure, vital signs
42. Supervise screening of the nutritional status of the population and/or community groups
43. Conduct assessment of the nutritional status of the population and/or community groups

44. Provide nutrition care for population groups across the lifespan, i.e., infants through geriatrics, and a diversity of people, cultures, and religions
45. Conduct community-based health promotion/disease prevention programs
46. Participate in community-based food and nutrition program development and evaluation
47. Supervise community-based food and nutrition programs

COMPETENCY STATEMENTS FOR EMPHASIS AREAS

All dietitian education supervised practice programs must offer at least one emphasis area. The emphasis areas are not intended to prepare specialists or advanced level practitioners as defined for credentialing purposes. Competencies for each emphasis area build on the core competencies and are designed to begin to develop the *depth* necessary for future proficiency in that area of dietetics practice. More experience in at least one area provides a model for learning throughout one's professional life.

For establishing an emphasis area, the program has the following options:

- Use one or more of the four defined emphasis areas; or,
- Develop a general emphasis by selecting a minimum of seven competency statements, relevant to program mission and goals, with at least one from each of the four defined emphasis areas. The selected competencies should build on the core competencies. General emphasis does not mean achievement of all competencies from all emphasis areas; or,
- Create a unique emphasis area with a minimum of seven competency statements, based on environmental resources and identified needs.

Nutrition Therapy Emphasis Competencies

1. Supervise nutrition assessment of individual patients/clients with complex medical conditions, i.e., more complicated health conditions in select populations, e.g., renal disease, multi-system organ failure, trauma
2. Integrate pathophysiology into medical nutrition therapy recommendations
3. Supervise design through evaluation of nutrition care plan for patients/clients with complex medical conditions, i.e., more com-

plicated health conditions in select populations, e.g., renal disease, multi-system organ failure, trauma

4. Select, monitor, and evaluate complex enteral and parenteral nutrition regimens, i.e., more complicated health conditions in select populations, e.g., renal disease, multi-system organ failure, trauma
5. Supervise development and implementation of transition feeding plans from the inpatient to home setting
6. Conduct counseling and education for patients/clients with complex needs, i.e., more complicated health conditions in select populations, e.g., renal disease, multi-system organ failure, trauma
7. Perform basic physical assessment
8. Participate in nasoenteric feeding tube placement and care
9. Participate in waivered point-of-care testing, such as blood glucose monitoring
10. Participate in the care of patients/clients requiring adaptive feeding devices
11. Manage clinical nutrition services

Community Emphasis Competencies

1. Manage nutrition care for population groups across the lifespan
2. Conduct community-based food and nutrition program outcome assessment/evaluation
3. Develop community-based food and nutrition programs
4. Participate in nutrition surveillance and monitoring of communities
5. Participate in community-based research
6. Participate in food and nutrition policy development and evaluation based on community needs and resources
7. Consult with organizations regarding food access for target populations
8. Develop a health promotion/disease prevention intervention project
9. Participate in waivered point-of-care testing, such as hematocrit and cholesterol levels

Foodservice Systems Management Emphasis Competencies

1. Manage development and/or modification of recipes/formulas
2. Manage menu development for target populations
3. Manage applied sensory evaluation of food and nutrition products
4. Manage production of food that meets nutrition guidelines, cost parameters, and consumer acceptance
5. Manage procurement, distribution, and service within delivery systems

6. Manage the integration of financial, human, physical, and material resources
7. Manage safety and sanitation issues related to food and nutrition
8. Supervise customer satisfaction systems for dietetics services and/or practice
9. Supervise marketing functions
10. Supervise human resource functions
11. Perform operations analysis

Business/Entrepreneur Emphasis Competencies

1. Perform organizational and strategic planning
2. Develop business or operating plan
3. Supervise procurement of resources
4. Manage the integration of financial, human, physical, and material resources
5. Supervise organizational change process
6. Supervise coordination of services
7. Supervise marketing functions

RESOURCES

Directory of Dietetics Programs: The *Directory of Dietetics Programs* is the complete listing of CAADE-accredited Coordinated and Internship Programs, CAADE-approved and accredited Dietetic Technician Programs, and CAADE-approved Preprofessional Practice and Didactic Programs in Dietetics. Advanced degree and specialty practice education programs also are listed. Copies of the *Directory* may be ordered from ADA Customer Service. Call 1-800-877-1600 ext. 5000 for price and ordering information.

Web Site: The ADA Web site includes a listing with selected information on CAADE-accredited/approved programs. The URL is http://www.eatright.org/caade.html.

For More Information Contact:

ADA Education and Accreditation Team
312/899-0040, ext. 5400
Fax: 312/899-4817
E-mail: education@eatright.org

SOURCE: Reproduced with permission from The American Dietetic Association, Commission on Accreditation for Dietetics Education.

Appendix F

Advanced Level Credentials in Nutrition

Credential	Who Grants? Associated Organization	Requirements to Attain
Advanced Level Credentials that Require Registration as a Dietitian (RD)		
Certified Specialist Pediatrics (CSP) Renal (CSR)	Commission on Dietetic Registration (CDR) American Dietetic Association (ADA)	RD for 3 years 4,000 hours of specialty experience (pediatric or renal) within last 6 years Successful completion of written exam CE in area of specialty Renew every 5 years
Fellow of the American Dietetic Association (FADA)	CDR ADA	RD Graduate degree 8 years of work experience beyond RD in multiple roles with diverse & complex responsibilities Peer review of portfolio Renew every 10 years
Certified Nutrition Support Dietitian (CNSD)	National Board of Nutrition Support Certification American Society for Parenteral and Enteral Nutrition	RD Recommend 2 years of nutrition support experience Successful completion of written exam Renew every 5 years

Credential	Who Grants? Associated Organization	Requirements to Attain

Advanced Level Credentials that do not Require Registration as a Dietitian (RD)

Credential	Who Grants? Associated Organization	Requirements to Attain
Certified Diabetes Educator (CDE)	National Certification Board of Diabetes Educators American Association of Diabetes Educators	Unrestricted license or registration (e.g., RN, RD) or be a health care professional with a minimum of a master's degree from a U.S. college or university in...nutrition... 2 calendar years of experience in direct diabetes patient and self-management education; within those 2 years or up to 5 calendar years prior to date of application..., must have worked a minimum of 1,000 hours in direct diabetes patient and self-management education; must be engaged in practice of direct diabetes patient and self-management education at time of application Successful completion of written exam Renew every 5 years
Specialist in Clinical Nutrition (MD, DO) Specialist in Human Nutrition (PhD)	American Board of Nutrition	MD or OD with primary board certification, and 1 year of postgraduate fellowship training in clinical nutrition or 2 years of postgraduate training in subspecialty training program with supervised experience with nutritional problems or PhD in nutrition or highly related field Letters of reference; successful completion of written exam PhD and 2 years postdoctoral training and experience in human nutrition of which 1 year must include clinical training/ patient consultation with supervision Letters of reference; successful completion of written exam
Certified Nutrition Support Physician	National Board of Nutrition Support Certification American Society for Parenteral and Enteral Nutrition	MD

continued

Credential	Who Grants? Associated Organization	Requirements to Attain
Certified Nutrition Support Nurse	National Board of Nutrition Support Certification American Society for Parenteral and Enteral Nutrition	RN Recommend 2 years of nutrition support experience Successful completion of written exam Renew every 5 years
Certified Nutrition Support Pharmacist	Board of Pharmaceutical Specialties	Current, active license to practice pharmacy 3 years practice (upon completion of a nutrition support residency or fellowship, this requirement is decreased to 1 year) Successful completion of written exam

Other Certification

Certified Nutrition Specialist (CNS) (not advanced-level)	Certification Board for Nutrition Specialists American College of Nutrition	Advanced degree in nutrition from regionally accredited program At least 1,000 hours supervised experience or at least 4,000 hours unsupervised experience; successful completion of written exam Renew every 10 years

NOTE: For additional information see Chernoff R, Bruner D, Fitz P, Gannon J, Glade M, Hausman P, Howell WH, Jensen G, Stallings V, Wallach S, Zeisel S. 1997. Credentials available in human clinical nutrition: A report of the Intersociety Committee on Nutrition Certification. *Am J Clin Nutr* 65:1562–1566.

Appendix G

U.S. Preventive Services Task Force Rating of Professionals to Deliver Dietary Counseling

COUNSELING TO PROMOTE A HEALTHY DIET

Intervention	Level of Evidence[a]	Strength of Recommendation[b]
Efficacy of Risk Reduction in the General Population		
Limiting intake of dietary fat (especially saturated fat)	I, II-2, II-3	A
Limiting intake of dietary cholesterol	II-2	B
Emphasizing fruits, vegetables and grain products containing fiber	II-2, II-3	B
Maintaining caloric balance through diet and exercise	II-2	B
Maintaining adequate intake of dietary calcium in women	I, II-I, II-2, II-3	B
Reducing intake of dietary sodium	II-3	C
Increasing intake of dietary iron	II-2, II-3, III	C
Increasing intake of beta-carotene and other antioxidants	II-2, II-2	C
Breastfeeding infants	I, II-2	A
Effectiveness of Counseling		
Counseling to change dietary habits		
Specially trained educators	I[c]	B
Primary care clinicians	III	C

[a] Quality of evidence: I = evidence obtained from at least one properly randomized

355

controlled trial; II-1 = Evidence obtained from well-designed controlled trials without randomization. II-2 = Evidence obtained from well-designed cohort or case-control analytic studies, perferably from more than one center or research group; II-3 = Evidence obtained from multiple time series with or without the intervention, dramatic results in uncontrolled experiments (such as the results of the introduction of penicillin treatment in the 1940s) could also be regarded as this type of evidence. III = Opinions of respected authorities, based on clinical experience; descriptive studies and case reports; or reports of expert committees.

b Strength of Recommendations: A = There is good evidence to support the recommendation that the condition be specifically considered in a periodic health examination; B = There is fair evidence to support the recommendation that the condition be specifically considered in a periodic health examination; C = There is insufficient evidence to recommend for or against the inclusion of the condition in a periodic health examination, but recommendations may be made on other grounds; D = There is fair evidence to support the recommendation that the condition be excluded from consideration in a periodic health examination; E = There is good evidence to support the recommendation that the condition be excluded from consideration in a periodic health examination.

c These trials generally involved specially trained educators such as dietitians delivering intensive interventions (e.g., multiple sessions, tailored materials) to selected patients with known risk factors.

SOURCE: USPSTF (U.S. Preventive Services Task Force). 1995. *Guide to Clinical Preventive Services, 2nd ed. Report of the U.S. Preventive Services Task Force*. Washington, D.C.: U.S. Department of Health and Human Services, Office of Public Health, Office of Health Promotion and Disease Prevention.

Appendix H

Summary of Cost Estimation Methodology for Outpatient Nutrition Therapy

SCENARIO ASSUMPTIONS

Baseline Utilization Scenario

Utilization in initial year and subsequent years to be consistent with selected previously published research and expert clinical judgment.

For example, Sheils and coworkers (1999) reported that from 1991 to 1996, the average utilization patterns for patients with diabetes reflected 464 nutrition sessions per 1,000 patient years. Using the estimated number of nutrition therapy visits per a 5-year period (seven for diabetes only, eight for diabetes with one other diagnosis, and nine for diabetes with two other diagnoses) and the NHANES III distribution between these categories (NCHS, 1997), the average number of visits per year is 1.64 per patient with diabetes. The actual rates provided by the two studies were 0.464 (28 percent utilization) and 0.193 (12 percent utilization). Thus, the baseline scenario was based on assumed utilization rate of 21 percent. This process was completed for each diagnosis.

Low Utilization Scenario

Utilization in initial year and subsequent years during the initial 5-year period may be lower that expected due to time needed to adjust healthcare system and physician referral patterns to new benefit. Using the diabetes example from above, the low utilization cost estimate used 12 percent as the assumed utilization rate.

High Utilization Scenario

Utilization in initial year and subsequent years is projected to be higher that any previous studies to account for possible financial incentives in new benefit and potential impact of new practice protocols that were not being consistently followed during time of data collection of previous studies. For example, the research leading to the recommended number of diabetic visits was published in 1995 and the current protocols were published in 1998. In addition, some nutrition is assumed to be included in the new diabetes self management benefit, so the full initial nutrition therapy may not be warranted for persons using this benefit. For example, the high utilization scenario used 30 percent as the assumed utilization rate.

COST ESTIMATE ASSUMPTIONS

- Conservative cost estimates (highest reasonable cost) were used.
- Dollars are expressed in nominal terms and not discounted.
- Medicare costs were provided by The Lewin Group, Inc. based on 1998 data from Office of the Actuary, Health Care Financing Administration.
- Both Medicare costs and projected Medicare projected reimbursement rates were assumed to grow at the rate of 3 percent per year.
- Reimbursement rates for nutrition therapy were assumed to be for individual sessions using rates established for diabetes care ($55.41 per session).
- Estimated Medicare reimbursement costs were computed by estimating total direct costs and subtracting 20 percent cost sharing.
- Future premium increases were estimated to be 25 percent of projected Medicare reimbursements.
- Even though some Medicare-eligible would have other insurance, these cost estimates assumed that Medicare would be the payor for all nutrition therapy sessions received by beneficiaries.
- Maximum number of nutrition therapy sessions were based on expert opinion and accepted protocols. They assume more sessions in year of initial diagnosis/referral than in subsequent years for most diagnoses. Even though most protocols are written for single diagnosis, patients usually present with combinations of diagnoses. Initial year treatments were estimated using highest number of sessions with an additional one visit per additional nutrition-related diagnoses.

• Assumed that all beneficiaries receiving nutrition therapy received the maximum estimated number of nutrition therapy visits.

• Assumed that all current Medicare beneficiaries would have disease prevalence similar to NHANES III data and that they would all become eligible for "newly diagnosed" benefit in the first year of coverage.

• Assumed that Medicare beneficiary population changed at constant rate over the 5-year period. The estimated number of new beneficiaries was based on estimates from Office of the Actuary, Health Care Financing Administration.

• All new beneficiaries were assumed to be treated as "initial year of diagnoses" for purposes of nutrition therapy. This assumes that previous health plan coverage did *not* offer nutrition as a covered benefit. (However some plans do; see discussion in chapter 14.)

ECONOMIC BENEFIT ASSUMPTIONS

Similar cost assumptions were used to quantify some potential economic benefits of nutrition therapy. Plus the following assumptions.

• Nutrition therapy is usually provided in a multidisciplinary and multi-modality treatment plan. Therefore clinical outcomes of nutrition alone are difficult if not impossible to quantify accurately. Expert opinion and research were used to estimate amount of benefit that could be reasonably attributed to nutrition therapy. For example, diabetes trials indicate that intensive therapy including nutrition led to 0.9 percent point reduction in HbA_{1c}, (e.g., 8.0 percent to 7.1 percent) however committee estimates for benefits were based on the assumption that 25 percent of this reduction might be reasonably attributed to nutrition therapy.

• Clinical trial results were adjusted downward since maximum benefits reported are not likely to be replicated when nutrition therapy is provided to a broader population in a less controlled manner. For example, clinical trials with intensive nutrition therapy yielded a 6 percent reduction in cholesterol, while these estimates of benefits were based on a 3 percent reduction.

• Economic benefits are likely for other diagnoses, however research showing quantifiable link between nutrition therapy and outcomes was not sufficient to prepare an estimate (e.g., for heart failure).

• Various methodologies were used to prepare estimates for each diagnosis, and it is not appropriate to simply add the estimates since they overlap and accommodate persons with multiple diagnoses.

• Economic benefits identified are not to be used as expected offsets for budget estimates.

- Some benefits are likely not to occur immediately (i.e., within the first 2 years after therapy is initiated) and may well occur after the 5-year period of these estimates.

Estimated Reimbursement Cost in Billions to Medicare Summed over 2000 to 2004 (after adjustment for copayment and premium increase)

	Baseline	Low	High
	$1.069 billion	$740 million	$1.97 billion

Estimated Potential Benefit in Millions to Medicare Summed over 2000 to 2004

	Baseline	Low	High
Diabetes	231	132	330
Hypertension	83	52	167
Dyslipidemia	89	54	154

Data were not available to permit estimating benefits of nutrition therapy for heart failure, pre-dialysis renal, and the one visit estimated for all remaining beneficiaries (over 65 years old without diagnoses and all beneficiaries under 65 years old) that were assumed to have other diagnoses that also could warrant referral for nutrition therapy.

REFERENCES

NCHS (National Center for Health Statistics). 1997. *Third National Health and Nutrition Examination Survey* (Series 11, No. 1, SETS version 1.22a). [CD-ROM]. Washington, D.C.: U.S. Government Printing Office.
Sheils JF, Rubin R, Stapleton DC. 1999. The estimated costs and savings of medical nutrition therapy: The Medicare population. *J Am Diet Assoc* 99:428–435.

Appendix I

Committee Biographical Sketches

Virginia A. Stallings, M.D., is chief, Nutrition Section, Division of Gastroenterology and Nutrition, the Children's Hospital of Philadelphia and professor of pediatrics, the University of Pennsylvania School of Medicine. Dr. Stallings is a member of the Food and Nutrition Board, Institute of Medicine, and an active member of the American Society for Clinical Nutrition. She holds a B.S. in nutrition and foods from Auburn University, an M.S. in human nutrition and biochemistry from Cornell University, and an M.D. from the University of Alabama School of Medicine. In addition, Dr. Stallings completed a clinical and research fellowship in pediatric nutrition at the Hospital for Sick Children in Toronto, Ontario.

Lawrence J. Appel, M.D., M.P.H., is associate professor of medicine, epidemiology, and international health of the Johns Hopkins University Medical Institutions. Dr. Appel has been the principal or coprincipal investigator in numerous studies that examined the effects of life-style modification, particularly nutrition interventions on blood pressure. In addition, Dr. Appel is the course director for critical appraisal of published clinical research and clinical trial—issues and controversies—at Johns Hopkins University. Dr. Appel holds a M.D. from the New York University School of Medicine and a M.P.H. from Johns Hopkins University.

Julia A. James is principal, Health Policy Alternatives, Inc. (HPA). Ms. James joined HPA as a principal in 1998 with more than 25 years in health services research, planning, and policy. Before joining HPA, she was the chief health policy analyst for the Senate Committee on Finance. In this capacity she was responsible for overseeing health policy issues within the jurisdiction of the committee, including Medicare, Medicaid, the State Children's Health Insurance Program, and health system reform issues. Prior to joining the Finance Committee staff in 1991, Ms. James was involved with health policy in the state of Oregon. She has experience in applying evidence-based medicine and cost-effectiveness analyses to health policy development. She received her B.A. from Oregon State University and has done graduate work in public administration at Portland State University and the Lewis and Clark Graduate School of Professional Studies.

Gordon L. Jensen, M.D., Ph.D., is associate professor of medicine, Division of Gastroenterology, Vanderbilt University Medical Center and adjunct associate physician, Department of Gastroenterology and Nutrition, Pennsylvania State Geisinger Health System. Dr. Jensen is currently chairman of the Clinical Practice Issues Committee for the American Society of Clinical Nutrition and is a member of the Board of Directors of the American Board of Nutrition. He also serves on the editorial board of the *Journal of Parenteral and Enteral Nutrition*. His current research interests include nutritional concerns of rural older persons, nutrition screening for risk in elderly populations, and obesity and function in older persons. He holds a B.S. in biology from the Pennsylvania State University, a Ph.D. in nutritional biochemistry from Cornell University, and an M.D. from Cornell University Medical College. Dr. Jensen completed internal medicine as well as fellowship training in hyperalimentation and nutrition at New England Deaconess Hospital.

Elvira Q. Johnson, M.S., R.D., C.D.E., is director, Clinical Nutrition Services, Cambridge Health Alliance. In this capacity, Ms. Johnson coordinates all clinical nutrition services throughout the alliance including Women, Infants, and Children, ambulatory, acute, long-term, and home care, and is charged with the task of improving the nutritional health of the community and reducing health care costs. She received the American Dietetic Association Foundation Award for Excellence in the Practice of Clinical Nutrition and was Employee of the Year for the City of Cambridge in 1995. She holds a B.S. from Rutgers University and an M.S. in nutrition and adult education from Boston University. In addition, she is a certified diabetes educator.

Joyce K. Keithley, D.N.Sc., R.N., is professor, Rush University, College of Nursing, Chicago, and adjunct assistant professor, University of Illinois, College of Nursing. Dr. Keithley has published several papers on nutritional topics such as enteral nutrition, obesity, and nutrition assessment. She holds a B.S.N. from the University of Illinois, an M.S.N from DePaul University, and a D.N.Sc. from Rush University. The specialty area for her D.N.Sc. was clinical nutrition and complex gastrointestinal surgery patients.

Colonel Esther F. Myers, Ph.D., R.D., F.A.D.A., is chief consultant to the U.S. Air Force Surgeon General for Nutrition and Dietetics, associate chief, Biomedical Sciences Corps for Dietetics, and flight commander, Nutritional Medicine at 60th Medical Group, Travis Air Force Base, California. Col. Myers was actively involved in the development of the Department of Defense outcome measurement system for indicators of outpatient nutrition services, focusing particularly on data to support management decisions on the effectiveness of various methods of nutrition counseling. She currently serves on the Health Services Research Committee of the American Dietetic Association. She received a B.S. from North Dakota State University, an M.S. in human nutrition and food management from the Ohio State University, and a Ph.D. in human ecology from Kansas State University.

F. Xavier Pi-Sunyer, M.D., M.P.H., is director of the Obesity Research Center and chief of endocrinology, diabetes and nutrition at St. Lukes-Roosevelt Hospital Center, and professor of medicine at the College of Physicians and Surgeons, Columbia University. Dr. Pi-Sunyer's research interests include the hormonal control of carbohydrate metabolism, diabetes mellitus, obesity, and food intake regulation. He is a past president of the American Diabetes Association, the American Society of Clinical Nutrition, and the North American Association for the Study of Obesity. He currently serves on the National Institute of Diabetes and Digestive and Kidney Diseases Task Force for the Prevention and Treatment of Obesity. Dr. Pi-Sunyer served on the past Institute of Medicine Committee on Opportunities in the Nutrition and Food Sciences. He holds a B.A. in chemistry from Oberlin College, an M.D. from Columbia University College of Physicians and Surgeons, and an M.P.H. from Harvard University.

Harold Pollack, Ph.D., is assistant professor, Department of Health Management and Policy, School of Public Health, University of Michigan, Ann Arbor. Dr. Pollack's main research interests include the targeting and cost-effectiveness of services for severely disadvantaged populations. He is a member of the American Economic Association and the American Public Health Association. Dr. Pollack holds a B.S.E. from Princeton University in electrical engineering and computer science, as well as an M.P.P. and a Ph.D. in public policy from Harvard University.

Carol Porter, Ph.D., R.D., F.A.D.A., is director, Nutrition Services and Dietetic Internship Program, University of California, San Francisco Medical Center. Dr. Porter's expertise includes the area of clinical nutrition management. Her current research interests include nutrition in the nursing home setting. She holds a B.A. and an M.S. in nutrition from the University of Iowa and a Ph.D. in nutrition from the University of California at Berkeley.

David B. Reuben, M.D., is chief, Division of Geriatrics and director, Multicampus Program in Geriatric Medicine and Gerontology, University of California at Los Angeles School of Medicine. Dr. Reuben's area of expertise includes gerontology and evidence based medicine. His research interests include geriatric nutrition screening and assessment. Dr. Rueben is a member of the Board of Directors of the American Geriatrics Society and a member of the Gerontological Society of America. He currently serves on the editorial board of the *Journal of the American Geriatric Society*. Dr. Reuben has served on a past IOM Committee to Advise the Hartford Foundation on Strengthening the Geriatric Content of Medical Training. He attended Emory College and received his M.D. from Emory University School of Medicine.

Robert S. Schwartz, M.D., is professor and attending physician, Division of Gerontology and Geriatric Medicine, Harborview Medical Center, University of Washington School of Medicine, Seattle. He is also a graduate faculty member in nutrition at the University of Washington. Dr. Schwartz's research interests include diet, exercise, obesity, and diabetes in the elderly. He is a member of the American Geriatrics Society, the Gerontological Society of America, and the American Society for Clinical Nutrition. In addition, he currently serves on the editorial board of the *Journal of the American Geriatric Society*. Dr. Schwartz holds a B.S. in zoology from the University of Michigan and an M.D. from Ohio State University, Columbus.

Annalynn Skipper, M.S., R.D., C.N.S.D., F.A.D.A., is codirector, Nutrition Consultation Service, Rush-Presbyterian, St. Luke's Medical Center and assistant professor, Department of Clinical Nutrition, Rush University. Ms. Skipper's area of expertise lies in the delivery of nutrition support and the management of a multidisciplinary nutrition support service. She has numerous publications on enteral and parenteral nutrition, including its practice in home care and the development of an outcomes database for patients receiving parenteral nutrition. She holds a B.S. from Tarleton

State University and an M.S. in nutrition from Texas Tech University. She has been a certified nutrition support dietitian since 1987.

Linda G. Snetselaar, Ph.D., R.D., is associate professor and chair, Preventive Nutrition Education, Department of Preventive Medicine and Environmental Health, University of Iowa. She is also a faculty member in the Department of Internal Medicine, Division of Endocrinology. Dr. Snetselaar has served as a principal or coprincipal investigator for several sentinel diet-related intervention studies including the Diabetes Control and Complications Trial, the Modification of Diet in Renal Disease study, Dietary Intake in Lipid Research, and the Women's Health Initiative. She has directed numerous counseling workshops for nutrition interventions. Her research interests include diet intervention in cardiovascular disease, renal disease, diabetes, and cancer. She holds an M.S. in nutrition and a Ph.D. in health sciences education, both from the University of Iowa.